MW01713475

Nursing Assistant

A Nursing Process Approach

9th Edition

Volume 2

Barbara R. Hegner, MSN, RN
(deceased)

Barbara Acello, MS, RN
Independent nurse consultant and educator

Esther Caldwell, MA, PhD
Consultant in Vocational Education (CA)

THOMSON
NELSON

Printed and bound in the United States
1 2 3 4 10 09 08 07

For more information contact
Thomson Nelson
1120 Birchmount Road,
Scarborough, Ontario, M1K 5G4.
Or you can visit our internet site at
http://www.nelson.com

This textbook is a Nelson custom publication. Because your instructor has chosen to produce a custom publication, you pay only for material that you will use in your course.

Cover images: Photo.com

ISBN-13: 978-0-17-646277-2
ISBN-10: 0-17-646277-5

Consists of:

Nursing Assistant
9th Edition
Barbara R. Hegner, Barbara Acello, Esther Caldwell
ISBN 1-4018-0633-3, © 2004

Contents

section **5**

Safety and Mobility

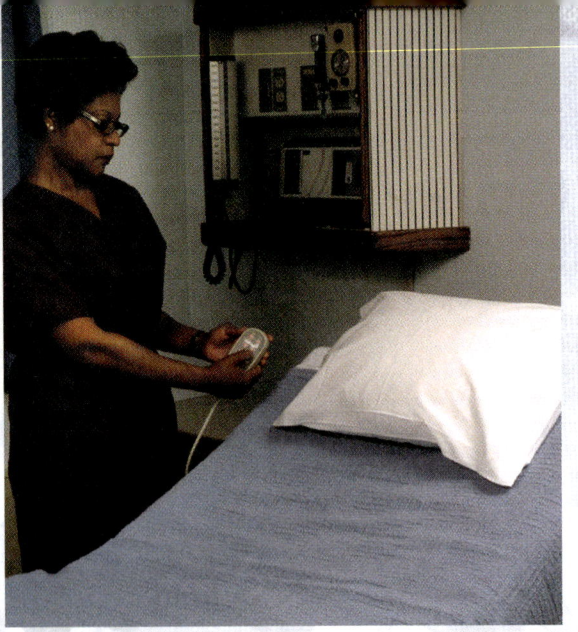

unit **14**

Environmental and Nursing Assistant Safety

objectives

After completing this unit, you will be able to:

- Spell and define terms.
- Describe the health care facility environment.
- Identify measures to promote environmental safety.
- List situations when equipment must be repaired.
- Describe the elements required for fire.
- List five measures to prevent fire.
- Describe the procedure to follow if a fire occurs.
- Demonstrate the use of a fire extinguisher.
- List techniques for using ergonomics on the job.
- Demonstrate appropriate body mechanics.
- List at least 10 guidelines for dealing with a violent individual.
- Describe the types of information contained in Material Safety Data Sheets (MSDS).

vocabulary

Learn the meaning and the correct spelling of the following words and phrases:

concurrent cleaning
environmental safety
ergonomics
incident
incident report
Material Safety Data Sheet (MSDS)
PASS
private room
RACE
semiprivate room
side rails
ward
workplace violence

INTRODUCTION

The hospital room is the patient's home while he or she is hospitalized (Figure 14-1). The room becomes the patient's world. Cheerful and pleasant surroundings give the patient a better sense of well-being. Consistent attention to safety helps foster feelings of security in this strange environment. *Both* aid in speeding recovery.

The nursing assistant helps keep the patient's unit safe and clean. All health care providers share the task of keeping the entire nursing unit safe and clean.

Environmental safety refers to the condition of an entire facility—patient rooms, hallways, and all departments. The environment includes:

- Temperature (heating and air conditioning)
- Air circulation
- Light
- Cleanliness
- Noise control
- Walls, ceilings, and floors
- Plumbing
- Electricity
- Equipment and furniture

Prevention of injuries to patients, visitors, volunteers, and staff members is of primary concern.

THE PATIENT ENVIRONMENT

In a health care facility, the basic patient unit consists of a/an:

- Hospital bed with rails (Figure 14-2)
- Bedside table
- Chair
- Reading lamp

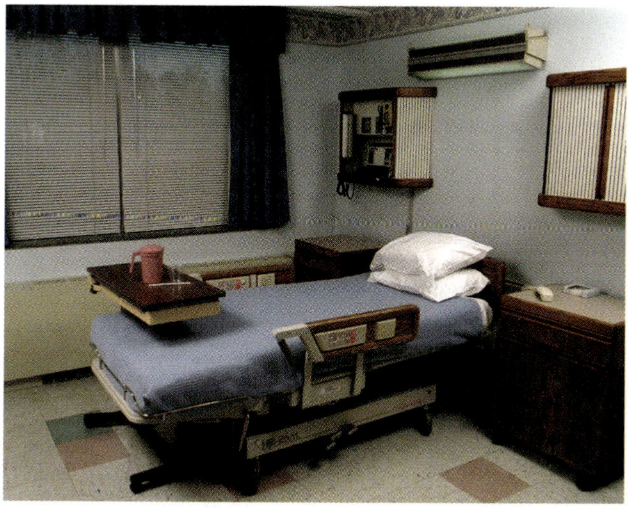

FIGURE 14-1 The patient's unit is his home during his stay in the hospital.

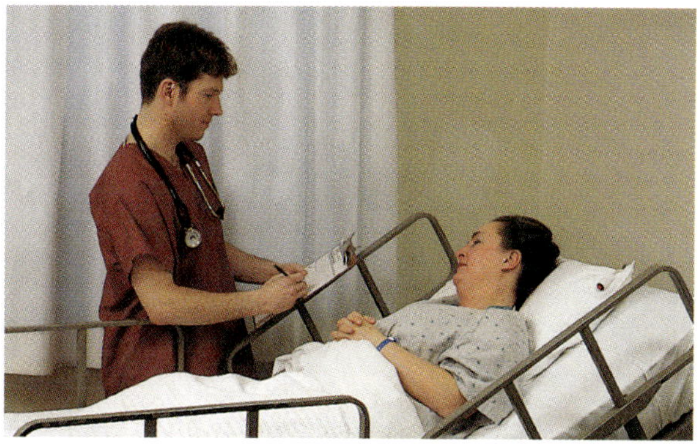

FIGURE 14-2 All hospital beds are equipped with side rails. These are split rails that can be raised and lowered in any combination.

- Waste basket
- Overbed table
- Signal cord

This equipment may be located in a single-, double-, or multiple-bed room. A **private room** contains only one bed. **Semiprivate rooms** contain two beds. **Wards** are multiple-bed rooms.

Each room is numbered. The beds are marked by letters or numbers. For example, Room 871 in a large medical center may be a four-unit ward. The beds are labeled A, B, C, D (or 1, 2, 3, 4). The patient in the fourth bed is in Unit 871–D or Unit 871–4.

The equipment from one unit should not be used by other patients. For home care, the same unit elements will be present, but they will be modified. For example, there may not be an adjustable hospital bed or an overbed table.

Hospital Beds

Hospital beds mostly have the same features, but there may be some differences. Hospital beds:

- Differ in the ways in which they operate. Some are controlled electrically (Figure 14-3). Others are operated by the turning of cranks or gatch handles (Figure 14-4).

OSHA *Alert*

Elevating the bed to a proper working height is one of the most important measures to use for protecting your back. If a gatch handle is used to elevate the bed, use good body mechanics by squatting down when you turn the handle. For patient safety, make sure you lower the bed when you leave the room.

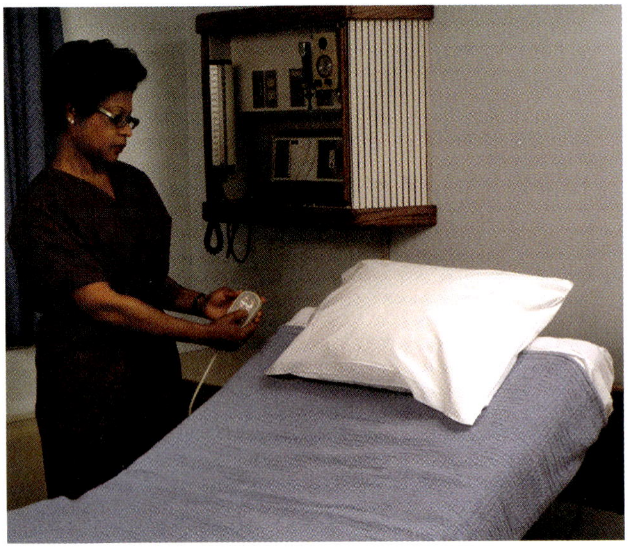

FIGURE 14-3 Electrically operated hospital beds may have foot controls, handheld controls, or controls mounted on the side to control the position of the bed.

- May be raised to a high horizontal position. In this position, there is less strain for those giving care. Beds must be returned to the lowest horizontal position when you leave the room.
- Are on wheels, to make it easy to move beds from one place to another. The wheels should always be locked unless the bed is being moved.
- Break in the middle so that the head may be raised.
- Break behind the knees to increase physical comfort for the bedridden patient.

Side rails are attached to the hospital bed. They protect the patient from falling. Side rails are considered to be restraints in some circumstances. Most health care facilities have policies, procedures, and guidelines describing their use. Potential benefits of side rails are that they:

- Provide support and a "handle" for the patient to use for turning and repositioning in bed.
- Provide a "handle" for getting into and out of bed.
- Give the patient a feeling of security.
- Reduce the risk of the patient falling out of bed when he or she is being transported in the bed.
- Provide access to bed and television controls that are part of the bed rail design.

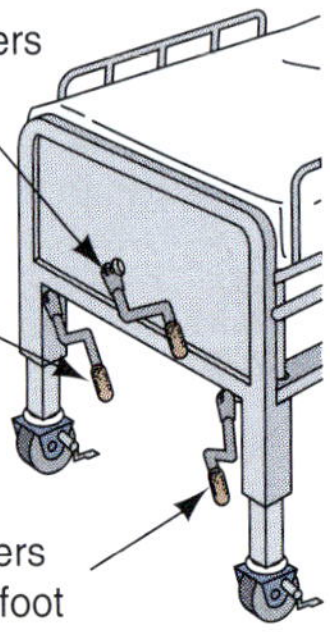

FIGURE 14-4 Gatch handles are used to change the position of nonelectric beds.

OSHA Alert

Always test the patient's ability to assist with moving procedures, unless contraindicated. The side rails are perfect tools for patients to use when moving in bed. When the patient uses the rail to assist in a move, your job is made easier and there is less strain on your back. Remember to lower the rail when you leave the room, according to facility policies or if indicated on the care plan.

The potential risks of side rails include:

- Strangulation, suffocation, bodily injury, or death when the patient or part of the patient's body becomes entrapped between the bars of the side rails or between the side rails and the mattress.
- Serious injuries if the patient climbs over the rails and falls from this height.
- Skin tears, bruises, cuts, scrapes.
- Agitation caused by a feeling of being trapped or caged in.
- Feelings of isolation or restriction.
- Sadness because of loss of independence and having to call for help.
- Actual loss of independence, such as the ability to get up to use the bathroom or to retrieve an item dropped on the floor.

Several types of side rails are used on hospital beds. One type is a single rail that runs the length of the bed. Split rails are more common in acute care hospitals. Each side of the bed has two half-rails. One or both can be raised, depending on the patient's needs and plan of care. When side rails are used, they:

- Should be checked and attached securely before you leave the bedside, unless ordered otherwise.
- Should be down only when beds are in the lowest horizontal position, or if a release form has been signed by the patient.
- Should never be used for the attachment of tubes such as IV lines or catheters. Raising and lowering the side rails could put undue stress on such tubes and even pull them out.
- Should never be used for the attachment of restraints.

The use of side rails may upset some patients. Sometimes it may be necessary to reassure the patient that her condition is not becoming worse. The patient should be told that the raising of side rails is hospital policy or is being done as a reminder of a new environment.

Temperature, Air Circulation, and Light

As you adjust and maintain the temperature, light, and ventilation, keep in mind the patient's condition, the patient's personal preference, and the needs of the other patients in the room.

- The best temperature is about 70 degrees. A lower temperature may cause chilling and a higher one may make the patient uncomfortable.
- Movement of air and the temperature may be controlled by opening windows at the top and bottom if air conditioning is not being used. (In some facilities the windows are sealed shut.)
- Patients can be shielded from drafts by screens or curtains.

In most hospitals and health facilities, rooms are automatically air-conditioned. The thermostat may be set from a central location, or set individually in each patient's room.

Lighting comes from several sources. There will be times when less light is desired. At other times, more light will be needed (Figure 14-5). Use as much light as needed to safely carry out your job. Be careful to shield other patients as much as possible.

Patients often find it difficult to sleep if lights are too bright. There should be only enough light at night to enable the staff to work safely.

- Rooms are equipped with lights above each bed. These illuminate a single patient bed.
- There may also be a ceiling light.
- Additional spotlights can be brought from the utility room when needed to provide extra light for delicate procedures.
- The best lighting is indirect; glare causes fatigue.
- Be sure to return extra lights as soon as you are finished, because added clutter in a room is hazardous.
- Be sure to turn ceiling lights off when leaving the room.

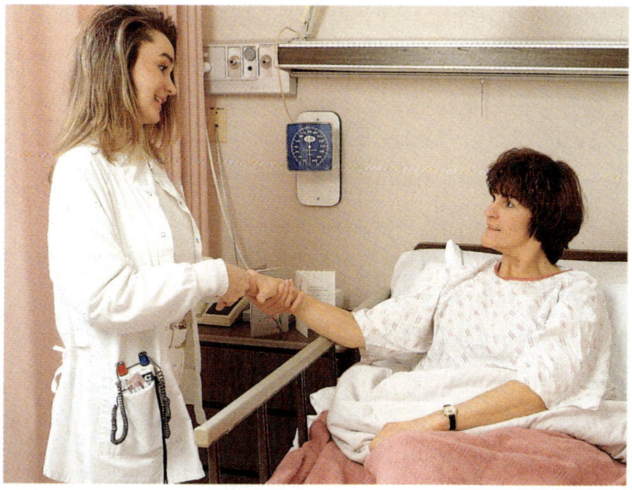

FIGURE 14-5 The overbed light can be adjusted to several different lighting levels.

INFECTION CONTROL *Alert*

Make sure clean and soiled items are separated in patient rooms and storage areas. Keep the lids tightly closed on trash cans and linen hampers. Avoid putting biohazard contaminated trash into open wastebaskets. Discard soiled items in a plastic bag or a covered trash can.

- Night lights are often left on for very ill or elderly patients.

Cleanliness and Noise Reduction

You are responsible for the cleanliness, quiet, and order of the patient units to which you are assigned. To contribute to the comfort of the patient:

- Speak quietly.
- Report squeaky equipment wheels that should be oiled.
- Avoid banging equipment and trays against other surfaces.
- Keep the area neat as you work. Check its overall appearance before you leave.
- Return equipment to its proper location after completing patient care.
- Do not turn the TV on or up while giving care to patients unless the patient asks you to do so.

You are responsible for keeping the patient supplied with fresh water, ice, disposable drinking cups, tissues, and straws. Make sure that all necessary pieces of equipment, such as the wash basin, emesis basin, bedpan, urinal, soap, and towels, are always available, clean, and in good condition (Figure 14-6). These items should always be stored in the bedside table.

INFECTION CONTROL *Alert*

When two or more patients share a room, make sure that all personal care items are labeled with each patient's name. Keep personal care items in the appropriate area. Store grooming supplies in a clean area. Avoid storing personal care equipment and supplies in community areas, such as bathrooms; storage in these areas increases the risk that personal care items will be used for the wrong patient(s).

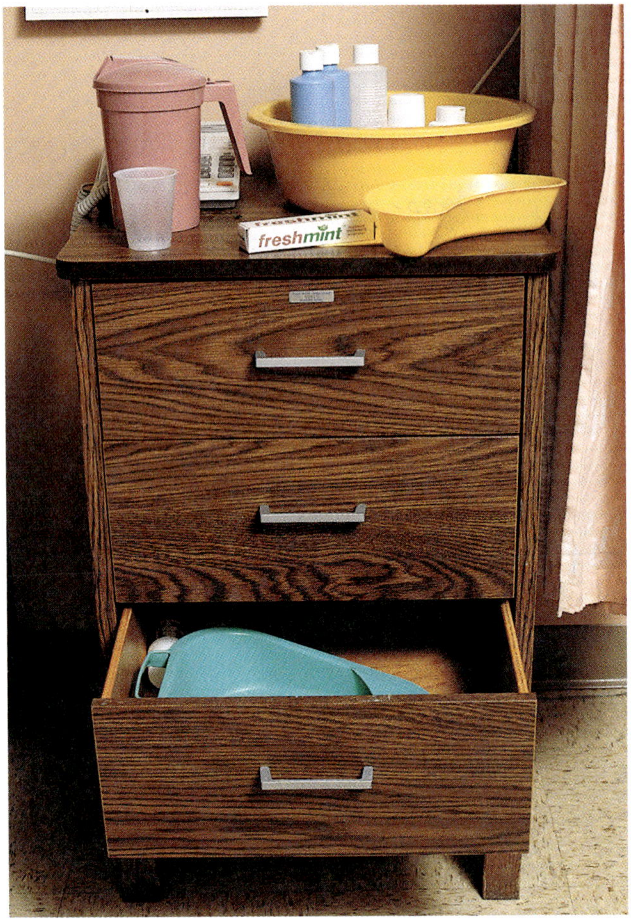

FIGURE 14-6 Personal care supplies are stored in the bedside stand. Items considered clean and dirty are stored in separate drawers.

SAFETY MEASURES

Safety is the responsibility of everyone. A safe environment is essential for both the patients and the staff. Safety must be a part of everything you do. This concern extends to the safety of the unit and the entire environment. The number of accidents involving patients and staff can be greatly reduced if simple measures are followed.

When an accident occurs in the health care facility, it is referred to as an **incident**. An incident is any unexpected occurrence or event that interrupts normal procedures or causes a crisis. Incidents can cause harm to a patient, employee, or any other person. If you see an incident or are involved in one, you need to report it to your charge nurse. The nurse fills out an **incident report** (Figure 14-7) after obtaining information from the persons involved. Prevention of incidents depends on employees:

- Knowing their jobs and following all policies and procedures related to safety
- Maintaining a safe environment
- Knowing the patients and implementing safety measures to decrease their risk of injury

AGE-APPROPRIATE CARE *Alert*

Besides the safety practices already discussed, keep sharp objects and plants away from children and patients who are mentally confused. If you are not sure about the safety of an item, check with the nurse.

Environmental Safety Conditions

Incidents can be prevented by keeping hallways and other walkways free of equipment and clutter. Most facilities require that all equipment that must be in the hall be kept on the same side of the hall. Report these situations promptly:

- Burnt-out light bulbs and light switches or electric plugs that do not work.
- Water leaks from faucets or pipes.
- Faucets or water fountains that do not flow properly.
- Loose or missing floor tiles.
- Windows that do not close tightly or are cracked or broken.
- Temperatures that are too hot or too cold and cannot be controlled within the room. (State licensing agencies have strict regulations regarding environmental temperatures.)
- Loose or missing ceiling tiles or leaks from the ceiling.
- Toilets that do not flush properly.

SAFETY *Alert*

Each state has laws governing the water temperature in patient care areas of the facility. In most cases, water temperature at sinks should not exceed 120°F. The regulators sometimes fail, sending excessively hot water into the facility. Water in bath and shower areas must be warm enough to comfortably bathe patients. Comfortable temperature for most people is 95°F to 105°F. Report water in bathing areas that does not warm up enough for comfortable bathing. Also report steaming water, or water that feels excessively hot at any faucet in a patient care area. Use bath thermometers to check water temperatures before giving patient care, whenever possible.

INCIDENT REPORT

Family Name	First Name	M.I.	Room No.	Hosp. No.

Address	City	State	Zip Code	Age	Sex M F

Date of Incident	Time a.m. p.m.	Place	Attending Physician

Status of person involved: Patient ______ Employee ______ Visitor ______ Other ______

Diagnosis: ______

Describe condition before incident: Disoriented ____ Senile ____ Sedated ____ Normal ____ Other ____

Was height of bed adjustable? Yes ___ No ___ Was bed up? Yes ___ No ___ Was bed down? Yes ___ No ___
Were bed rails ordered? Yes ___ No ___ Were they present? Yes ___ No ___ Were they up? Yes ___ No ___
Were they down? Yes ___ No ___ Other ______

Describe incident entirely, include part of body injured and treatment:

Vital Signs: Temp ______ Pulse ______ Resp ______ Blood Pressure ______

Indicate on diagram location of injury

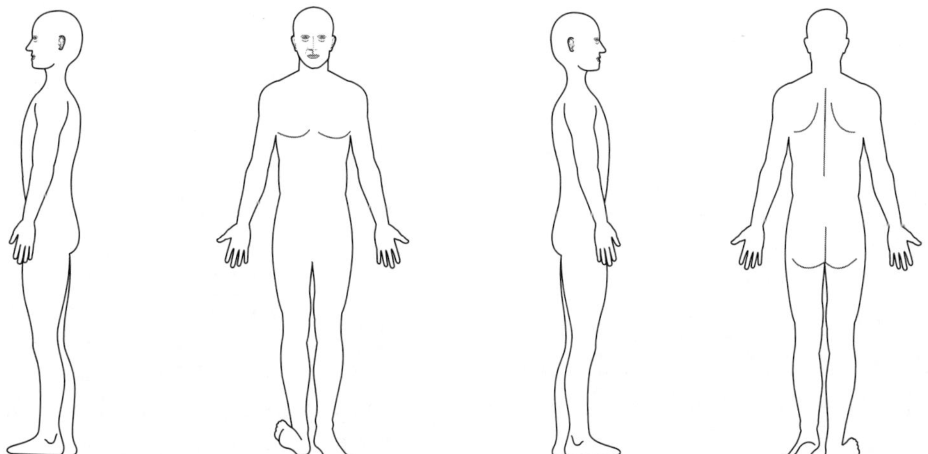

– over –

FIGURE 14-7 A special report is completed any time an incident occurs. *continues*

Was physician called? Yes _______ No _______ Time __________ a.m. p.m.

Who responded? ____ Time ____________ a.m. p.m.

Attending physician _____ On-call physician _____

Statement of physician ____

____

____

____

____

Was family called? Yes _______ No _______ Time __________ a.m. p.m. Who: ____________________

Give names, addresses, and phone numbers of any who witnessed incident ____________________

____

____

____

A copy of this report will be sent to Patient's physician.

Date of Report ____________________ Signed ____

Signature and title of person preparing report

Nursing Office Review of Incident: Date ________________ Signed ____________________

Comments: ____

____

____

____

____

____

FIGURE 14-7 *continued*

Equipment and Its Care

The daily or **concurrent cleaning** of equipment is an important part of your job. It contributes to the safety of your patient. The housekeeping department maintains environmental cleanliness. However, spills must be mopped up immediately to avoid falls.

In most health care facilities, equipment is tagged when it needs repair (Figure 14-8). That equipment is not to be used again until the tag is removed. Facility policy differs as to who is responsible for applying and removing the tag. Reporting broken or nonfunctioning equipment is the responsibility of everyone.

You can prevent accidents related to equipment by:

1. Reporting needed repairs promptly. Possible hazards include:
   - lost screws
   - frayed straps
   - loose wheels
   - broken control knobs
   - latches that do not hook
   - side rails that do not fasten correctly
   - faulty brakes on wheelchairs and stretchers
   - frayed electrical cords
2. Reporting immediately if call lights (signal cords) are not working.
3. Disposing of equipment in proper containers. Facilities must dispose of sharps, such as needles and blades, in special containers.
4. Never handling broken bits of glass with your hands. Put on gloves. Large pieces can be picked up with forceps. Broken glass can also be cleaned up using a brush or broom and a dustpan (Figure 14-9).
5. Always knowing what you are handling and the proper method for its disposal.
6. Inspecting mechanical lifts (Figure 14-10) carefully before using. Check:
   - Handle, to make sure legs open and close safely

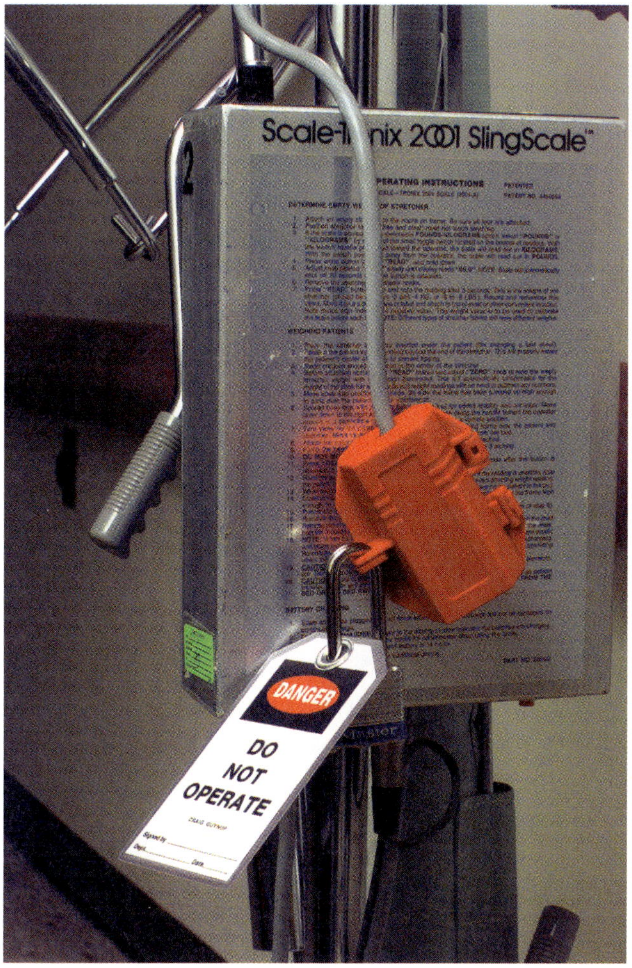

FIGURE 14-8 Unsafe electrical equipment is tagged and locked until it can be repaired.

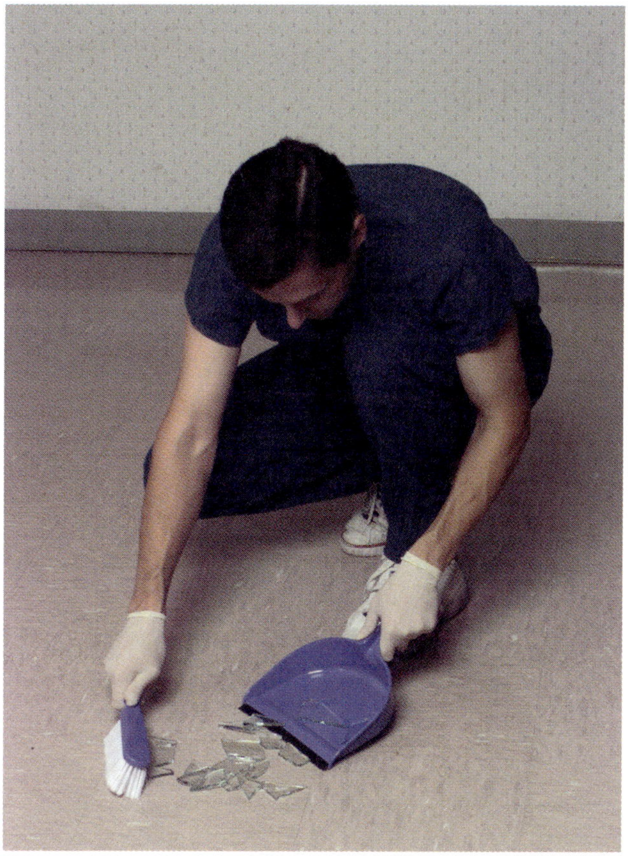

FIGURE 14-9 Never handle broken glass. Sweep it with a broom and dustpan or use an instrument to pick up large pieces. Wear gloves. Discard the glass in the proper container.

OSHA *Alert*

Handle needles, razors, and other sharp objects with care. Needles are never cut, bent, broken, or recapped by hand. After using a sharp object, dispose of it in a puncture-resistant "sharps" container. Avoid overfilling the sharps container. Seal the cap when it is three-quarters full. The cap is designed so it cannot be snapped back off after it is closed. The sealed sharps container is stored until it can be picked up with the biohazardous waste. The biohazardous waste disposal area is used for discarding items contaminated with blood or body fluids. Special precautions are taken to contain waste in this area.

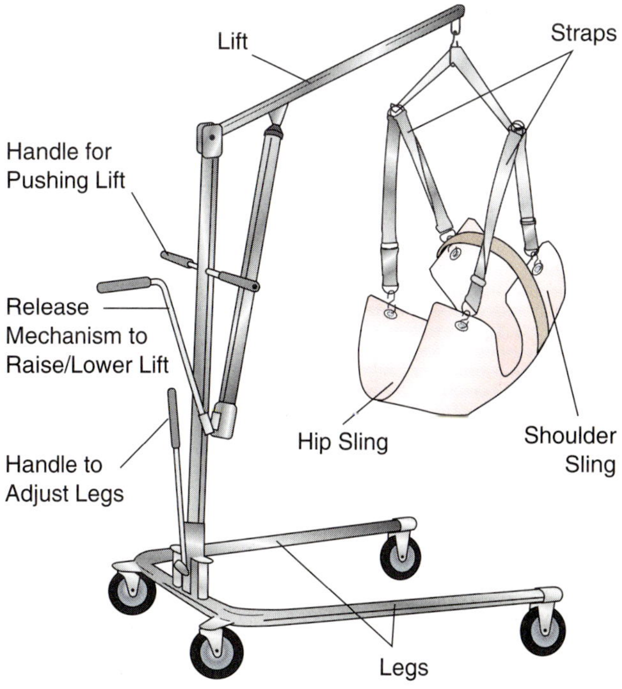

FIGURE 14-10 Carefully examine the mechanical lift before using it.

OSHA Alert

The mechanical lift is an important device for back safety. Using the mechanical lift for patients who are large or difficult to move is safer for both the patient and the nursing assistant. However, you should never use the hydraulic mechanical lift alone. Make sure one or more other workers are available to assist you.

- Release mechanism for raising and lowering lift
- All straps and chains for frayed areas or clasps that do not close correctly
- Sling, to be sure it is the right sling to use with that lift and that there are no frays or tears
- For hydraulic fluid on the floor—do not use the lift if fluid is present

7. Making sure that equipment and supplies are stored properly. Never block a doorway with equipment. Items in boxes should not be stored on the floor.

FIRE SAFETY

It is a scientific fact that if three elements are present in the right proportions (Figure 14-11), there will be a fire. The three elements are heat, fuel, and oxygen.

It is the responsibility of every staff member to know and regularly practice the fire and evacuation plans for the facility.

- Role-play the emergency procedures until you are completely secure. Remember that in any emergency the welfare and safety of the patients are most important.

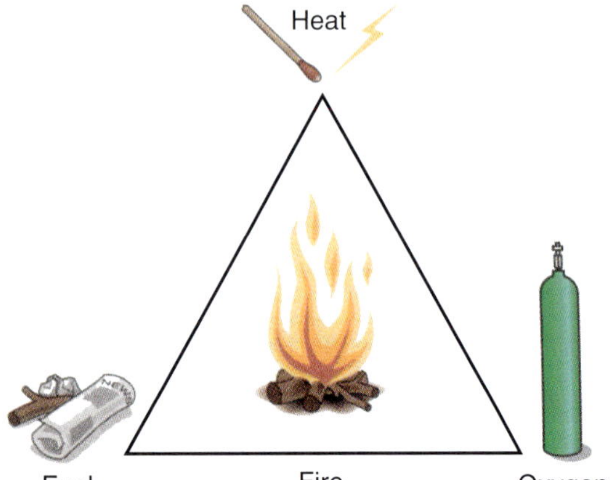

FIGURE 14-11 The fire triangle shows the elements needed to start a fire.

- Learn the location of escape routes and the location and operation of all fire control equipment (Figure 14-12), such as:
  - Fire alarms
  - Extinguishers
  - Sprinklers
  - Fire doors
  - Fire escapes
- Know and practice fire drill procedures. These are conducted on a regular basis by each facility. Many patients could be injured during a fire because of the confusion and their inability to help themselves.
- Keep alert to all possible fire hazards. Report them immediately to the proper authorities.

Fire Hazards

Some possible fire hazards include:

- Frayed electrical wires
- Overloaded circuits
- Plugs that are not properly grounded
- Accumulated clutter such as papers and rags
- Improper protection during oxygen therapy
- Uncontrolled smoking; most health care facilities prohibit smoking throughout the facility
- Matches left where children or others have unauthorized access to them
- Smoking in rooms where oxygen is in use

Fire Prevention

You and every staff member can do a great deal to prevent the disaster of fire. In general:

- Check for frayed electrical wires.
- Do not overload circuits with too many electrical cords.
- Do not use a lightweight electrical cord with equipment that draws a heavy power load.
- Use three-prong grounded plugs.
- Do not allow clutter to accumulate in doorways or traffic lanes.
- Empty wastepaper cans in proper receptacles.

SAFETY Alert

Avoid stacking linen and supplies on upper shelves closer than 18 inches to the ceiling. If supplies are stacked close to the ceiling, the sprinkler system will not be effective during a fire.

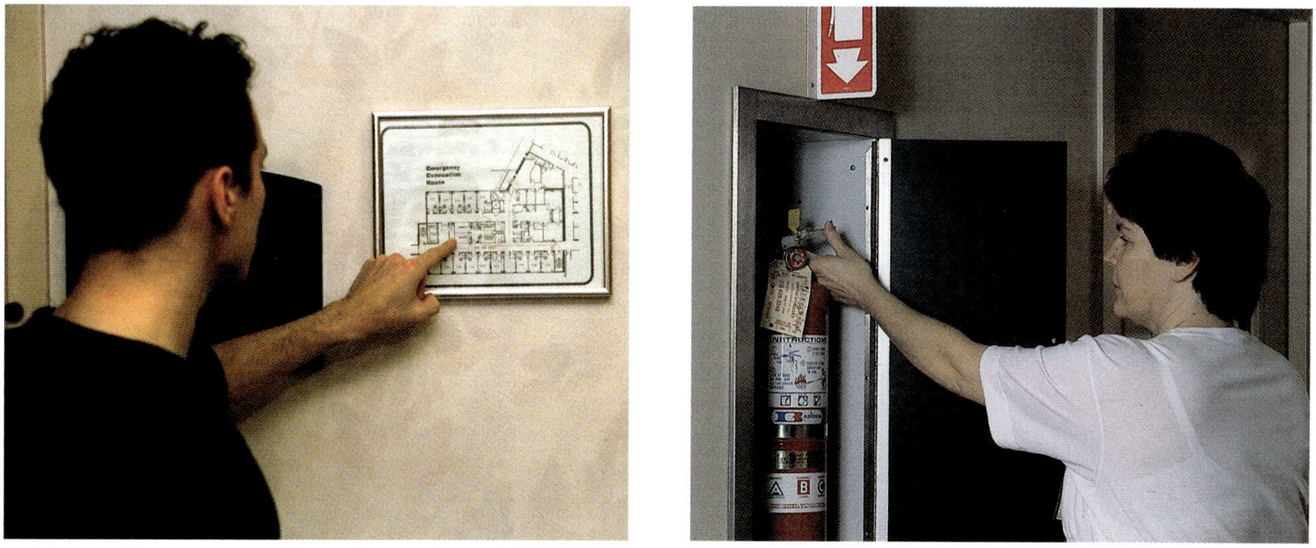

FIGURE 14-12 All personnel must be familiar with the evacuation plan, the location of fire extinguishers, and how to use them.

- Do not store oily rags or paint rags.
- Report any possible hazards right away.
- Report smoke and/or burning smells.
- Keep all fire exits clear of equipment and debris.
- Know and practice fire drill safety.
- Do not let visitors give cigarettes to patients.

Smoking

Smoking in bed should never be permitted. Smoking should be strictly limited to specific areas, if it is permitted at all. Most health care facilities do not permit smoking by anyone in any area.

This applies to patients, visitors, and staff alike. Ashtrays should be large. The use of matches should be watched. Smoking materials are usually stored at the nurse's station. Patients who do not have smoking privileges should not have smoking materials. If you notice that a patient who is not allowed to smoke has smoking materials, collect the materials and inform the nurse. Some patients may need direct supervision whenever they smoke.

Oxygen Precautions

The use of oxygen presents a specific hazard. When oxygen is in use:

- Never permit smoking, lighted matches, or open flames in the area.
- Do not use flammable liquids such as oils, alcohol, nail polish, aftershave, lotions, perfume, or hair spray.
- Do not use electrical equipment such as radios, hair dryers, electric razors, heating pads, or toys.
- Post a sign indicating that oxygen is in use.
- Use cotton blankets and gowns for the patient.

SAFETY Alert

Oxygen is a prescription item, like a medication. Using oxygen is safe as long as you follow facility policies and safety guidelines. Never change the fittings from one type of oxygen bottle to another. Make sure you use the correct adaptor and plug for the unit. Make sure the oxygen cylinder is secure in an upright position. If it is accidentally knocked over, it has the potential to turn into a missile and cause great damage. If you have reason to believe that an oxygen tank or liquid oxygen canister is leaking, remove the patient from the room and close the door. Report the problem to the proper person. Never attempt to carry or move an oxygen cylinder or canister if it is leaking.

SAFETY Alert

Bed linen can absorb oxygen. Any time oxygen is in use, avoid sparks. Static electricity can start a fire.

- Wear cotton uniforms and nonwool sweaters when providing care.
- Be certain there are no cigarettes, matches, or lighters in the room.
- Do not adjust the liter flow.

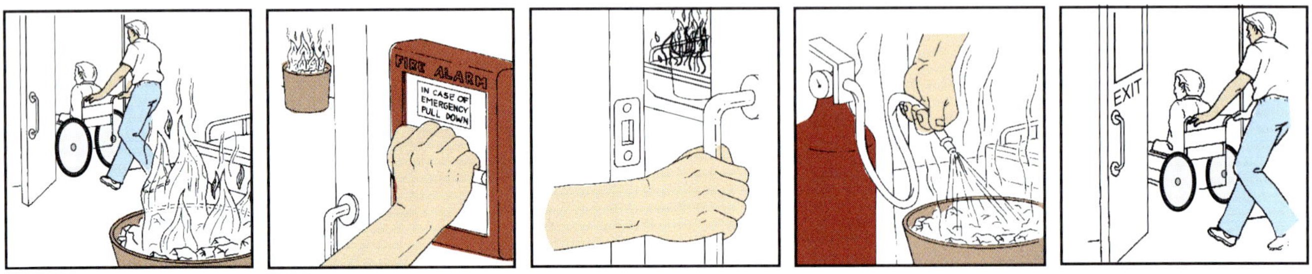

Remove **A**ctivate **C**ontain or **E**xtinguish or **E**vacuate

FIGURE 14-13 Remember the sequence of critical actions in case of fire.

In Case of Fire

You must be familiar with the fire policies and procedures for your facility. In case of fire, keep calm. Be sure those in immediate danger are moved to safety, then sound the alarm according to facility policy. Follow the evacuation plan as you have practiced. The patients may be confused and frightened. Therefore, the staff must be calm and in control. In a fire emergency, remember **RACE** as defined here (Figure 14-13):

- **R** = Remove patients. Move patients to safety. Patients who can walk can be escorted. In some cases, they may be called upon to assist others to escape routes. Patients may need to be moved in their beds out of the danger areas. If a person is unable to walk and the bed cannot be moved, bedsheets may be used as cradles and the patient pulled to safety.
- **A** = Alarm. Sound the alarm. Use the intercom, emergency signal bell, telephone, or fire alarm as directed by facility policy. Give the location and type of fire.
- **C** = Contain fire. Close windows and doors (Figure 14-14) to prevent drafts, which cause the fire to spread more rapidly.
- **E** = Extinguish fire or evacuate the area.

Follow the fire emergency plan for your facility:

- Keep calm. Be prepared to follow directions when a person in authority takes charge.
- Shut off air conditioning and other electrical equipment.
- Shut off oxygen.
- Do not use elevators.

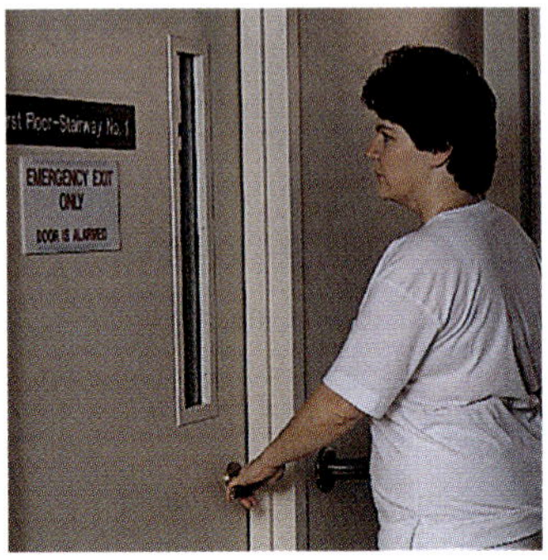

FIGURE 14-14 Fire doors slow the spread of fire when closed.

SAFETY *Alert*

Health facilities are built with safety features that prevent fires from spreading. These safety features include doors that close automatically when the fire alarm sounds, an automatic sprinkler system, smoke detectors, and fire exits. Many materials used on the floors, doors, walls, and furnishings are fire-rated. This means that they will take longer to burn. Nevertheless, fire prevention is an important responsibility. Despite the built-in safety features, health care facilities catch on fire. Many lives can be lost.

SAFETY *Alert*

When a fire occurs, patients are removed from immediate danger. After the alarm is sounded, the fire is contained by closing doors and windows. Patients are moved behind closed doors to keep them safe. Closing doors and windows slows the spread of fire. The hallways are cleared of patients and pieces of equipment that will burn. If the fire is large and spreading rapidly, patients may be evacuated from the building.

Use of a Fire Extinguisher

If you have been trained in the use of a fire extinguisher, you may use it on small fires.

- Fire extinguishers should be carried upright.
- Remove the safety pin.

SAFETY Alert

Smoke from a fire is very dangerous. If you are in a smoke-filled area, stay as close to the floor as possible. If you can crawl to an exit, cover your mouth and stay on your knees. The floor has the most oxygen available, because smoke rises. Before entering a room, touch the door with the *back* of your hand. *If the door is hot to the touch, do not open it.* If you are trapped in a room and the door is hot to the touch, stay in the room and place wet blankets or towels under the door to keep the smoke out. Opening the door could cause the fire to enter explosively.

- Push the top handle down.
- Direct the hose at the base of the fire.

Remember the letters **PASS**.

P—PULL the pin
A—AIM the nozzle at the base of the fire
S—SQUEEZE the handle
S—SWEEP back and forth along the base of the fire

OTHER EMERGENCIES

There may be other disasters for which you and your facility must be prepared. Tornadoes, hurricanes, floods, earthquakes, and bomb threats are examples of such disasters. Each facility has its own policies. Be sure you are familiar with them.

In all emergency situations, get patients to safety, follow your facility's policy, and keep calm.

VIOLENCE IN THE WORKPLACE

Episodes of violence in the workplace are increasing in our society. Hospitals and other health care facilities are not exempt from violence incidents. Serious violence has occurred in both rural and urban communities. Many facilities have violence prevention training programs. The goal of this training is to eliminate or reduce worker exposure to conditions that can lead to injury. OSHA has developed guidelines for preventing violence in the health care facility and many employers use these guidelines to implement safety programs and train their employees.

Workplace violence is any physical assault, threatening behavior, or verbal abuse that occurs in the workplace. The workplace includes, but is not limited to, the facility buildings and the surrounding perimeters, including parking lots, field locations, clients' homes, and traveling to and from work assignments. Workplace violence includes:

- Beatings
- Stabbings
- Suicides and attempted suicides
- Shootings
- Rapes
- Psychological traumas
- Threats or obscene telephone calls
- Intimidation
- Verbal or physical harassment
- Being followed, sworn at, or shouted at

Violence in the workplace can be committed by strangers, patients, coworkers, or personal acquaintances. Some of the potential causes of health care facility violence are:

- The prevalence of handguns and other weapons
- Use of hospitals by the criminal justice system for criminal holds and the care of disturbed, violent individuals

SAFETY Alert

Although rare in some parts of the country, a tornado can occur anywhere. A *tornado watch* means that conditions are favorable for a tornado to develop. A *tornado warning* means that a tornado is actually in the area. Patients are not evacuated during a tornado watch. Someone is designated to monitor the weather in case the situation changes. During a tornado warning, you will help with the evacuation of patients. This means that all patients will be moved to the basement, if the facility has one. In multiple-story buildings, patients are moved to the lowest level. Frequently patients are moved to a strong area in the center of the building. Patients should not be moved to areas where there are windows, as flying glass may cause serious injuries. Evacuation must be done very quickly, as tornadoes strike with little warning. If patients cannot walk, they are moved in wheelchairs or beds. You may be instructed to cover patients with blankets to protect them from flying debris. You may also be required to close the room doors, fire doors, windows, and curtains facing the direction of the oncoming tornado. If there is enough time, open the doors, windows, and curtains on the opposite side of the building. Do not go near the windows during the storm.

- Acute and chronically mentally ill patients
- Individuals who abuse alcohol and drugs
- The availability of controlled substances in the facility, making it a likely target of robbery
- The increasing number of gangs and gang members in many communities
- Unrestricted movement of the public in health care facilities
- Drug and alcohol abuse
- Distraught family members and other individuals who become angry and frustrated
- Low staffing levels, particularly during meals and at other times when staff is busy caring for patients and unable to observe activity in the hallways
- Poorly lit parking lots, garages, and ramps
- Lack of staff awareness of risk factors
- Failure to use safety precautions, such as locking doors and reporting suspicious individuals

guidelines *for* Violence Prevention

Follow all facility policies and procedures involving safety and security. Other things you can do to prevent potential incidents are:

- Participate in continuing education programs to learn how to recognize and manage escalating agitation, assaultive behavior, or criminal intent.
- Attend classes on cultural diversity that offer sensitivity training on racial and ethnic issues and differences.
- If you are responsible for a secured area, control access to the area and keep it locked. Avoid propping locked doors and windows open. Never disable a door alarm.
- Do not leave keys unattended. Never share security alarm codes with unauthorized persons.
- Close shades or curtains at night.
- Report assaults or threats of assaults to the nurse manager immediately.
- Avoid wearing scarves, necklaces, earrings, and other jewelry that could cause injury if a patient or other individual attacks you.
- Do not carry valuables or large sums of cash to work.
- Avoid remote, dark areas when you are alone.
- Report lights that are burned out and locks that are not working.
- Exercise caution in elevators, stairwells, and unfamiliar areas. Immediately leave the area if you believe a hazard exists.
- Use the "buddy system" if personal safety may be threatened.
- If a patient or other person is "acting out," or you believe you may be assaulted, do not let the person come between you and the exit.
- Keep your head up, look ahead, and be aware of your surroundings.
- If your facility has security personnel, request that they escort you in dark or potentially dangerous areas. If no security personnel are on duty, ask other staff members to accompany you.
- Park in well-lighted areas. Always lock your car after parking. Look in the car before getting in, then lock the doors after you get in. Do not roll windows down to speak with individuals approaching your car.
- Report suspicious individuals or other potential safety hazards to the proper person. Never approach a suspicious person by yourself.

guidelines *for* Dealing with a Violent Individual

- Remain calm and avoid raising your voice, which may further agitate the person.
- Speak slowly, softly, and clearly.
- Call for help, if possible, or send someone to get help.
- Move away from heavy or sharp objects that may be used as weapons.
- Monitor your body language and avoid movements that could be challenging, such as placing your hands on your hips, moving toward the person, pointing your finger, or staring directly at the person. However, focus your attention on the person so you know what he or she is doing at all times.

continues

guidelines *continued*

- Position yourself at right angles to the person. Avoid standing directly in front of him or her. Maintain a distance of 3 to 6 feet.
- Position yourself so that an exit is accessible. Never let the person come between you and the exit.
- Avoid making sudden movements.
- Listen to what the person is saying. Encourage the person to talk, and communicate that you genuinely care and will try to help. Acknowledge that you understand that he or she is upset. Break big problems into smaller, manageable ones.
- Avoid arguing and defensive statements. Accept criticism in a positive way. If you sincerely feel criticism is unwarranted, ask clarifying questions.
- Ask the person to leave and return when he or she is calmer.
- Ask questions to help regain control of the conversation.
- Avoid challenging, bargaining, or making promises you cannot keep.
- Describe the consequences of abusive behavior.
- Avoid touching an angry person.
- If a weapon is involved, ask the person to place it in a neutral location while you continue talking. Avoid trying to disarm the person, which may put you in danger.

NURSING ASSISTANT SAFETY

The work performed by nursing assistants requires a great deal of lifting and moving of patients, objects, and equipment. It is important that you use your body correctly to avoid injury.

Ergonomics

The word **ergonomics** means adapting the environment and using techniques and equipment to prevent injury to the body. If certain risk factors are present, it is more likely that an ergonomic (work-related) problem will occur. These risk factors include:

1. Performing the same motion or motion pattern every few seconds for more than two to four hours at a time.
2. Being in a fixed or awkward posture for more than a total of two to four hours.
3. Using forceful hand exertions for more than two to four hours at a time.
4. Doing heavy lifting, unassisted, for more than one to two hours.

Here are several ergonomic techniques you can use to reduce the risk of having an incident:

1. Use correct body mechanics at all times, both at work and when you are off duty.
2. Raise beds to a comfortable working height (remember to lower the beds when you finish your task).
3. Use mechanical lifts when you need to transfer very heavy and/or dependent patients from the bed or chair and back.
4. Use back supports if your employer requires them or if this is your preference. The use of back supports is controversial, but many nursing assistants find them helpful (Figure 14-15).
5. Get another person to help when you need to transfer a patient who cannot bear his own weight fully.
6. Use a cart to move heavy items.

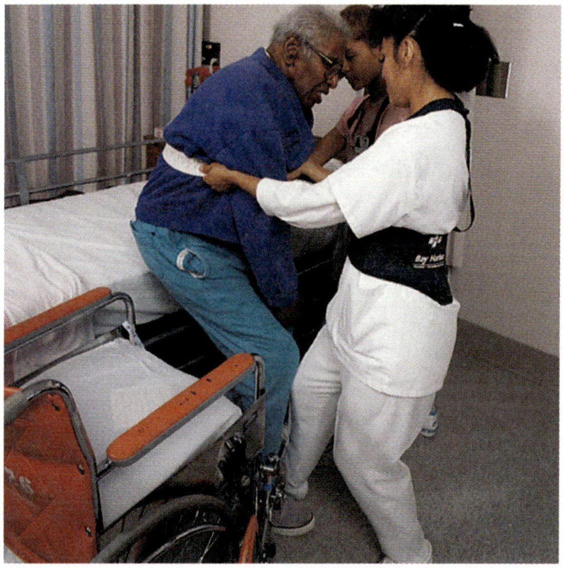

FIGURE 14-15 Some employers require employees to wear back support belts when lifting and moving patients.

OSHA Alert

The back support belt works by keeping your spine in good alignment. You are less likely to be injured if your spine is straight and you are using good body mechanics. Do not lift more than you would if you were not wearing the belt. Using a back support belt does not make you stronger.

If you follow these eight commandments for lifting, you will greatly decrease the risk of injuring yourself.

1. Plan your lift and test the load (Figure 14-16A).
2. Ask for help (Figure 14-16B).
3. Get a firm footing (Figure 14-16C).
4. Bend your knees (Figure 14-16D).
5. Tighten your abdominal muscles (Figure 14-16E).
6. Lift with your legs (Figure 14-16F).
7. Keep the load close (Figure 14-16G).
8. Keep your back upright (Figure 14-16H).

Warming up before working is another way to maintain a healthy body. The exercises shown in Figures 14-17A through 14-17J can be performed before each work shift. Check with your physician before beginning any exercise program.

Remember that you can avoid many problems if you also:

- Exercise every day.
- Eat a nourishing, well-balanced diet.
- Get adequate sleep.
- Avoid alcohol, cigarettes, drug use, and too much caffeine.
- Wear comfortable shoes with good support.

SAFETY *Alert*

Have you ever heard the expression, "When your feet hurt, you hurt all over"? Most experienced health care workers will tell you this old adage is true. Buying a sturdy pair of athletic shoes or duty shoes is one of the best investments you will make in your uniform. Make sure that the shoe soles are appropriate for the floor surface in your facility. In most cases, this means having a nonslip sole. Having proper footwear will make you feel better and reduce your risk of falls and injuries.

Hazards in the Work Environment

All health care facilities have hazards in the work environment that can potentially cause injury to employees. Many of these items are chemicals that you may have in your own home (chlorine bleach, for example). On a nursing unit you might find cleaning supplies, disinfectants, and other

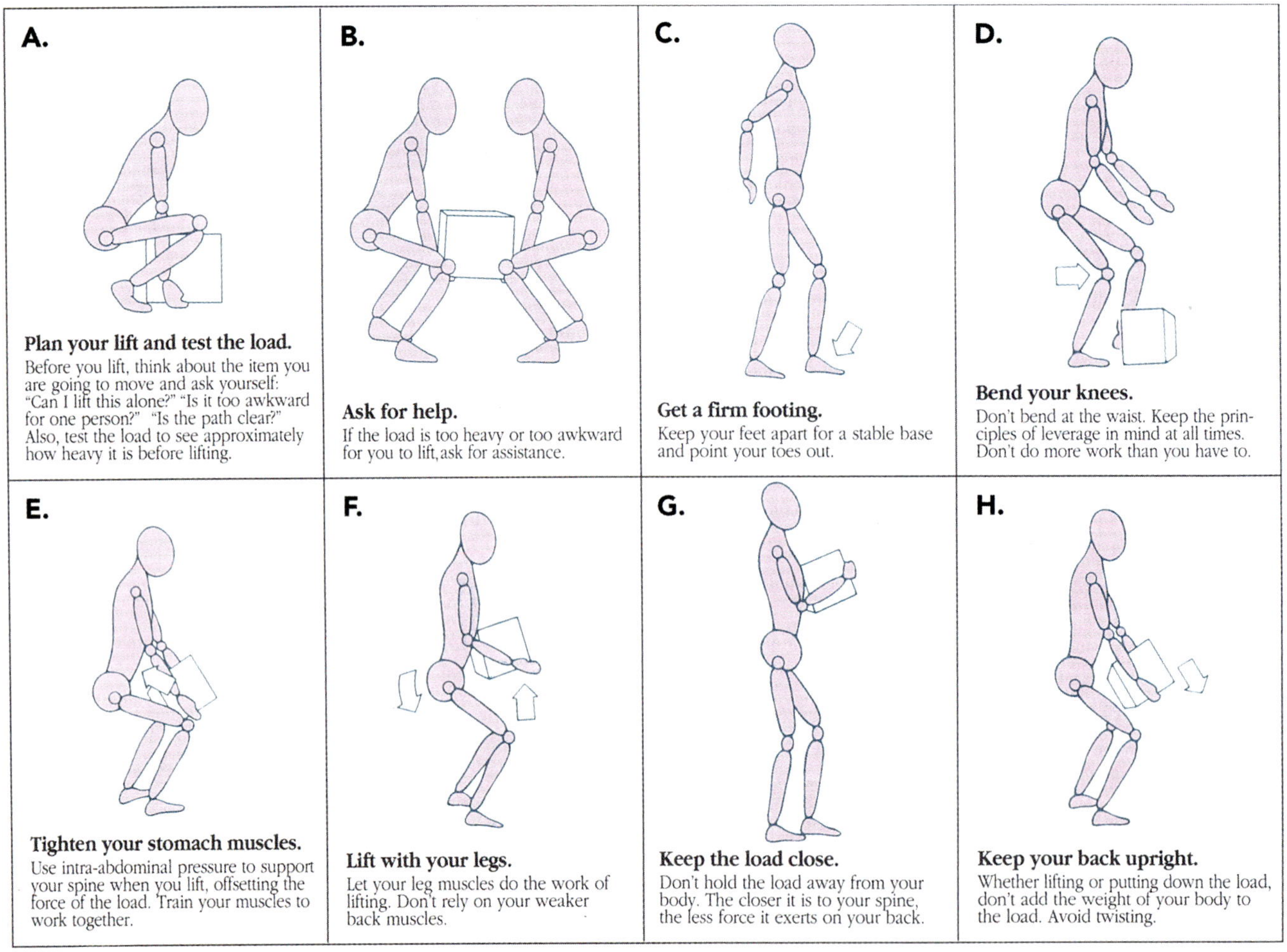

FIGURE 14-16 Eight rules for lifting. *(Reprinted with permission from Ergodyne Corporation, St. Paul, MN)*

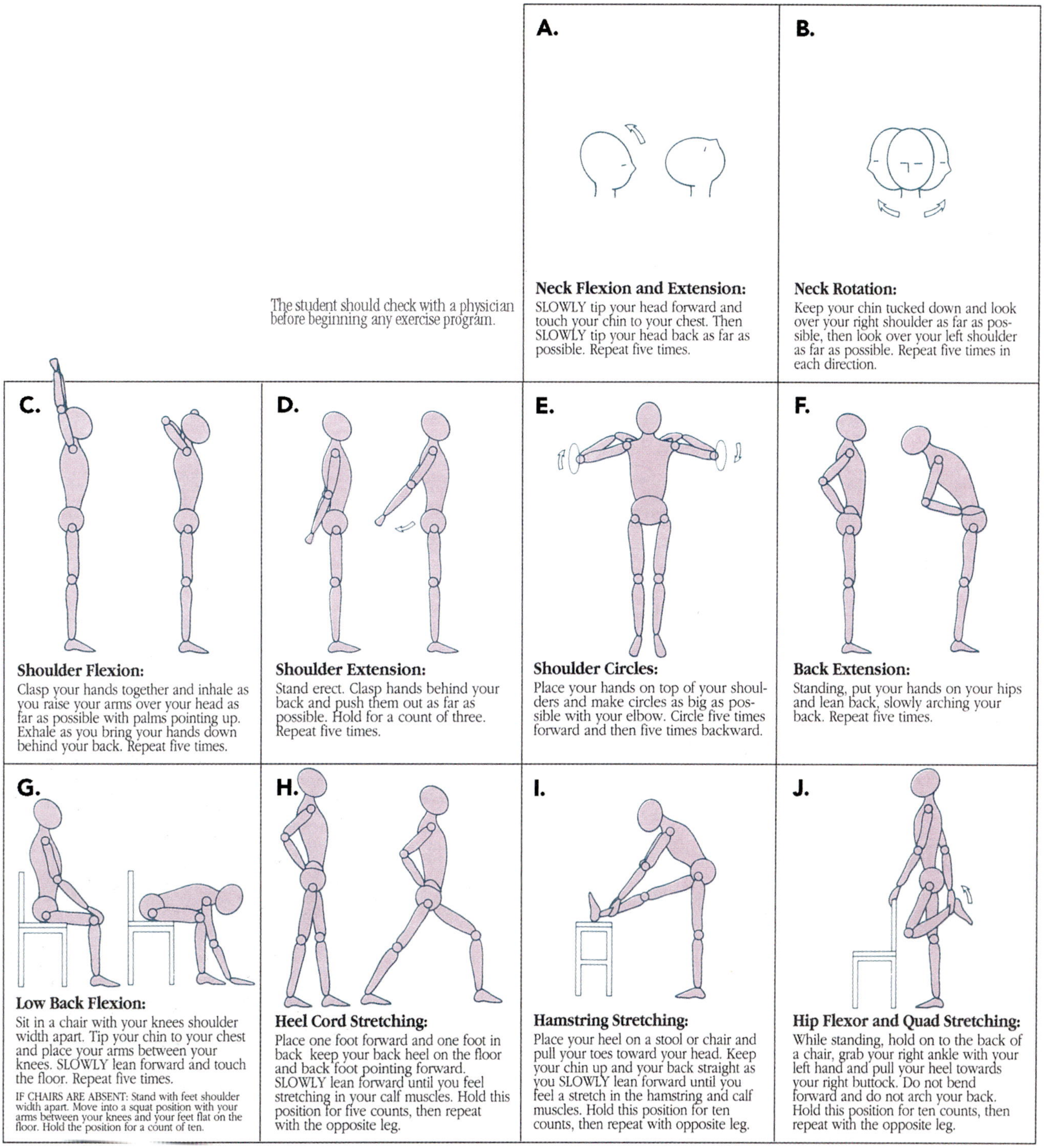

FIGURE 14-17 Warming up before work can help prevent injuries. *(Reprinted with permission from Ergodyne Corporation, St. Paul, MN)*

products that are considered hazardous. Injuries can be prevented if you know what the hazards are and how to protect yourself and others. The Occupational Safety and Health Administration (OSHA) is a section of the Department of Labor under the federal government. OSHA is responsible for employee safety. OSHA requires that all manufacturers of these items supply **Material Safety Data Sheets** (**MSDS**) with any hazardous products they sell. The MSDS provide hazard communications that explain:

- What precautions to take in the presence of a hazard (for example, wearing personal protective equipment)
- Instructions for safe use of the potentially dangerous substance
- How to clean up and dispose of the hazardous product
- First aid measures to use if exposure occurs

OSHA has also established other rules for a safe environment. Employers are required to inform employees of:

- The location of the MSDS
- The hazards that exist in the work environment and where they are in the building
- The location of information related to the hazards
- How to read and understand chemical labels and hazard signs
- What type of personal protective equipment should be worn while working with these chemicals, and where the personal protective equipment is stored
- How to manage spills and where cleaning equipment is stored

All hazardous products must be kept in their original containers with the original labels intact and legible. Health care facilities must keep all chemicals in locked cupboards.

OSHA *Alert*

Many chemicals can be hazardous to both patients and nursing assistants. Always use chemicals according to the directions on the label. Make sure they are properly diluted and that containers and surfaces are properly rinsed. Never repackage chemicals into unmarked containers. Use only the original container or special, small containers provided by the manufacturer. Chemicals should always be under your visual control, meaning you can see them. If you cannot see a chemical, it should be stored in a locked area. Wear utility gloves when using chemicals for cleaning procedures. Many chemicals will cause defects in the examination gloves used for patient care. This can irritate your hands, and the chemicals may be absorbed through your skin. Wear eye protection if there is a possibility of splashing or spraying chemicals during a cleaning procedure. Learn the locations of your facility's MSDS sheets, eye wash station, and body wash station.

REVIEW

A. Multiple Choice.

Select the one best answer for each of the following.

1. The patient's name is Phe Quan. She is in Room 116-D. From this information, you know that she is occupying a bed in a
- **a.** private room.
- **b.** rehabilitation department.
- **c.** semiprivate room.
- **d.** ward.

2. Side rails should be up and secure when
- **a.** the bed is at the lowest horizontal height.
- **b.** the patient has a catheter.
- **c.** leaving the patient after care, unless there is a signed release.
- **d.** the patient does not have an order for restraints.

3. The best room temperature is approximately
- **a.** 45°F.
- **b.** 65°F.
- **c.** 70°F.
- **d.** 78°F.

4. Which of the following represents a fire hazard?
- **a.** Frayed electrical wire
- **b.** Using three-prong plugs
- **c.** Supervised smoking
- **d.** Using UL-approved items

5. Ashtrays should be emptied into
- **a.** a plastic container.
- **b.** a metal container.
- **c.** a paper sack.
- **d.** the open wastebasket.

6. Which of the following contributes to unsafe conditions in the facility?
- **a.** Equipment sitting in the halls
- **b.** Chemicals in locked cupboards
- **c.** Allowing patients to smoke with supervision
- **d.** Teaching patients how to use assistive devices such as canes and walkers

7. When oxygen is in use, you should not
- **a.** use cotton blankets on the patient's bed.
- **b.** remove cigarettes from the room.

c. adjust the liter flow.
d. post a sign on the door.

8. Every staff member should know
   a. the facility fire procedure.
   b. the RACE procedure.
   c. the distance from the fire department to the facility.
   d. how to extinguish a fire by aiming the extinguisher at the top of the flames.
9. The word that means adapting the environment to prevent body injury is
   a. body mechanics.
   b. incident.
   c. ergonomics.
   d. RACE.
10. One principle of good body mechanics is to
   a. bend from the waist when lifting.
   b. keep your feet close together when lifting.
   c. use the strong muscles of your arms for lifting.
   d. keep the load as far from your body as possible.
11. Material Safety Data Sheets (MSDS) are required to include information that
   a. describes how to repackage the product.
   b. explains first aid measures to use if exposure occurs.
   c. describes how to use the product.
   d. lists other approved uses of the product.
12. When dealing with a potentially violent individual, the nursing assistant should
   a. speak loudly and clearly.
   b. maintain a distance of 2 feet.
   c. listen to what the person is saying.
   d. attempt to touch the person gently.

B. Completion.

Choose the correct word from the following list to complete each statement in questions 12–20.

body mechanics	mechanical lift
call light	Material Safety Data Sheets (MSDS)
ergonomics	OSHA
hips and knees	RACE
incident	

13. Using your body correctly while you are working is called ______.
14. Basic rules for lifting include bend from the ______ and not from the waist.
15. An unexpected situation that can cause harm to an employee, a patient, or a visitor is called (a, an) ______.
16. Adapting the environment and using techniques and equipment to prevent body injury is called ______.
17. You should use a ______ when you need to transfer very heavy or dependent patients.
18. All patients must have access to a ______ because it may be the only way they have to summon help.
19. All manufacturers must supply ______ with the hazardous products they sell.
20. The section of the federal government that oversees employee safety is called ______.
21. The acronym used to remember the sequence of critical actions in case of fire is ______.

C. True/False.

Mark the following true or false by circling T or F.

22. T F The bed should be left in the lowest horizontal position when the patient is sleeping.
23. T F Side rails are restraints in certain circumstances.
24. T F There should always be enough light to enable staff to work safely.
25. T F Noise and clutter are very disturbing to most people.
26. T F Needed repairs should be reported immediately.
27. T F The signal cord is the patient's way of letting the staff know that he is in need.
28. T F It is all right to play while at work as long as no one gets hurt.
29. T F You are responsible for knowing and practicing fire drill procedures.
30. T F In case of a fire, follow your own plan of action.
31. T F It is wise to use an elevator during a fire emergency.

D. Nursing Assistant Challenge.

Mary Hernandez is a new nursing assistant at Community Memorial Hospital. She has just completed her CNA course. Consider the information she needs to receive in orientation in order to be a safe and efficient worker.

32. What information does Mary need to learn about the facility to prevent fires and to follow correct procedure in the event of a fire?
33. Mary will need information on equipment she will be working with. What items of equipment is she likely to be using on her job?
34. Discuss everything Mary can do to prevent work-related injuries.
35. What chemicals is she likely to be using?

EXPLORING THE WEB

Description	Location
Ergonomics articles	http://www.hill-rom.com
Safety/hygiene	http://www.delmarhealthcare.com/olcs/white/pnotes.asp (see Chapter 20)
Back Belts: Do They Prevent Injury?	http://www.cdc.gov/niosh/backbelt.htm
Back Care for Nurses	http://www.phil-e-slide.com http://www.spineuniverse.com
Back Injury Prevention	http://www.twcc.state.tx.us
Back Injury Prevention Guide for Health Care Providers	http://165.235.90.100/DOSH/dosh_publications/backinj.pdf
Back Safety	http://www.mmhospital.org
Example Safety Program and Policies	http://www.costaffing.com
Fire Safety	http://www.nfpa.org
Health and Safety Info	http://www.healthsafetyinfo.com
Hospital Linx	http://www.hospitaladminlinx.com
International Association for Healthcare Safety and Security	http://www.iahss.org
Material Safety Data Sheets	http://www.phys.ksu.edu
Occupational Safety and Health Administration (OSHA)	http://www.osha.gov
–Ergonomics for the Prevention of Musculoskeletal Disorders: Guidelines for Nursing Homes	http://www.osha.gov/ergonomics/guidelines/nursinghome/index.html
–OSHA Ergonomics Recommendations	http://www.osha.gov/ergonomics/index.html
Risk Management Foundation	http://www.rmf.harvard.edu
Safe Patient Movement and Handling	http://www.va.gov
Safety Alerts	http://www.safetyalerts.com
Safety Info	http://www.safetyinfo.com
University of Michigan Risk Management	http://www.umich.edu

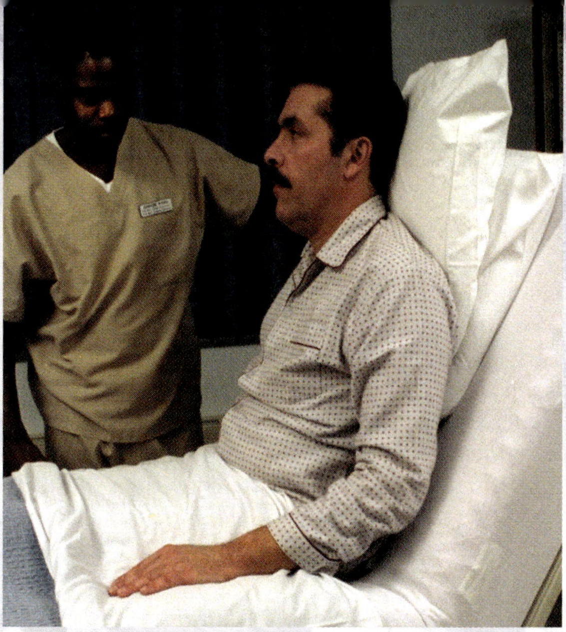

unit 15

Patient Safety and Positioning

objectives

After completing this unit, you will be able to:

- Spell and define terms.
- Identify patients who are at risk for having incidents.
- List alternatives to the use of physical restraints.
- Describe the guidelines for the use of restraints.
- Demonstrate the correct application of restraints.
- Describe two measures for preventing these types of incidents: accidental poisoning, thermal injuries, skin injuries, and choking.
- List the elements that are common to all procedures.
- Describe correct body alignment for the patient.
- List the purposes of repositioning patients.
- Demonstrate these positions using the correct supportive devices: supine, semisupine, prone, semiprone, lateral, Fowler's, and orthopneic.
- Demonstrate the following procedures:
  - Procedure 14 Turning the Patient Toward You
  - Procedure 15 Turning the Patient Away from You
  - Procedure 16 Moving a Patient to the Head of the Bed
  - Procedure 17 Logrolling the Patient

vocabulary

Learn the meaning and the correct spelling of the following words and phrases:

ambulate
aspiration
body alignment
chemical restraint
contracture
draw sheet
enabler
Fowler's position
high Fowler's
laceration
lateral
mobility
orthopneic position
orthotic devices (orthoses)
physical restraint
postural support
pressure ulcer
procedure
prone
semi-Fowler's
semiprone
semisupine
Sims' position
spasticity
splint
supine
supportive device
transfer
trochanter roll
turning (moving) sheet

PATIENT SAFETY

In Unit 14, you learned how to maintain a safe environment and how to avoid personal injuries. The prevention of patient injuries is another very important part of your job as a nursing assistant. Patients in health care facilities are at risk for incidents, because they may:

- Have impaired **mobility** (ability to move about) due to an injury, disease, or surgery
- Be receiving medications that affect mental status, balance, and coordination
- Be disoriented because of the change in environment or because of a medical disorder
- Have impaired hearing or impaired vision

Because of these risk factors, most incidents involving patients in any health care setting are falls. Falls may occur because the patient:

- Misjudges the distance from the bed to the floor
- Feels weak or dizzy when trying to get up
- Changes position too rapidly and loses balance when trying to stand up
- Encounters hazards when walking
- Is walking in a poorly lit area

USE OF PHYSICAL RESTRAINTS

In the past, restraints were often used routinely as a preventive measure to avoid falls. Research has shown that side rails and restraints do not necessarily accomplish this purpose. In fact, many falls occur with side rails up and restraints intact. This can result in serious injury and even death. There are two types of restraints: physical restraints and chemical restraints. **Chemical restraints** are medications that affect the patient's mood and behavior. As a nursing assistant, you will be more concerned with the use of physical restraints. **Physical restraints** are defined as any technique or device that is attached or next to the patient's body that the patient cannot easily remove and that restricts freedom of movement and normal access to the body. OBRA (1987) clearly states when and how chemical and physical restraints may be used in a long-term care facility. The Residents' Rights state that "residents have the right to be free from physical and chemical restraints." According to this definition, many devices qualify as restraints if the patient does not have the physical or mental ability to remove the device readily. These guidelines have been implemented in acute care facilities as well. Physical restraints are to be used only when the safety of the

guidelines *for*

Preventing Patient Falls

- Always leave the bed in its lowest horizontal position when you have finished giving care.
- Keep brakes locked on bed wheels at all times except when the bed is being moved.
- Check to see whether the side rails are to be raised. Make sure they are attached securely.
- Check and adjust protruding objects such as bed wheels or gatch handles.
- Do not block or clutter open areas with supplies and equipment.
- Wipe up spills immediately.
- Encourage patients to use the rails along corridor walls when walking (Figure 15-1).
- Monitor patients for signs of weakness, fatigue, dizziness, and loss of balance.
- Monitor patients for safe practice if they independently:
  - propel their wheelchairs
  - **transfer** (get out of bed)
  - **ambulate** (walk)

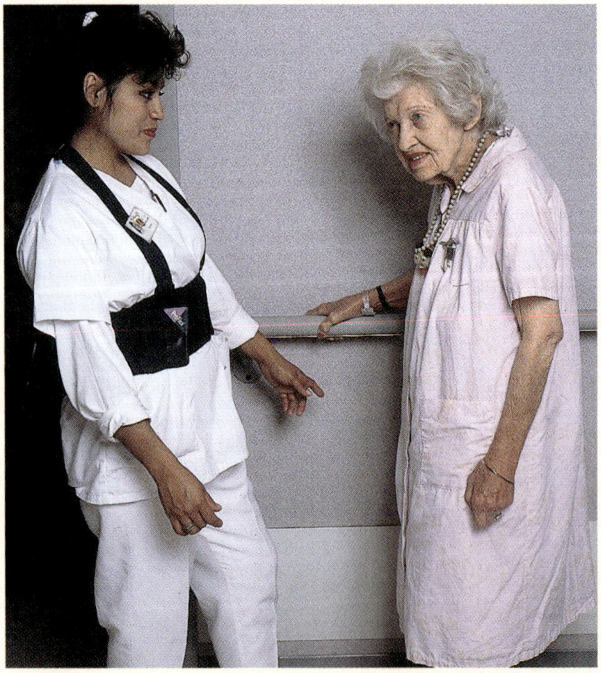

FIGURE 15-1 Encourage patients to hold rails on corridor walls when walking.

continues

guidelines *continued*

- Provide adequate lighting.
- Eliminate noise and other distractions that may increase confusion and create anxiety.
- Avoid leaving patients alone in the tub or shower unless you are given specific permission to do so.
- Check patients' clothing for fit and safety. Loose shoes and laces, long robes, and slacks increase the risk of falling. Footwear should be appropriate for the floor surface. In general, this means using nonskid shoes (Figure 15-2) on tile floor surfaces. For carpeted floors, consult the physical therapist if there is a question about appropriate footwear for the patient. Nonskid shoes may stick to the carpeting, causing falls. A leather or synthetic shoe sole may be more appropriate for a carpeted surface.
- Care for the patient's physical needs promptly. Many incidents occur when patients attempt to get out of bed to go to the bathroom.
- Always use the correct techniques for transferring and walking patients.
- Use a gait belt when assisting patients to transfer or ambulate.
- Follow the care plan when assisting patients with transfers and ambulation.

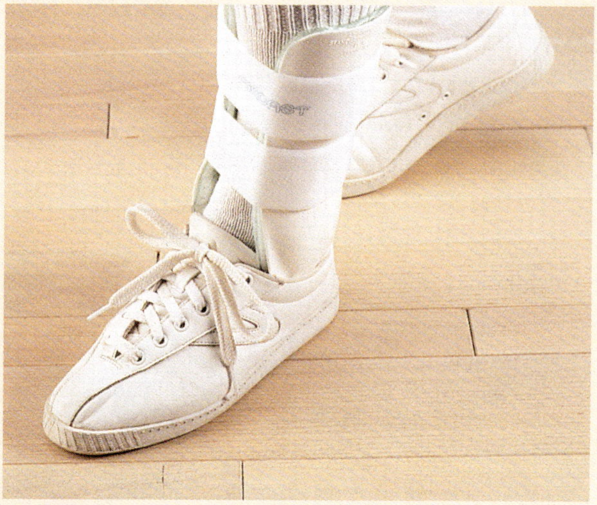

FIGURE 15-2 Patients should wear nonskid shoes for transfers and walking on tile floors. *(Aircast® ankle stirrup is provided by Sammons Preston, Inc., a Bissell® HealthCare Company. Reprinted with permission.)*

patient or other persons is at risk. Before a restraint is used, the staff must:

- Document all patient behavior indicating the need for a restraint.
- Document all actions that were taken as an alternative to restraints.
- Consult with the patient and the family or legal guardian when alternatives are unsuccessful and obtain their approval and consent to apply a restraint (Figure 15-3).

Examples of physical restraints include:

- Wrist/arm (Figure 15-4) and ankle/leg restraints
- Vests (Figure 15-5)
- Jackets (Figure 15-6)
- Hand mitts (Figure 15-7)
- Geriatric and cardiac chairs (Figure 15-8)
- Wheelchair safety belts, bars, and tables (Figure 15-9)
- Bed rails (if they meet the definition of a restraint)

Restraints are medical devices. They should never be used as a form of punishment, or for the convenience of the nursing staff. Patients have been seriously injured and died as a result of restraint use, so restraint application must be considered very seriously and avoided whenever possible. Other potential complications of restraints are listed in Table 15-1.

Before restraints are used, the staff must assess the patient's capabilities and the reasons for use of the restraint. If the cause of the patient's problem can be identified and corrected, the need for a restraint may be eliminated. For example, if restraints are being considered to prevent falls,

SAFETY *Alert*

The vest is a very secure restraint used for patients at high risk of injury. It looks like a vest and crosses over in the front. Other similar restraints are pulled over the head. These are called by different names, such as *jacket* or *poncho*, but the principles of application are the same for all three devices. Years ago, health care providers were taught to cross the vest restraint over the patient's back. Some personnel still apply vests in this manner, but doing so is not safe. Crossing the vest in the back can cause choking and other serious injury. A vest restraint that fits properly, and is crossed in front according to manufacturers' directions, will safely and securely hold the patient.

Physical Restraint Informed Consent

Patient's name ______________________________

Method of physical restraint used ______________________________

The reason the physical restraint is needed ______________________________

____

Times when restraint will be applied ______________________________

Alternatives tried ______________________________

In compliance with federal and state regulations, this facility is committed to limiting of the use of physical restraints only to situations necessary to maximize a patient's physical, mental, and psychological well-being. It is the policy of this facility that, if physical restraints are deemed necessary, the least restrictive method will be applied for the shortest amount of time possible.

Physical restraints will be used by this facility only when it has been determined that they are required to treat a patient's medical symptoms or a therapeutic intervention, as ordered by a physician, and based on (1) a documented assessment, by an appropriate health professional, of the patient's capabilities; the physical condition or mental treatment that requires the use of physical restraints; the less restrictive measures or therapeutic interventions that have proved ineffective; and the specific physical restraint most effective for the patient's condition; and (2) demonstration by the care planning process that using a physical restraint as a therapeutic intervention will promote the care and services necessary for the patient to attain or maintain the highest practicable physical, mental, or psychosocial well-being.

This patient has been assessed regarding his or her need for appro-priate physical restraint. He or she will be reassessed at least quarterly or as his or her needs change throughout the stay at this facility. A report will be made each quarter as to the effectiveness of the physical restraint in maximizing the patient's physical, mental, or psychosocial well-being. Ongoing assessments help to further this goal. The duration of consent for the use of this physical restraint is good only until the next annual assessment of the patient's needs, or if there is a need for more restrictive physical restraints. At those times, a new informed consent will be required.

The benefits of physical restraints include the prevention of injuries to oneself or to others, enhancement of functional abilities, reduced potential for falling, and continued provision of medically necessary procedures. Potential complications associated with physical restraints include incontinence, decreased range of motion, decreased ability to ambulate, symptoms of withdrawal or depression, or reduced social contact. This facility will monitor the use of physical restraints daily and respond to any developing complications to physical restraint use.

By virtue of my signature, I state that I received, read, and had an opportunity to discuss any questions I may have regarding the application of physical restraints in this facility. I give consent for the use of physical restraints when the benefits outweigh the identified risks in accordance with this informed consent. I understand that I can revoke consent for this physical restraint at any time. I further consent to physical restraint reduction as soon as feasible.

____

(Signature of Patient or Authorized Individual) (Date)

____

(Signature of Witness) (Date)

[ ] Patient unable to sign.

FIGURE 15-3 Many facilities obtain written consent from the patient or responsible party before applying a restraint.

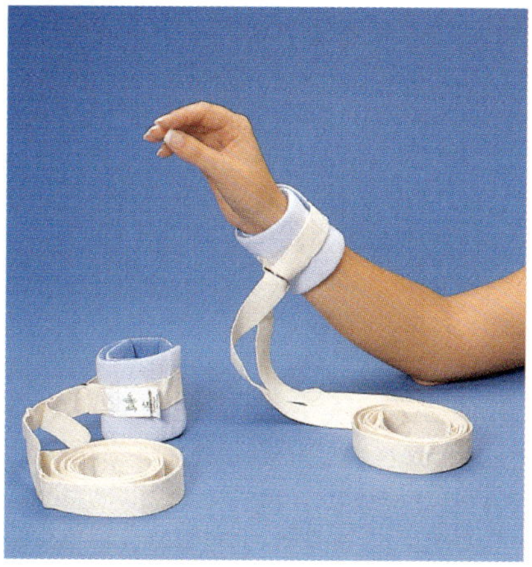

FIGURE 15-4 Wrist restraints may be used to prevent the patient from pulling on IVs and other tubes.

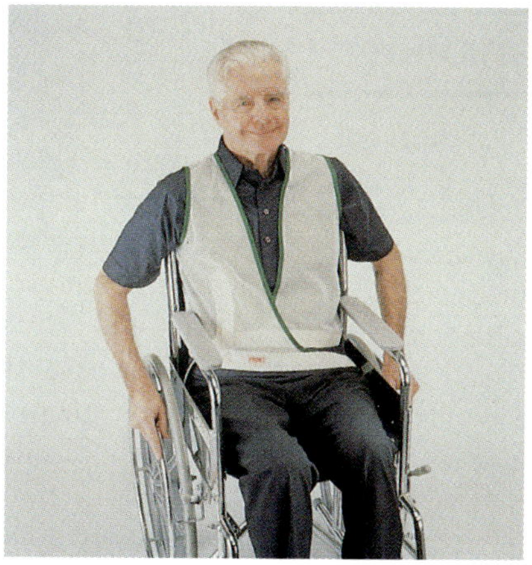

FIGURE 15-5 Vest restraints must be applied as pictured here, with the straps crossed over in front of the patient.

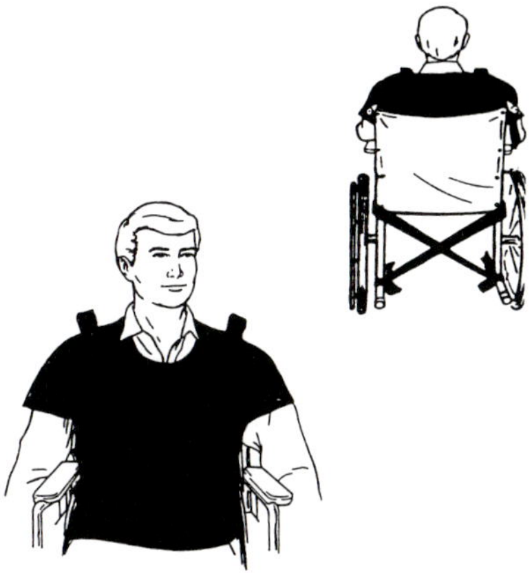

FIGURE 15-6 Jacket restraint.

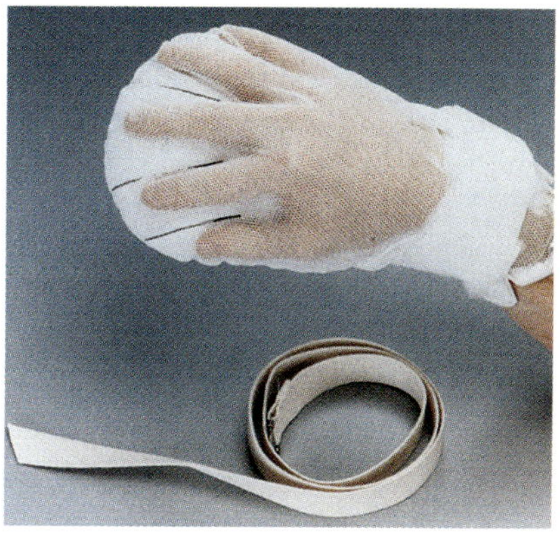

FIGURE 15-7 Hand mitts may be applied to keep the patient from injuring himself or pulling on tubes.

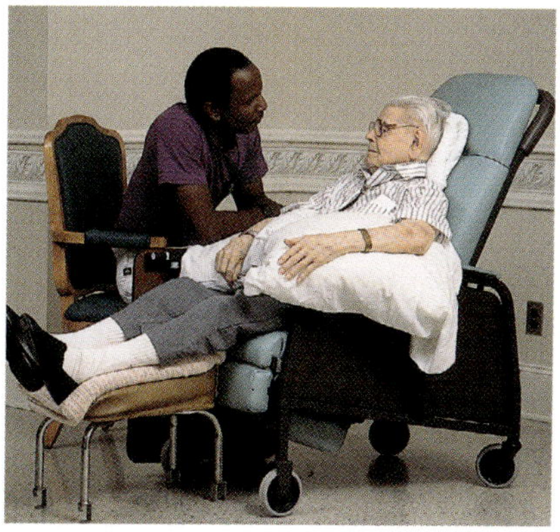

FIGURE 15-8 Geriatric chairs are restraints in some circumstances.

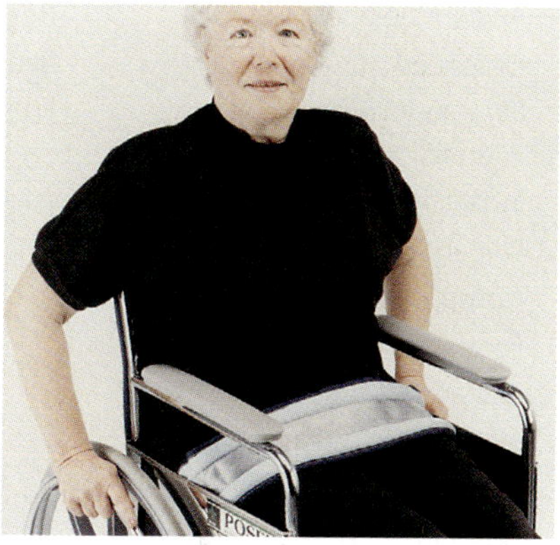

FIGURE 15-9 Wheelchair safety belts, bars, and tables are considered restraints if the patient does not have the physical or mental ability to remove them.

(Figures 15-4, 15-5, 15-6, 15-7, and 15-9 are all courtesy of J.T. Posey Co., Inc., Arcadia, CA.)

the patient's individual risk factors associated with falls are assessed. If some risk factors can be eliminated or modified, this reduces the risk of falls, and restraints may not be necessary. For example, an unsteady male patient gets up to use the bathroom at night, but does not call for help. His risk of falls can be modified by making sure a urinal is within reach and emptied regularly.

If a patient is a danger to himself or others, or requires emergency medical treatment, restraints may be appropriate. However, less restrictive alternatives to restraints must be considered first. Many alternative devices are available to use instead of restraints. If a restraint is determined to be the best approach, it is applied. However, an ongoing assessment of the factors creating the need for restraints is necessary, and personnel must work to reduce or eliminate the need for the restraint.

If restraints are indicated, the least restrictive restraint required to keep the patient safe should be selected. The restraint should be used as infrequently as possible. Using restraints requires careful assessment, planning, and monitoring. Studies have proven that it takes more time to care for patients in restraints than to care for patients who are not restrained. The physician must agree to the use of restraints and write an order before they can be used. The care plan will provide information about the type of restraint to use, the time the restraint is to be applied, and other special information and instructions.

Enablers. **Enablers** are devices that empower patients and assist them to function at their highest possible level. For example, a patient in a wheelchair is unable to sit up straight to feed herself, so she is fed by staff. If a supportive

TABLE 15-1 COMPLICATIONS OF RESTRAINTS

Potential Physical Problems	Potential Psychosocial Problems
Decreased independence	Worsening of behavior problems
Pressure ulcers	Withdrawal, loss of social contact
Weakness	Depression
Decreased range of motion	Forgetfulness
Muscle wasting	Fear
Contractures (frozen, deformed joints)	Anger
Loss of ability to ambulate	Shame
Edema of ankles, lower legs, feet, fingers	Agitation
Decreased appetite, weight loss	Mental confusion
Dehydration	Combativeness
Acute mental confusion	Restlessness
Distended abdomen	Sense of abandonment
Urge to void frequently, dribbling	Frustration
Incontinence	Loss of self-esteem
Urinary tract infection	Depression
Constipation	Screaming, yelling, calling out
Fecal impaction	
Lethargy	
Shortness of breath	
Pneumonia	
Bruising, redness, cuts, skin tears	
Falls	
Impaired circulation	
Blood clots	
Choking	
Death	

device is applied to correct her posture and allow her to feed herself, the device is an enabler. Devices used as enablers that maintain body position and alignment are commonly called **postural supports**. Used correctly, they give patients a higher degree of independence and enable them to perform tasks they were previously unable to do. In this case, using the restraint improves the patient's self-esteem.

The wheelchair lap tray (Figure 15-10) is a restraint alternative that is also used as an enabler. The tray is simple to use: it is attached to the back of the wheelchair with Velcro® straps. Patients can lean on it, and its surface can hold personal items or reading and writing supplies. A tray may enable the patient to feed himself by moving the food closer so he can reach it. The tray also reminds the patient not to stand up. If the tray allows the patient to perform a task, it is an enabler. If it is used strictly to keep the patient in the chair, and he does not have the physical or mental ability to remove the tray, it is considered a restraint. If the tray can be removed by the patient, it is a restraint alternative.

Side Rails as Restraints. By definition, side rails are restraints. They can also be an enabler. Many patients pull on them to position and turn themselves in bed. Some patients may feel more secure if the rails are up. Side rails must always be up for patients who are restrained in vests, belts, and extremity restraints in bed.

Studies have shown that serious injuries can occur if patients attempt to climb over side rails and fall. This is a common cause of hip fractures in confused elderly patients. Leaving the rails down may be a much safer alternative. Alarms are available that sound if the patient attempts to get up. If side rails are used, monitor the patient frequently.

When side rails are used, it is important to check the space between the rail and the mattress. Hospital beds are permanent pieces of equipment that are used for years. Mattresses wear out and are replaced. There have been cases of injury and death in which patients became trapped between the mattress and side rails because the replacement mattress was not the same size as the original. Patients at high risk for entrapment include those with conditions such as confusion, restlessness, lack of muscle control, or a combination of these factors. Make sure that the gap between the mattress and the side rail is not large enough to cause injury. Figure 15-11 shows areas of potential entrapment.

Facilities and commercial manufacturers have developed many excellent alternatives to the use of side rails. Each patient's care plan or critical pathway will provide instructions regarding use of restraints, side rails, or alternative devices. Before applying restraints or raising the rails, ask yourself if the risks associated with their use presents less danger than other available options, including making the environment as safe and user-friendly as possible. Other possible alternatives to the use of side rails are:

- Keeping the bed in the lowest possible position with the wheels locked.
- Beds that can be raised and lowered close to the floor.
- Placing mats on the floor next to the bed, so that if a fall occurs, the patient will fall on a padded surface instead of the hard floor.
- Anticipate reasons why the patient might get up, including need to use the bathroom, hunger, thirst, restlessness, and pain. Meet these needs promptly and provide calm interventions when you are in the room.
- Using side rail bolster cushions (Figure 15-12).
- Pressure-sensitive bed and chair alarms that sound when a patient attempts to get up (Figures 15-13A, 15-13B, 15-13C).

Each health care facility has policies addressing when side rails may be used. Know and follow your facility policies.

The Vail Bed. A Vail bed (Figure 15-13D) is a useful alternative for confused adult patients who try to climb over the side rails. It is not used for mentally alert patients. This bed looks somewhat like a canopy bed or adult crib.

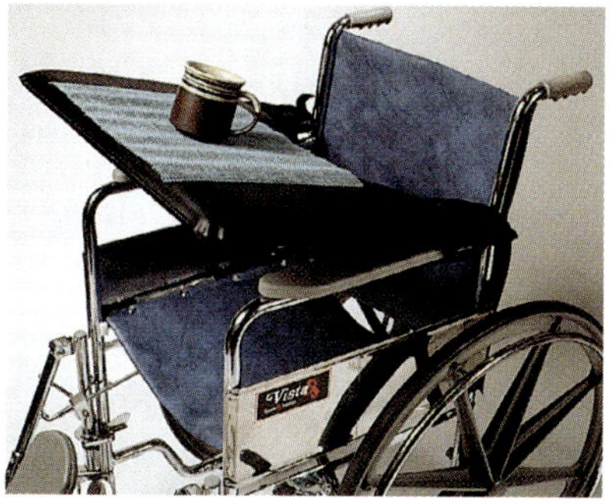

FIGURE 15-10 The lap tray is an enabler if it improves function, permitting the patient to eat independently. This tray is lined with gripper, a nonslip surface that holds the dishes in place. The tray is a restraint if it is used to keep the patient in the chair and he cannot remove it by himself. *(Courtesy of Skil-Care Corporation, Yonkers, NY, (800) 431-2972.)*

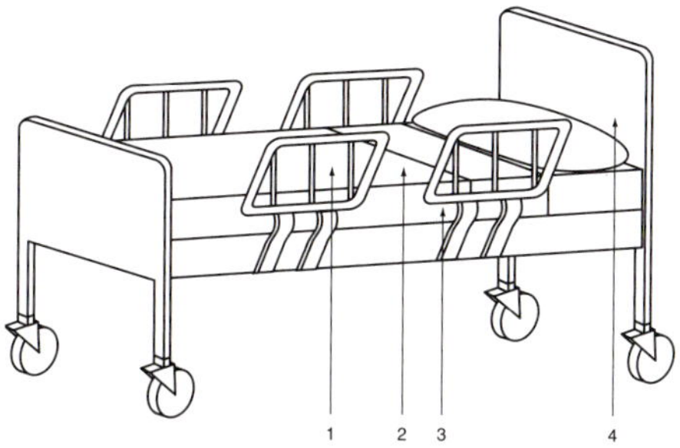

FIGURE 15-11 Entrapment between the mattress and side rails occurs in one of the following ways (numbers 1–4 in the diagram): (1) through the bars of an individual side rail; (2) through the space between split side rails; (3) between the side rail and mattress; or (4) between the headboard or footboard, side rail, and mattress.

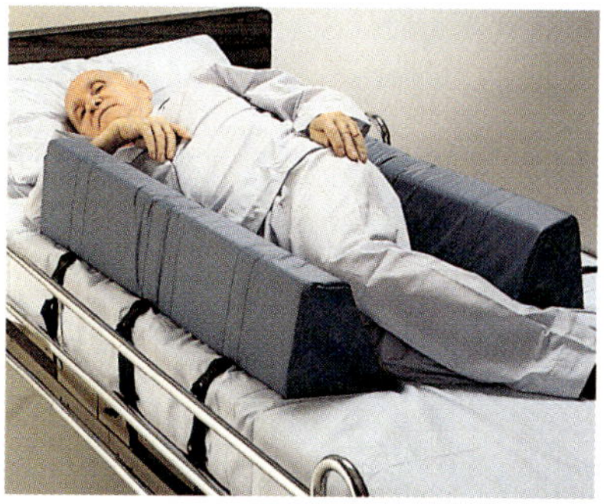

FIGURE 15-12 Bed control bolsters are a good option to use in place of side rails. *(Courtesy of Skil-Care Corporation, Yonkers, NY, (800) 431-2972.)*

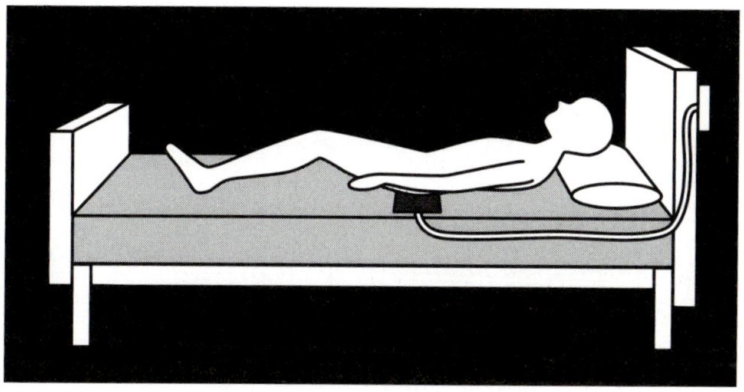

FIGURE 15-13A The pressure-sensitive pad is placed under the sheet. When the patient attempts to stand, an alarm sounds. *(Courtesy of RN+ Systems, Boulder, CO, (800) 727-1868.)*

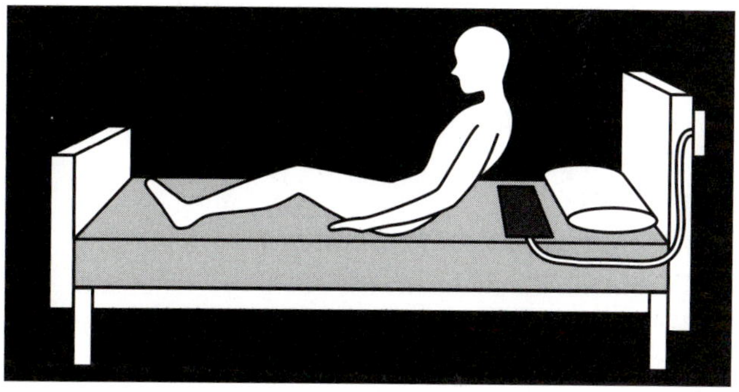

FIGURE 15-13B This pressure-sensitive pad is placed under the sheet beneath the patient's shoulders. When he lifts his upper body off the pad, the alarm will sound. *(Courtesy of RN+ Systems, Boulder, CO, (800) 727-1868.)*

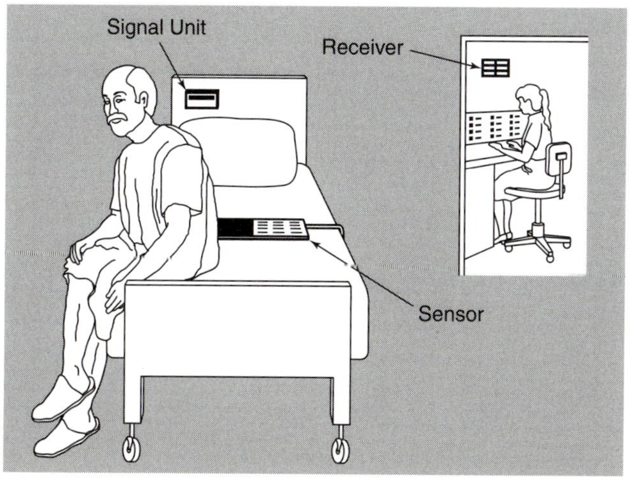

FIGURE 15-13C The pressure-sensitive pad is placed under the sheet. The signal unit is placed in the room. When the patient relieves pressure from the pad, a distinctive alarm sounds at the desk. The alarm sound is optional in the patient's room. *(Courtesy of RN+ Systems, Boulder, CO, (800) 727-1868.)*

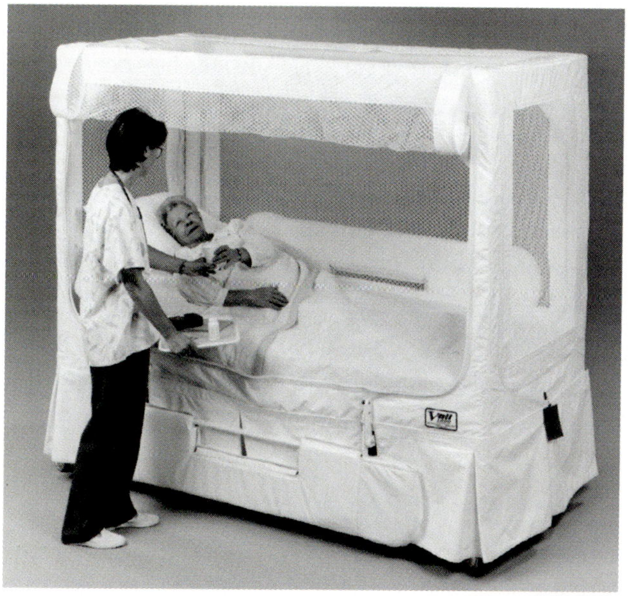

FIGURE 15-13D The Vail bed keeps patients safe without restricting mobility. *(Photo courtesy of Vail Products, Inc.)*

The top and sides are surrounded by netting. From the inside, the netting seems to fade out and is not perceived as a barrier. The patient views the room as though looking through a screen door. The patient can move about in the bed without becoming entangled or falling out of bed. The netting protects the caregiver if the patient becomes aggressive. The bed is accessible from all sides through special zippers in the netting that open only from the outside. Patients should not be left unattended with the covers unzipped. Pediatric versions of this bed are also available for infant and child patients.

Alternatives to the Use of Restraints

Alternatives to restraints should be tried before restraints are applied. Restraints are used only as a last resort in situations where the patient may harm himself or others. Nursing assistants can take a number of actions to help reduce the need to use restraints.

1. Care for patients' personal needs promptly.
   - Take patients to the bathroom regularly.
   - Provide adequate food and fluids to prevent hunger and thirst.
   - Report signs and symptoms of pain or illness promptly.
   - Follow all instructions for positioning and for assisting patients with exercise.
   - Be sure that patients have their eyeglasses and hearing aids if they need them.
   - Answer call signals promptly.
   - Check patients often to see if they need anything.
   - Provide appropriate exercise and activities.
2. Know which patients are at risk for falling. Monitor these patients regularly during your shift.
3. Observe patients who walk and transfer independently. Sometimes falls occur because patients use incorrect and unsafe methods. Report these situations and learn how to teach patients the correct way.
4. Report immediately any physical or mental change that could increase the risk of an incident, such as:
   - Disorientation (patient does not know time, place, or self)
   - Complaints of dizziness
   - Problems with balance and coordination
5. Maintain a safe, quiet, calm, environment.
6. Provide comfortable chairs. Use supportive devices as necessary.
7. A number of security devices are available that are designed to prevent falls and eliminate the need for restraints. These devices include:
   - Special sensors attached to a patient's wrist, leg, or wheelchair. The sensor will set off an alarm if the patient tries to leave the unit or building.
   - Special sensors (a pad) placed in the patient's bed or chair that will set off an alarm if the patient attempts to rise.

SAFETY *Alert*

When applying restraints to a patient in a chair, make sure the patient's hips are all the way back on the seat. Most restraints are designed to keep the hips down, so they must be applied in a manner that accomplishes this. The straps are usually inserted between the seat and the armrest. A common mistake is threading the straps through the armrest. Patients in wheelchairs frequently try to stand or slide their hips toward the front of the seat while restrained, causing injury. Threading the straps through the armrest places the restraint straps around the abdomen and fails to keep the hips down. If the patient attempts to stand or slides forward, the chair may tip, or another injury may occur. Attention to the manufacturer's directions for strap placement in the wheelchair is very important for preventing injuries.

LEGAL *Alert*

The law is very clear regarding the use of restraints. It specifies that restraints must be applied according to manufacturers' directions. Each manufacturer determines the best way to apply its restraints. The directions for restraint application are sent to the government, which approves the instructions. There are many restraint manufacturers, so you must become familiar with the directions for applying the type of restraints used in your facility. You must also consider the size of the restraint. Restraints come in different sizes. Each manufacturer lists weight and size guidelines for its restraints. Some restraints are color-coded so you can tell the size at a glance. Using a restraint that does not fit the patient correctly is dangerous. Applying the correct size is very important.

guidelines *for*

The Use of Restraints

There are a few situations in which a patient may need a restraint, no matter how many alternatives are tried. When restraints are necessary, these guidelines must be followed:

1. A physician's order must be obtained by the nurse before restraints may be used. The order must indicate the type of restraint to use and the reason for its use. Try the least restrictive device first.
2. Use the right type and size of restraint. All restraints must be applied according to manufacturer's directions.

   Check the device before use—do not use if it is frayed, torn, has parts missing, or is soiled. Restraints are put on over clothing, never next to bare skin. When applying a restraint to a female patient, make sure the breasts are not under the strap to the restraint.
3. Even if the patient does not seem to understand, always explain what you are doing. After application, check the fit of the device. You should be able to slip the width of three fingers between the restraint and the patient's body. The device should never restrict breathing.
4. The straps should be positioned so the patient is unable to reach them. The restraint straps should be smooth. Avoid twisting. Pad the restraint if necessary to prevent irritation to the skin.
5. Tie restraint straps with slip knots for quick release in an emergency.
6. The patient should always have access to the signal light. Check every 15 minutes for the patient's comfort and safety. Make changes as needed.
7. When the patient is restrained in a wheelchair, the brakes should be locked when the chair is parked. The large part of the small front wheels of the chair should face forward. This changes the center of gravity of the chair, making the chair more stable and preventing tipping.
8. Release the restraint at least every 2 hours for at least 10 minutes to:
   - Check for irritation or poor circulation
   - Change the patient's position
   - Exercise—ambulate the patient or do passive range-of-motion exercises
   - Take the patient to the bathroom
   - Change incontinent patients and cleanse their skin
   - Provide fluid or nourishment
   - Attend to any other needs

   Document each of these actions.
9. Maintain good body alignment whether the patient is in bed or a chair.
10. When restraints are used in bed:
    - There must be full side rails on the bed, and they must be raised
    - The patient should always be positioned in the middle of the mattress
    - Always secure the restraint to the movable part of the bed frame (Figure 15-14)
11. Do not use restraints in moving vehicles or on toilets unless you are sure the device is intended for that use by the manufacturer.

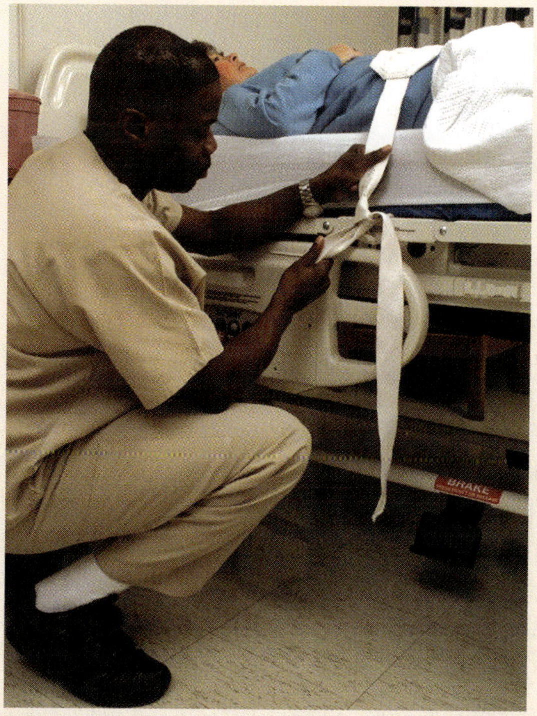

FIGURE 15-14 Always tie restraints to the movable part of the bed frame.

Many commercial devices are available to use in place of restraints. Sometimes clothing or other items can be used as restraint alternatives. For example, a male patient who pulls at his urinary catheter can be fitted with boxer shorts. A patient with a feeding tube in the abdomen can be covered with a t-shirt or abdominal binder. A patient with an intravenous infusion (IV) in the arm can wear a long-sleeved shirt. Covering the medical device may be all that is necessary to keep the patient from pulling on it. Previously, wrist restraints would have been used to keep the patient from dislodging tubes. Giving the patient something to hold, such as a Nerf® ball, will occupy the hands and serve as a distraction.

The nursing assistant plays an important role in knowing the patients' needs and making recommendations for restraint alternatives. Making sure the patient is in touch with his or her environment reduces agitation and confusion. Simply ensuring that she can see or hear well may improve mental orientation. Other observations that will help eliminate the need for restraints are:

- Does the patient see and hear well? Does the patient normally wear glasses? Is she wearing them now? Are they clean? Does the hearing aid work? Are the patient's ears plugged with wax? Sometimes behavior problems, balance problems, and other safety concerns arise because the patient is out of touch with the environment. Applying these simple corrective devices may eliminate the need for a restraint.
- Is the patient able to make her needs known? Sometimes unsafe behavior is caused by an unmet need, such as hunger, thirst, or need to use the bathroom. Discovering the unmet need and meeting it may help you avoid using a restraint.
- Does noise or confusion in the environment cause the patient to become agitated? Noise can be caused by other patients or staff, the public address system, radios, or television. Eliminating the noise may stop the behavior.
- Does the behavior occur during a certain time of day, during a certain activity, or when a specific person is providing care?
- Does the patient seem uncomfortable? Physical pain, hunger, thirst, or need to use the bathroom can cause unsafe behavior.
- Does the patient seem lonely or isolated? Bored? Boredom, loneliness, or looking for a misplaced item can cause unsafe behavior.
- Does the patient try to get out of bed or chair without help? Is the patient steady on her feet? Does she normally use a cane or walker? Is she using it now? Is the call signal available, and does the patient know how to use it? Would the patient benefit from use of an alarm that sounds when she stands up? Would use of an alarm remind the patient to sit down, alert the staff, and eliminate the need for a restraint?

If you observe a condition that causes confusion or agitation, or discover an approach that is effective in eliminating or reducing the need for restraints, inform your nurse manager. Other common restraint alternatives are pictured in Figure 15-15 through Figure 15-21.

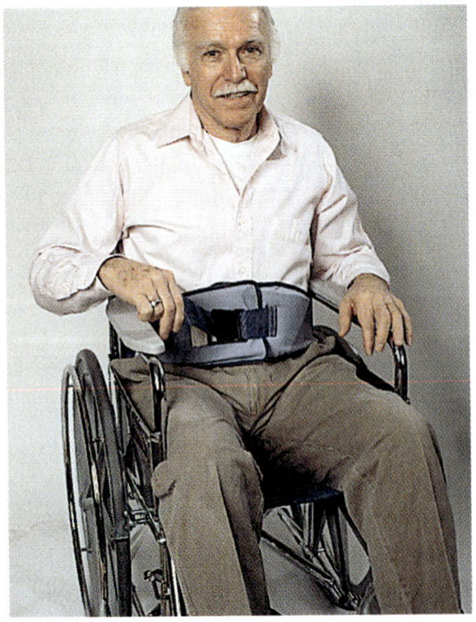

FIGURE 15-15 The self-release belt serves as a reminder to call for help before rising. It is not a restraint if the patient has the physical and mental ability to release the Velcro® fastener. *(Courtesy of Skil-Care Corporation, Yonkers, NY, (800) 431-2972.)*

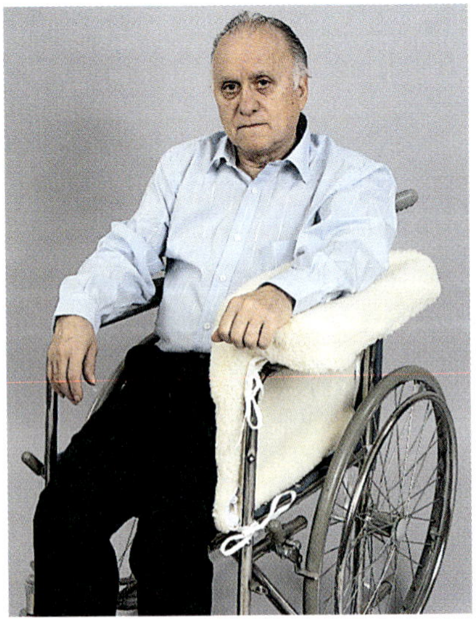

FIGURE 15-16 Some patients lean to the side, necessitating restraint to keep them upright in the chair. The lateral armrest supports and keeps the patient upright, making restraint unnecessary. *(Courtesy of Skil-Care Corporation, Yonkers, NY, (800) 431-2972.)*

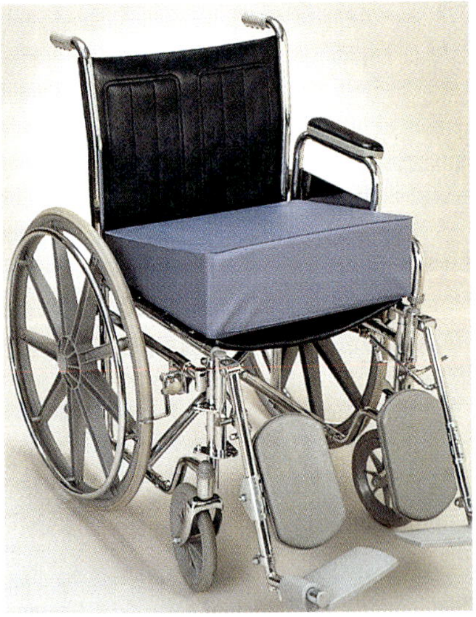

FIGURE 15-17 Some patients slide forward to the edge of the chair, and must be restrained to keep their hips back. The wedge cushion prevents sliding. A piece of gripper can be placed on top of the wedge for additional security. *(Courtesy of Skil-Care Corporation, Yonkers, NY, (800) 431-2972.)*

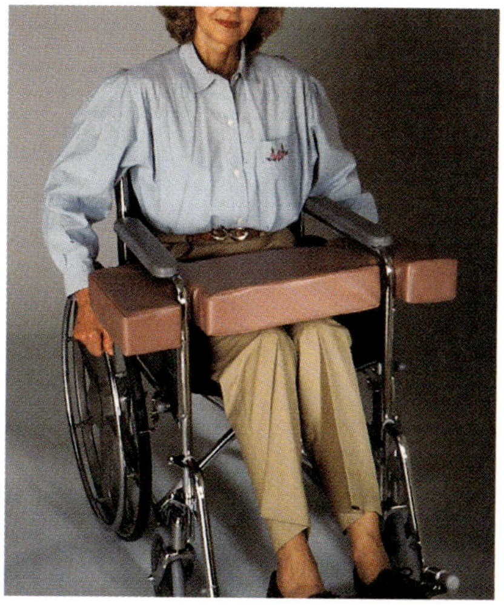

FIGURE 15-18 The lap buddy is foam covered with vinyl. It is lightweight and comfortable and may be used in place of a heavier tray. It is a restraint if the patient cannot remove it. *(Courtesy of Skil-Care Corporation, Yonkers, NY, (800) 431-2972.)*

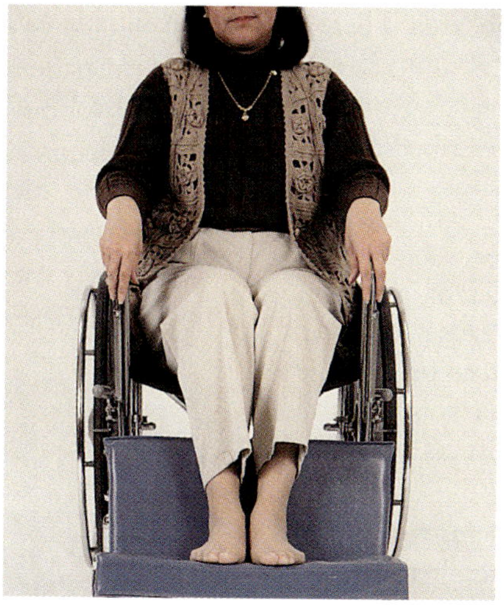

FIGURE 15-19 The patient's feet must be supported when she is sitting in a chair. The footrest elevator keeps the patient's legs from dangling and prevents her from sliding forward in the chair. *(Courtesy of Skil-Care Corporation, Yonkers, NY, (800) 431-2972.)*

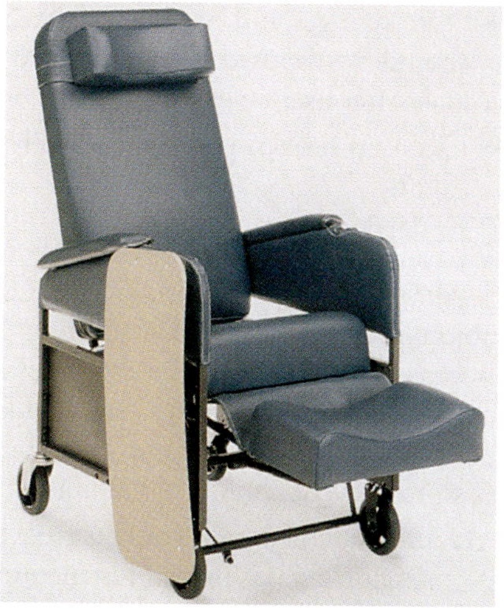

FIGURE 15-20 The geriatric chair can be used as a recliner for patient comfort. If the patient cannot stand, the chair is a restraint when in the reclining position. The tray is locked across the lap to prevent rising. It cannot be removed independently, and is considered a restraint. *(Photo courtesy of Hill-Rom® Long-Term Care Division.)*

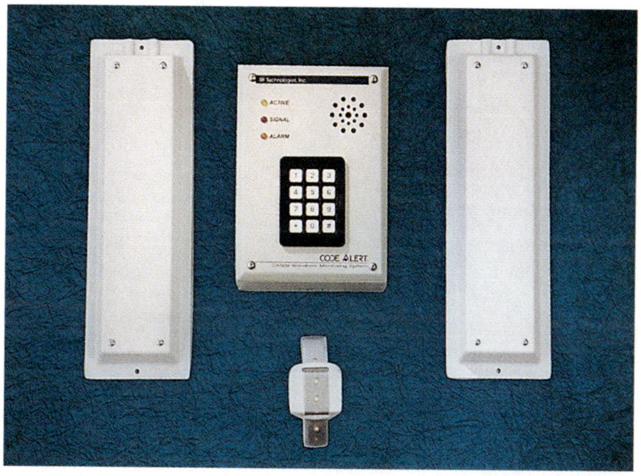

FIGURE 15-21 The magnetic sensor bracelet is used to allow cognitively impaired patients to wander within the unit. The door alarm will sound if the patient tries to exit. *(©1996, RF Technologies. Used with permission.)*

PREVENTION OF OTHER INCIDENTS

Many situations can result in an incident that may harm the patient. Incidents can be prevented when all staff members are aware of appropriate preventive measures.

Accidental Poisoning

Many common items, such as household chemicals, shaving lotion, plants, and cologne, are poisonous if ingested. Food kept in a bedside table may spoil and also cause illness. Patients who are disoriented may eat or drink any of these items. To prevent accidental poisonings:

- Keep all chemicals and cleaning solutions in locked cupboards.
- Store patients' personal food items in the refrigerator in dated labeled containers.

Thermal Injuries

Thermal injuries are those caused by heat or cold and result in burns. To prevent thermal injuries:

- Follow procedures accurately when administering warm or cold treatments.
- Check water temperatures before helping a patient into the bathtub or shower. Turn the hot water on last and turn it off first.
- Check food temperatures before feeding patients. Using a microwave oven to reheat food can be dangerous because of the uneven temperatures the oven produces.
- Store smoking materials in a safe place and supervise patients while they smoke. (Most health care facilities do not allow smoking by anyone.)

Skin Injuries

Skin injuries include **lacerations** (cuts or breaks in the skin) and punctures. To prevent these injuries:

- Store knives, scissors, razors, and tools in locked cupboards.

- Store syringes and needles in locked cupboards. These should be disposed of in a sharps container immediately after use.
- Clean up broken glass immediately, as described earlier.

Choking

Aspiration is the accidental entry of food or a foreign object into the trachea (windpipe). This causes choking. Because swallowing becomes less efficient as people age, choking occurs more often in the elderly. Persons who are disoriented or who have impaired consciousness are also at risk. To prevent choking or aspiration:

1. Be aware of which patients have problems with swallowing. Follow all instructions when helping with feeding:
   - Cut food into small pieces.
   - Feed slowly.
   - Offer fluids carefully between solid foods.
   - If the patient has had a stroke, place the food in the unaffected side of the mouth.
   - Use thickeners for liquids if ordered.
2. Place patients upright in good body alignment before meals. Have them remain in this position for at least 30 minutes after eating.
3. At the end of the meal, give oral care to patients who are known to keep food in their mouths. Food may remain in the mouth for several minutes after a meal and be accidentally aspirated if the patient coughs or goes to sleep.
4. Know the procedure to clear an obstructed airway. (See Unit 51.)

INTRODUCTION TO PROCEDURES

Caring for patients safely means that you must faithfully and carefully carry out specific routines. The normal manner of carrying out a task is called a **procedure**.

As you progress in your studies, you will learn the procedures for many nursing assistant tasks. You have already been introduced to the procedures for washing your hands and using PPE. The procedures that follow give you step-by-step directions for carrying out tasks that involve patients.

Certain things must be done before you begin patient care procedures. These actions are called *preprocedure* or beginning procedure actions. At the end of each patient care procedure, you will carry out a standard series of procedure completion actions.

Beginning Procedure Actions

At the beginning of each procedure, do the following:

- Wash your hands thoroughly (Figure 15-22A). You may use an alcohol-based hand cleanser, if permitted by your facility.
- Assemble equipment.
- At the patient's room, knock and pause before entering (Figure 15-22B).
- Introduce yourself and identify the patient by checking his or her identification bracelet (Figure 15-22C).
- Ask visitors to leave the room and inform them where they may wait.

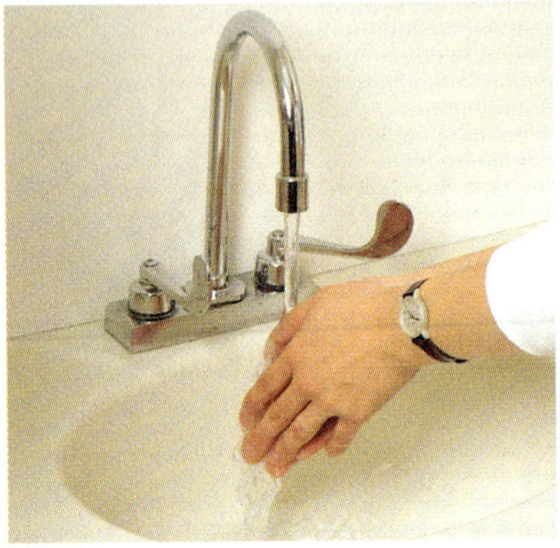

FIGURE 15-22A Wash your hands.

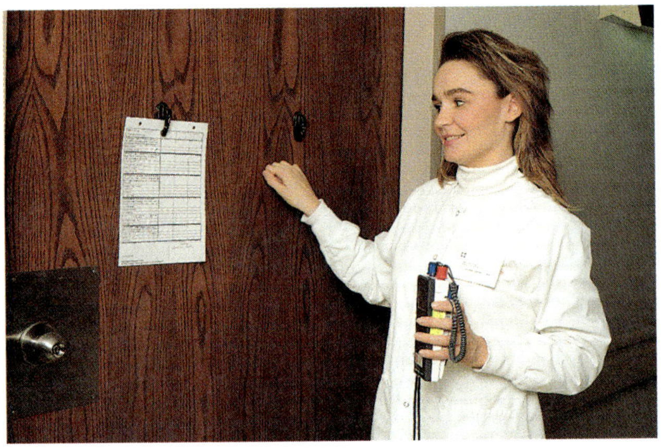

FIGURE 15-22B If the door is closed or the privacy curtains are drawn, knock or speak before entering. Allow enough time for the patient to respond.

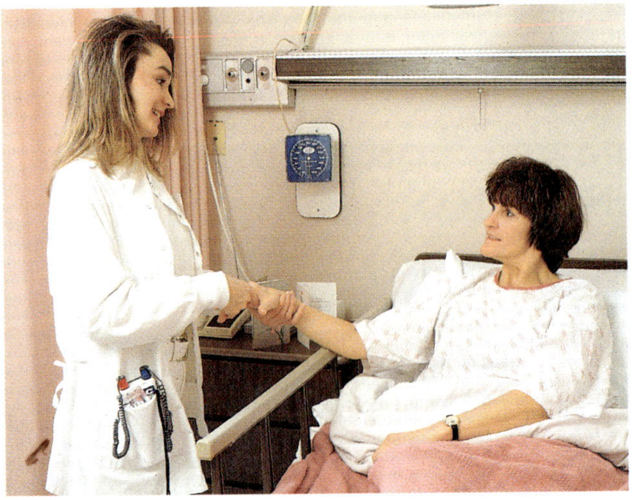

FIGURE 15-22C Identify the patient.

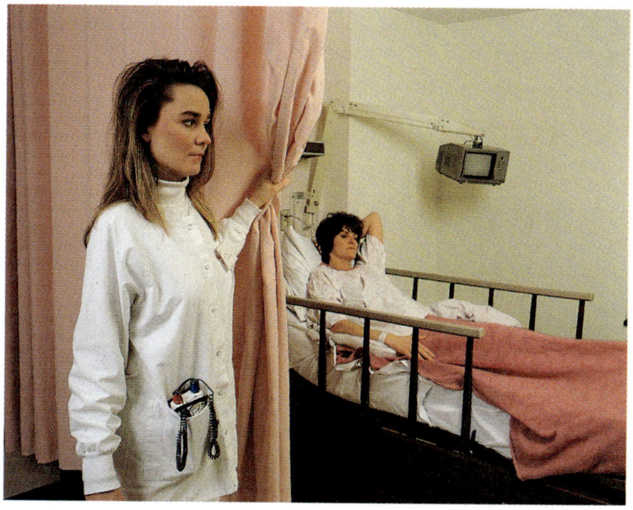

FIGURE 15-22D Draw the curtains for privacy. If the bed is near a window, also close the window curtains.

- Provide privacy (Figure 15-22D).
- Explain what will happen and answer questions.
- Allow the patient to assist as much as possible.
- Raise the bed to a comfortable working height.
- Lower the side rail on the side where you are working.
- Position the patient for the procedure. Ask an assistant to help, if necessary, or support the patient with pillows and props. Make sure the patient is comfortable and can maintain the position throughout the procedure.
- Drape the patient for modesty.
- Set up the equipment for the procedure at the bedside. Open trays and packages. Position items so that you can reach them conveniently. Avoid putting a container for soiled items in a place where you must cross over clean items to use it.
- Carry out precaution gowning and gloving.

COMMUNICATION *Highlight*

Communicate with the patient throughout the procedure. Whenever possible, use age-appropriate terms and explanations. Talk to the patient even if he or she is young, confused, may not understand, or cannot communicate verbally. Use gestures and body language to demonstrate, whenever possible. Continue to talk and smile throughout the procedure, regardless of the patient's age or level of understanding. This is important for the patient's well-being, and shows that you care. Remember that you also communicate with touch. Handle the patient gently to prevent injury and communicate caring.

- Use standard precautions when contact with blood, body fluids, mucous membranes, or nonintact skin is likely.

Procedure Completion Actions

When a procedure is completed, do the following:

- Remove gloves.
- Position the patient comfortably.
- Replace the bed covers, then remove any drapes used.
- Return the bed to the lowest horizontal position.
- Elevate the side rails, if used, before leaving the bedside.
- Leave signal cord (Figure 15-23A), telephone, and fresh water where the patient can reach them.
- Perform a general safety check of the patient and the environment.
- Open privacy curtains.
- Remove and discard personal protective equipment, if used, according to facility policy.
- Care for equipment following facility policy.
- Wash your hands (Figure 15-23B). You may use an alcohol-based hand cleanser if permitted by your facility. Do not use an alcohol product if you have protein substances on your hands.

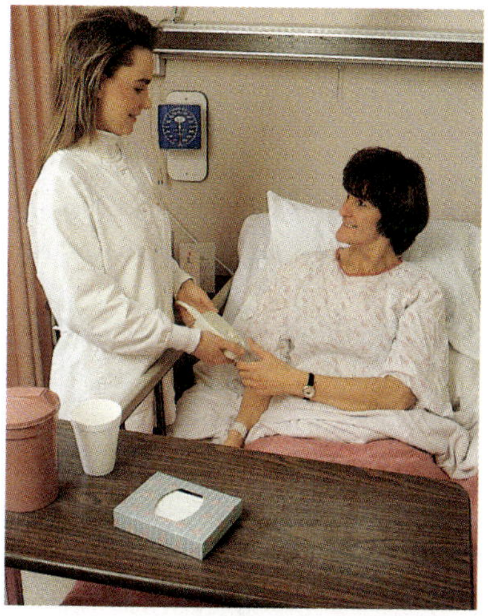

FIGURE 15-23A Lower the bed and place the signal cord within the patient's reach.

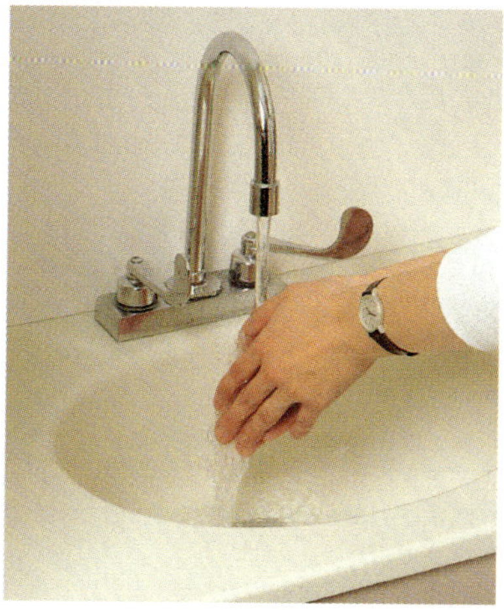

FIGURE 15-23B Wash your hands.

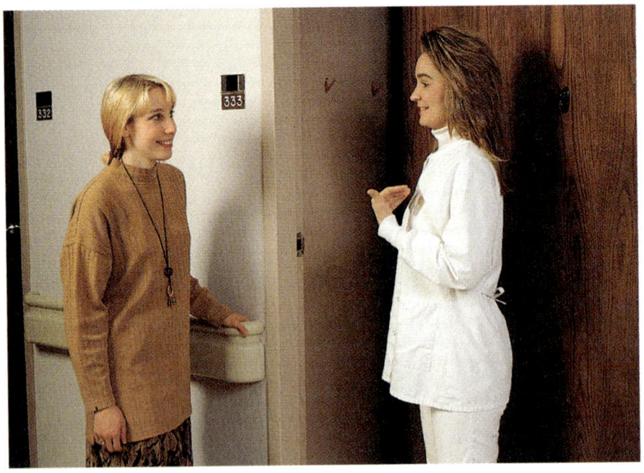

FIGURE 15-23C Let visitors know when they may reenter the room.

- Let visitors know when they may reenter (Figure 15-23C).
- Report completion of task (Figure 15-23D).
- Document action and your observations.

Note: Where there are open lesions, wet linen, or possible contact with patient body fluids, blood, secretions, excretions, mucous membranes, or nonintact skin, wear disposable gloves during the procedure. Put on gloves before contact with the patient or linen. Dispose of gloves according to facility policy after they are removed. **ALWAYS APPLY STANDARD PRECAUTIONS.**

So much handwashing may seem unnecessary, because of the short length of time that you are with the patient. Just remember that your hands can transmit germs. Patients already weakened by disease have a much lower resistance to germs.

Because the beginning procedure and procedure completion actions are the same for each patient care procedure, they are not restated in this book as individual steps with each procedure. Rather, a general reference is made to these steps at the beginning and end of each procedure. You must, however, learn and faithfully complete each of these steps for each patient care procedure you perform.

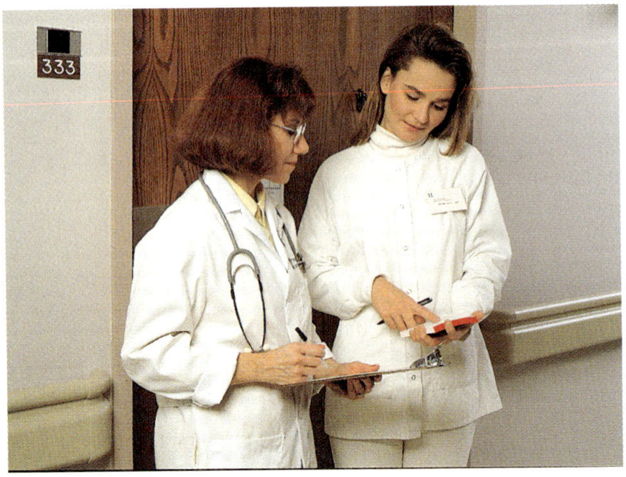

FIGURE 15-23D Report and document your actions and the patient's response.

BODY MECHANICS FOR THE PATIENT

Body mechanics for the patient are very similar to those for the health care team. Although the patient probably is not doing any lifting, good posture habits should not be neglected. Good posture for the patient means that moving in bed, getting out of bed, standing, and walking are done safely.

Bed patients sometimes find it hard to stay in a position; they tend to slide toward the foot of the bed when the head of the bed is elevated (Figure 15-24). Patients who are dependent are not able to change their position. These patients need extra help to gain and maintain proper alignment. Remember to:

- Get help.
- Use turning or lifting sheets.
- Change the patient's position frequently, at least every two hours.

Body Alignment and Positioning

Body alignment means maintaining a person in a position in which the body can properly function. Patients who are weak, have impaired consciousness, are disoriented, or are

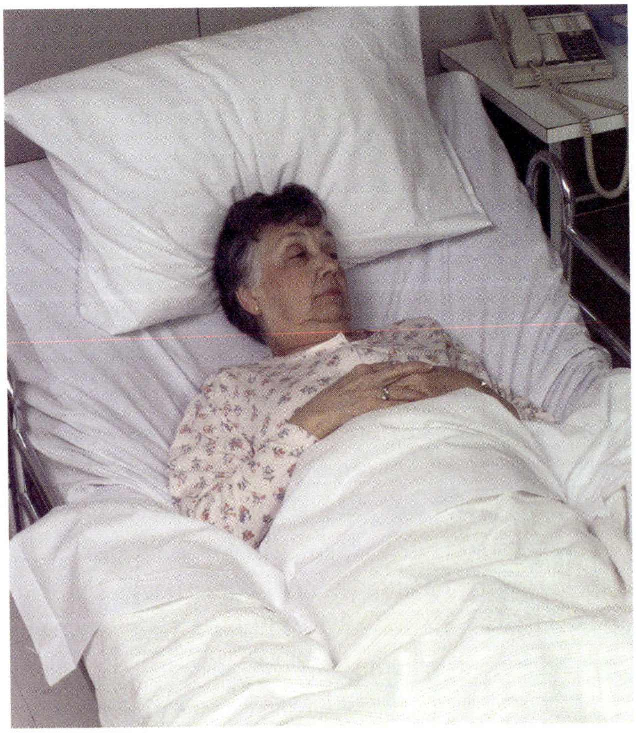

FIGURE 15-24 Patients frequently slide down in bed, causing poor body alignment.

in pain have problems keeping good alignment. Body alignment is maintained by moving, turning, and positioning the patient in a manner that:

- Helps the patient feel more comfortable
- Relieves strain
- Helps the body function more efficiently
- Prevents complications like contractures and pressure ulcers

Complications of Incorrect Positioning

Complications can occur when body alignment is not maintained or when the patient's position is not changed often enough. The two most common complications are pressure ulcers and contractures. **Pressure ulcers** (bedsores) result when unrelieved pressure on a bony prominence interferes with blood flow to the area. Pressure ulcers are dangerous and expensive to treat. (These are discussed in Unit 24.) **Contractures** occur when a joint is allowed to remain in the same position for too long (Figure 15-25). The muscles stiffen and shorten (atrophy), preventing the joint from full movement. The joint becomes fixed in a bent position (position of flexion). Contractures are permanent and can interfere with mobility.

Contractures can begin to develop within as little as four days of immobility and inactivity. After approximately 15 days, the patient loses the ability to move the joint freely. Contractures interfere with the patient's ability to move, complicate all nursing care, and interfere with proper positioning of the patient. Contractures promote the development of pressure ulcers and make treatment of existing pressure ulcers difficult. The contractures cause bony prominences to suffer reduced blood flow. Some studies have shown a relationship between the presence of contractures and the development of pressure ulcers. Contractures are a serious complication of immobility, making movement and activity painful and difficult. Voluntary movement of the contracted joint becomes impossible as the contracture worsens. Contractures can be prevented, and some can be reversed, with proper care. (Additional preventive measures for contractures are discussed in Unit 40).

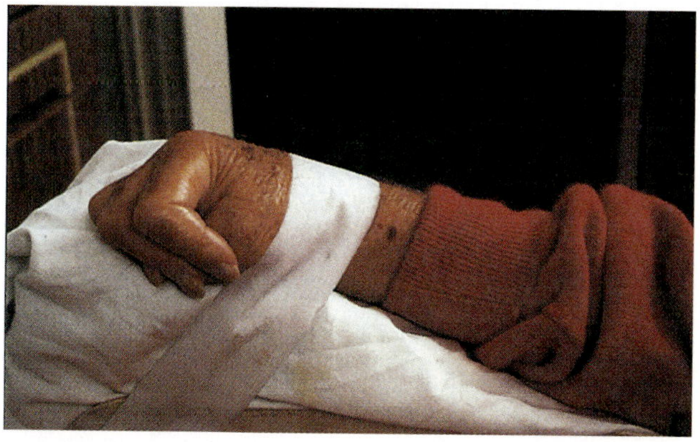

FIGURE 15-25 Contractures occur when joints are allowed to remain in the same position for too long.

Supportive Devices

Supportive devices are used to maintain proper body alignment and position in the bed or in a chair. Supportive devices include:

- Pillows and/or folded sheets, bath blankets, or mattress pads to support the trunk and extremities
- Splints and other specially designed **orthotic devices** (**orthoses**). Orthoses restore or improve function and prevent deformity.
- Special boots or shoes that are worn in bed to keep the feet in alignment (Figure 15-26A)
- Bed cradles, which prevent pressure on the feet from the bed covers (Figure 15-26B)
- Footboards to maintain foot alignment

A folded pillow placed between the soles of the feet and the foot of the bed, or a pillow resting against the footboard

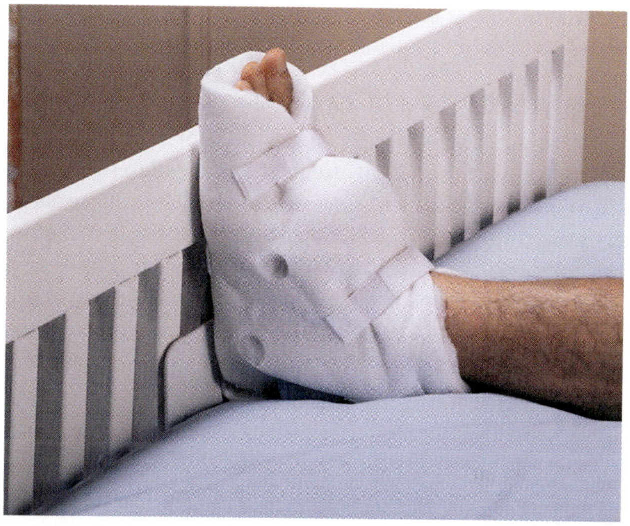

FIGURE 15-26A Special boots will maintain the ankles and feet in good alignment. *(Bunny boot support is provided by Sammons Preston, Inc., a Bissell® HealthCare Company. Reprinted with permission.)*

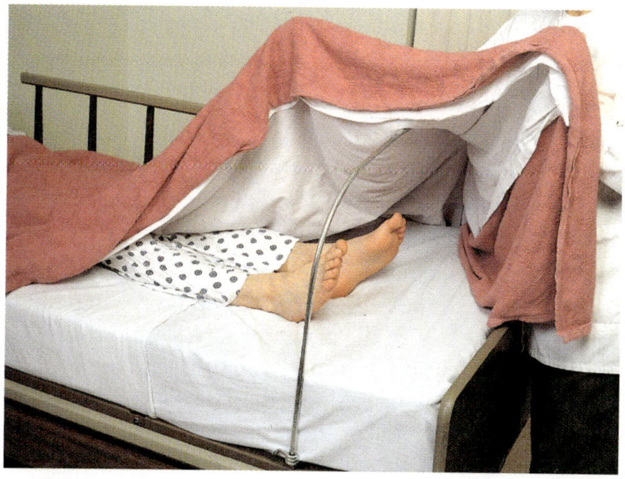

FIGURE 15-26B Bed cradles prevent pressure on the feet from the bed covers.

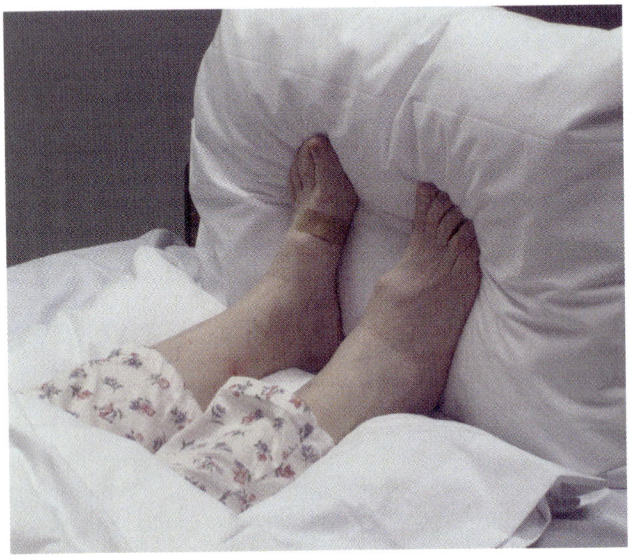

FIGURE 15-27 Footboards or a pillow resting against the footboard may be used to maintain good alignment and prevent contractures.

(Figure 15-27), can take the place of a footboard alone. In some cases, a footboard may be harmful. For example, a footboard against the soles of the feet can stimulate **spasticity** (involuntary muscle contraction) in the legs and possibly cause skin breakdown from the rubbing of the feet against the footboard. Special shoes are sometimes worn in bed to maintain the feet in correct alignment. In most cases, ankle contractures can be avoided by doing passive range-of-motion exercises consistently (Unit 40).

Many other commercial products can be used as supportive devices. Remember that a supportive device is also a restraint if it is attached or next to the patient's body, if the patient cannot easily remove it, and if it restricts freedom of movement and normal access to the patient's body.

Basic Body Positions

There are four basic positions, with variations for each one. These are:

- **Prone** (on the abdomen), with a variation of **semiprone**
- **Supine** (on the back), with a variation of **semisupine**
- **Lateral** (on either side), with a variation of **Sims' position**
- **Fowler's position**, with variations of **high Fowler's**, **semi-Fowler's**, and **orthopneic position**

Changing a patient's position involves these steps:

1. Moving the patient into proper body alignment. You may need to move the patient up in bed or to one side of the bed. If the patient will be positioned on his left side, move him to the right side of the bed. If the patient will be positioned on his right side, move him to the left side of the bed. That way he will not be too close to the edge of the bed after he is turned.
2. Turning the patient onto the back, onto the abdomen, or to the side.
3. Placing the patient's trunk and extremities in proper position and maintaining alignment with the use of supportive devices.

MOVING AND LIFTING PATIENTS

Lifting, moving, and transporting patients is a major responsibility of the nursing assistant. Using proper body mechanics and following safety rules will protect both you and your patients from injury. *Always* ask the nurse whether help is needed to lift or move a patient before pro-

OSHA Alert

Your spine is one of the most important parts of your body, enabling you to maintain an upright position, move freely, stand, and walk. The vertebrae protect your spinal cord, a column of nerves connecting your brain with the rest of your body. Your organs would not function without it. Keeping your spine healthy is a vital concern for nursing assistants. Unfortunately, back injuries from improper lifting and moving are common in health care workers. These are often caused by using improper lifting and moving techniques. Other contributing factors are rushing to get things done and not asking for help from others. Pay attention to your body and your position. Your back must last a lifetime.

SAFETY Alert

Using a lifting or turning sheet is better for the patient because it prevents injury to the skin. It prevents pain that sometimes occurs when you pull on the patient's body. It also reduces the risk of back injury in nursing assistants. When moving a patient on a sheet, make sure you have enough help. Two or three assistants may be necessary. Usually, two assistants are needed to reposition the patient's torso. A third may also be needed to prevent friction and shearing on the feet if the patient is being pulled up in bed.

ceeding with your assignment. Never be afraid to ask for help. By exercising caution, you are also preventing potentially serious injuries. Always check the care plan to see if there are special positioning instructions.

A **turning sheet** or **draw sheet** (folded large sheet or half sheet) may be placed under a heavy or helpless patient to make moving easier. The sheet must extend from above the shoulders to below the hips to be effective.

Procedures 14 to 17 should be followed when you are lifting or moving patients. As you practice these procedures, keep in mind the 10 basic rules of good body mechanics that were discussed in Unit 14.

PROCEDURE 14

TURNING THE PATIENT TOWARD YOU

1. Carry out each beginning procedure action.
2. Lower the side rail nearest to you. Cross the patient's far leg over the leg that is nearest to you.
3. Cross the far arm over the patient's chest. Bend the near arm at the elbow, bringing the hand toward the head of the bed.
4. Place your hand nearest the head of the bed on the patient's far shoulder. Place your other hand on the patient's hips on the far side. Brace your thighs against the side of the bed.
5. Roll the patient toward you (Figure 15-28A). Do it slowly, gently, and smoothly. Help the patient bring the upper leg toward you and bend it comfortably.
6. Put up the side rail. Be sure it is secure.
7. Go to the opposite side of the bed.
8. Place your hands under the patient's shoulders and then the hips. Pull toward the center of the bed (Figure 15-28B). This helps the patient maintain the side-lying position. Make sure the patient is not lying directly on the lower arm. The lower shoulder should be tipped slightly, so pressure is not centered directly over the joint.
9. Make sure the patient's body is properly aligned and safely positioned.
10. A pillow may be placed behind the patient's back. Secure it by pushing the near side under the patient to form a roll.
11. If the patient is unable to move independently, position the arms and legs. Support them with pillows between the shoulders, hands and knees, and ankles to prevent friction and contractures (Figure 15-28C). If the patient has an indwelling catheter, make sure the tubing is not between the legs, to prevent undue stress on the catheter and to prevent pressure ulcers.
12. Carry out each procedure completion action.

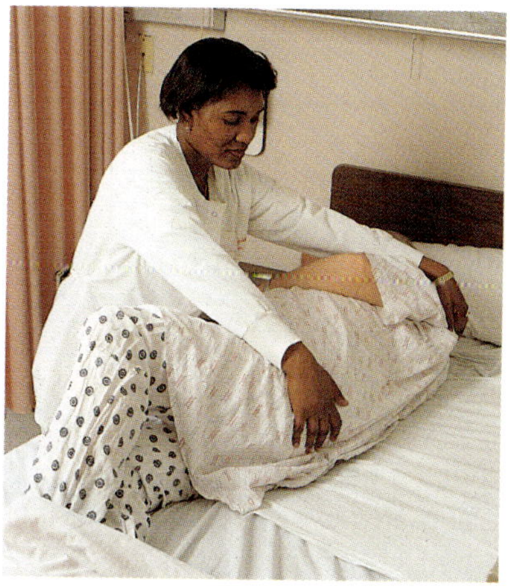

FIGURE 15-28A Place one hand on the patient's far shoulder and the other hand on the patient's hip, then turn the patient toward you.

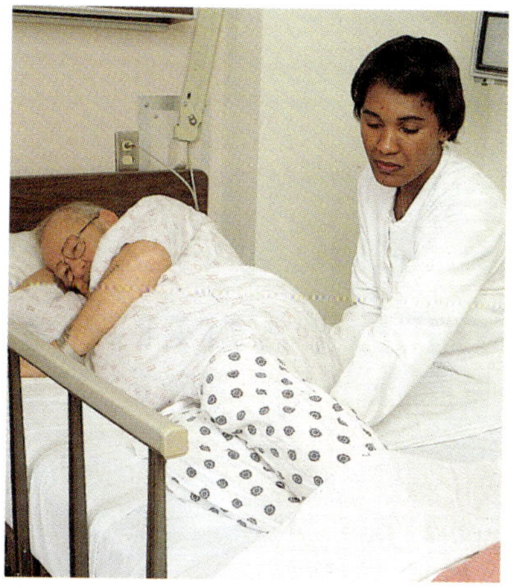

FIGURE 15-28B Move the patient to the center of the bed, keeping your back straight.

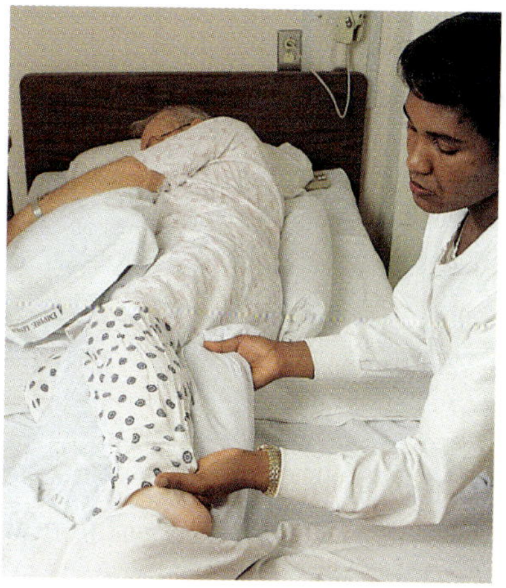

FIGURE 15-28C Place pillows to support the patient's body and maintain good alignment.

PROCEDURE 15

TURNING THE PATIENT AWAY FROM YOU

1. Carry out each beginning procedure action.
2. Lower the near side rail. Be sure the side rail on the opposite side of the bed is up and secure.
3. Have the patient bend his knees, if able. Cross the arms on the chest.
4. Place your arm nearest the head of the bed under the patient's head and shoulders. Place the other hand and forearm under the small of his back. Bend your body at the hips and knees. Keep your back straight. Pull the patient toward the edge of the bed.
5. Place your forearms under the hips and pull them toward you.
6. Move the ankles and knees toward you by placing one hand under the ankles and one under the knees.
7. Cross the near leg over the other leg at the ankles.
8. Roll the patient slowly and carefully away from you (Figure 15-29) by placing one hand under the shoulder and one hand under the hips.
9. Place your hands under the head and shoulders. Draw them back toward the center of the bed.
10. Move the hips to the center of the bed, as in step 5.
11. Place a pillow for support behind the back.
12. Make sure that the patient's body is in a good position. Support the upper leg with a pillow. Place the lower arm in a flexed position. Support the upper arm with a pillow.
13. Replace the side rail on near side of the bed. Return the bed to the lowest position.
14. Carry out each procedure completion action.

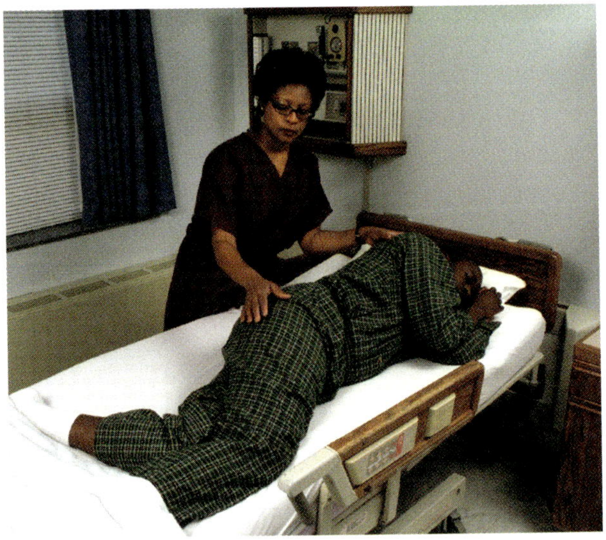

FIGURE 15-29 Roll the patient away from you.

PROCEDURE 16

MOVING A PATIENT TO THE HEAD OF THE BED

1. Carry out each beginning procedure action.
2. Ask a coworker to assist from the opposite side of the bed.
3. Lock the wheels of the bed. Raise the bed to comfortable horizontal working height. Lower side rails.
4. Lower the head of the bed if the patient can tolerate this position. Remove the pillow. Place it at the head of the bed, on its edge, for safety.
5. Lift top bedding and expose the draw sheet. Loosen both sides of the draw sheet.

continues

PROCEDURE 16

continued

6. Roll the draw sheet edges close to both sides of the patient's body (Figure 15-30).
7. Face the head of the bed. Grasp the draw sheet with the hand closest to the foot of the bed.
8. Position your feet 12 inches apart, with the foot that is farthest from the bed edge forward.
9. Place your free hand and arm under the neck and shoulders, cradling the head from both sides.
10. Bend your hips slightly.
11. Together, on a count of three, raise the patient's hips and back with the draw sheet, while supporting the head and shoulders. Move the patient smoothly toward the head of the bed.
12. Replace the pillow under the patient's head.
13. Tighten and tuck in the draw sheet. Adjust the top bedding.
14. Carry out each procedure completion action.

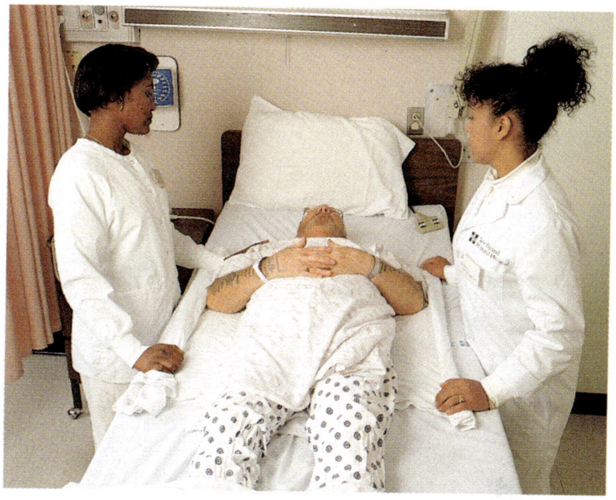

FIGURE 15-30 Using an overhand grasp, roll both edges of the turning (moving) sheet close to the patient's sides.

PROCEDURE 17

LOGROLLING THE PATIENT

Note: *This procedure is performed when the patient's spinal column must be kept straight, such as following spinal surgery or spinal cord or vertebral column injury. It is a good procedure to use with any dependent patient.*

1. Carry out each beginning procedure action.
2. Get help from another nursing assistant.
3. Raise the bed to waist-high horizontal position. Lock the wheels.
4. Lower the side rail on the side opposite to which the patient will be turned. Both assistants should be on the same side of the bed.
5. One assistant places hands under the patient's head and shoulders. The second person places hands under the hips and legs. Then move the patient as a unit toward you.
6. Place a pillow lengthwise between the legs. Fold the patient's arm over the chest.
7. Raise the side rail. Check for security.
8. Go to the opposite side of the bed and lower the side rail.
9. Turning the patient to side may be done by:
   a. Using a turning sheet that was previously placed under the patient.
      - Reach over the patient, grasping and rolling the turning sheet toward the patient (Figure 15-31 A).
      - One nursing assistant should be positioned beside the patient to keep the shoulders and hips straight.
      - A second assistant should be positioned to keep the thighs and lower legs straight.
   b. If a turning sheet is not in position, the first assistant should position hands on the patient's far shoulder and hips.
      - Second assistant positions hands on the patient's far thigh and lower leg.

continues

PROCEDURE 17

continued

10. At a specified signal, roll the patient toward both assistants in a single movement, keeping the spine, head, and legs straight. If a turning sheet is used, grasp the sheet and move the patient as a unit, onto her side (Figure 15-31B).
11. Place additional pillows behind the back to maintain the patient's position. A small pillow or folded bath blanket may be permitted under the patient's head and neck. Leave a pillow between the legs. Position small pillows or folded towels to support the arms.
12. Carry out each procedure completion action.

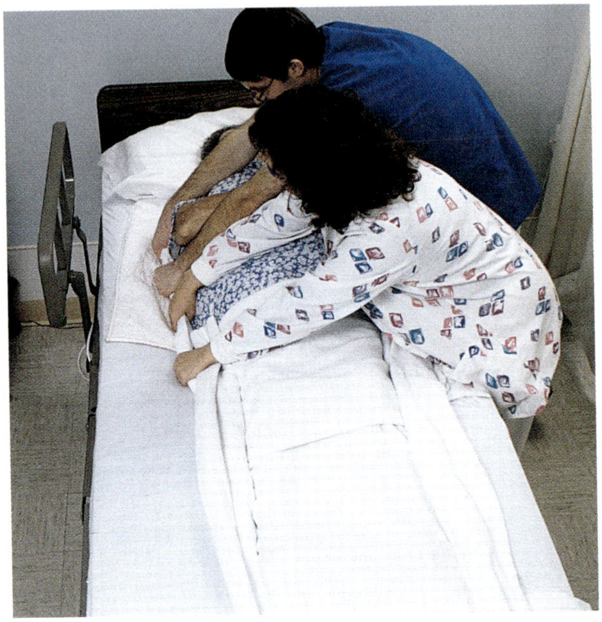

FIGURE 15-31A Roll the turning sheet against the patient.

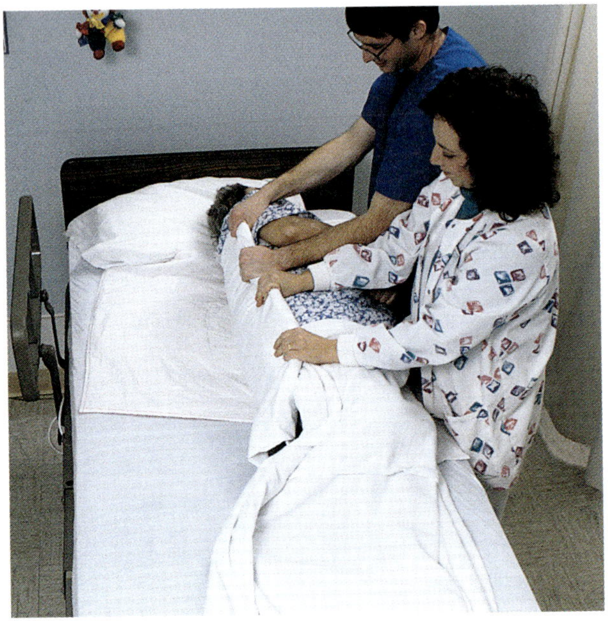

FIGURE 15-31B Pulling together, turn the patient to the side in one smooth motion.

Positioning the Patient

After you have turned and moved the patient into proper body alignment, you can place pillows and other supportive devices to help the patient maintain the position. Directions are given here for the basic four positions and their variations.

Supine Position (Figure 15-32A).

1. Start with the bed flat and the patient lying on the back. The patient's head should be about 2 to 3 inches from the head of the bed.
2. Place a pillow under the patient's head. It should extend about 2 inches below the patient's shoulders, with the head in the middle of the pillow.
3. Place a **trochanter roll** along the affected hip or along both hips if the patient has little control over the legs. A trochanter roll is devised by rolling a bath blanket into a shape about 12 inches long. The roll should be just long enough to reach from above the hip to above the knee (Figure 15-32B). The trochanter roll prevents external rotation (Figure 15-32C) of the hip.
4. Place pillows under the legs to reach from above the back of the knee to the ankle so that the ankles and heels do not rub on the sheets.

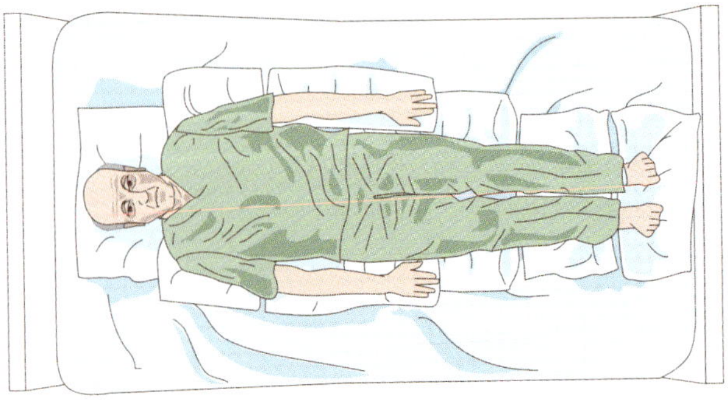

FIGURE 15-32A Supine position.

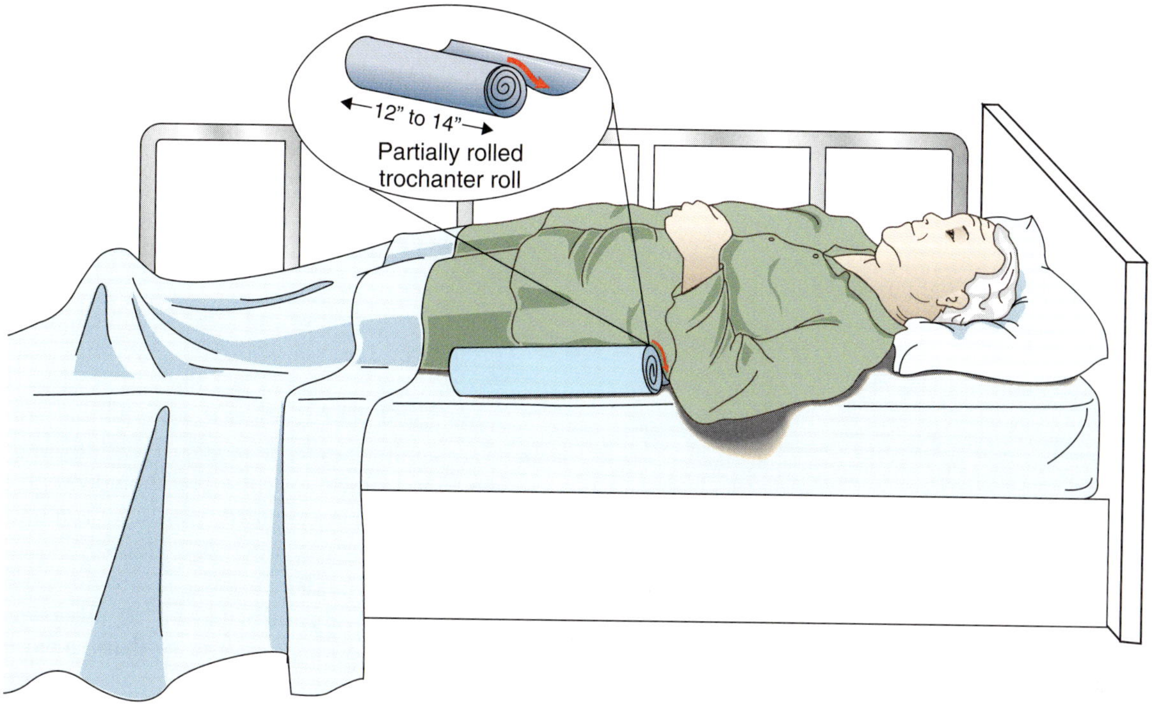

FIGURE 15-32B The trochanter roll should extend from above the hip to just above the knee.

5. If the care plan so indicates, position the footboard or place a folded pillow to support the patient's feet. The ankles should be at 90° angles.

6. Extend the patient's arms and place small pillows to reach from the elbow to below the wrist. The hand should be in alignment with the wrist and the palm should be down (Figure 15-32D).

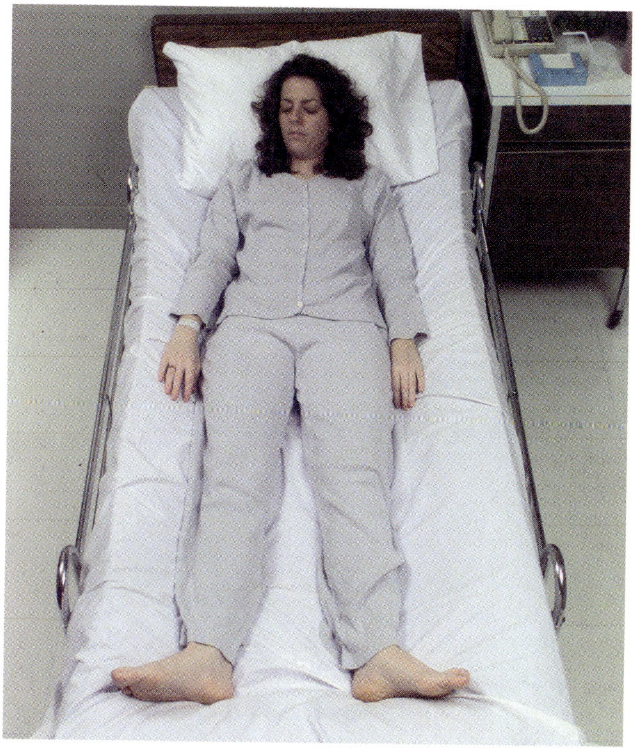

FIGURE 15-32C A correctly placed trochanter roll prevents external rotation of the hip.

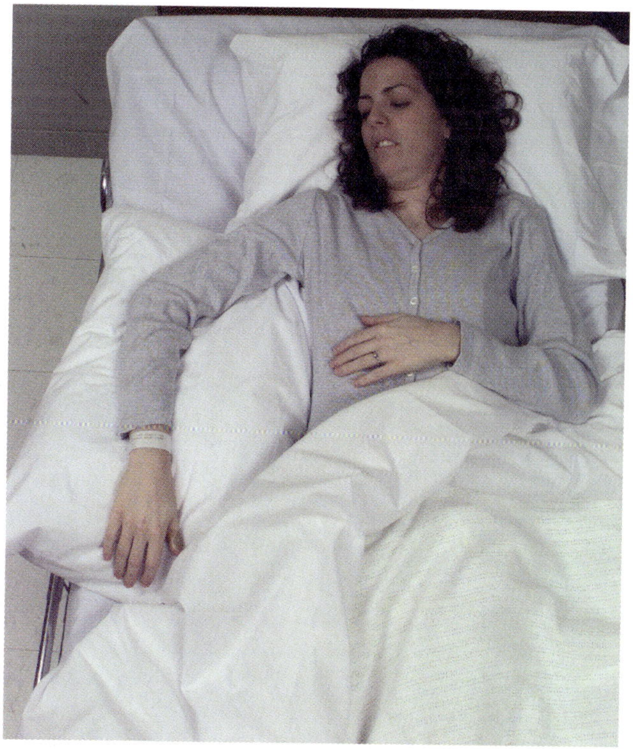

FIGURE 15-32D Pillows support the wrist and arm in good alignment and are more comfortable for the patient.

Semisupine Position (Figure 15-33). Start with the patient in supine position. Roll the trunk and shoulder away from you so that there is a 45° angle between the patient's back and the bed.

1. Place a pillow behind the back for support.
2. Bring the left shoulder forward. Flex the elbow of the left arm and place the lower left arm, palm up, on a pillow.
3. Flex the elbow of the right arm and bring the forearm across the chest with palm down.

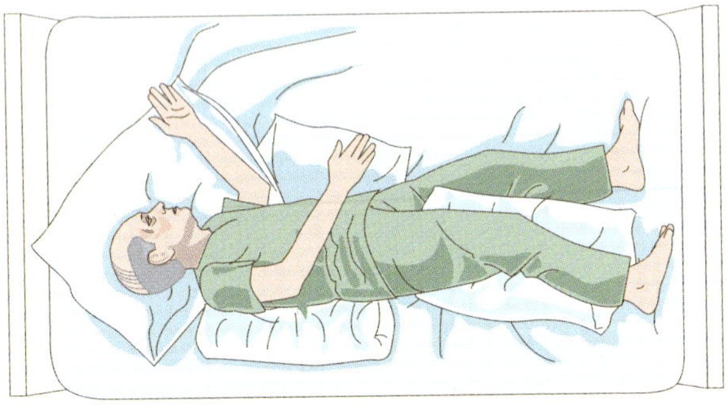

FIGURE 15-33 Semisupine position is a variation of supine that is very comfortable and prevents pressure on the major pressure points.

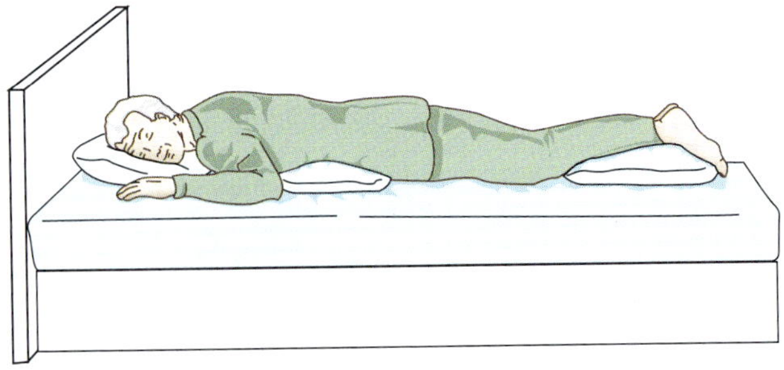

FIGURE 15-34A Prone position.

4. Extend both legs. Place the right leg a little behind the left leg. Support the right leg with two pillows folded in half that extend from groin to ankle.

Prone Position (Figure 15-34A). Start with the bed flat and the patient lying on the abdomen with the head turned to either side, spine straight and legs extended.

1. Place a small pillow under the head so that it extends to the patient's shoulders and 5 to 6 inches beyond the face.
2. Place a small pillow under the abdomen. This relieves pressure on the back and reduces pressure against a female patient's breasts. An alternate method is to roll a towel and place it under the shoulders.
3. Place a pillow under the arms to reach from the elbow to below the wrists. The shoulders and elbows may be flexed or extended, whichever is more comfortable for the patient (Figure 15-34B).
4. Place a pillow under the lower legs to prevent pressure on the toes. The patient may be moved down in bed before starting the procedure, so that the feet extend over the end of the mattress. This allows the foot to assume a normal standing position (Figure 15-34C).

Semiprone Position (Figure 15-35). This position relieves pressure on the hips. Breathing is easier in this position than in the full prone position. Directions are for the patient lying on the left side.

1. Extend the patient's left arm and tuck it slightly beneath the patient's body.
2. Place a pillow in front of and at right angles to the patient's chest.
3. Flex the patient's right knee and hip. Support with pillows that are parallel to the leg.
4. Grasp the patient's left arm from the back of the patient. Turn the patient onto the chest facing away from you. Gently pull his left arm toward you and push on the hip.

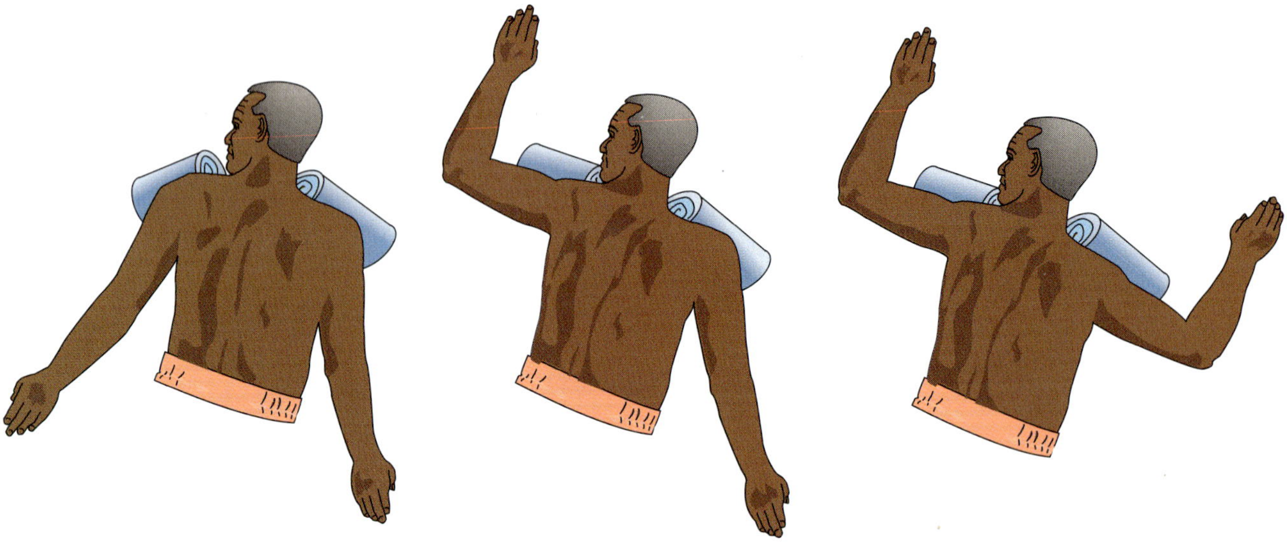

FIGURE 15-34B Position the arms in the way most comfortable for the patient.

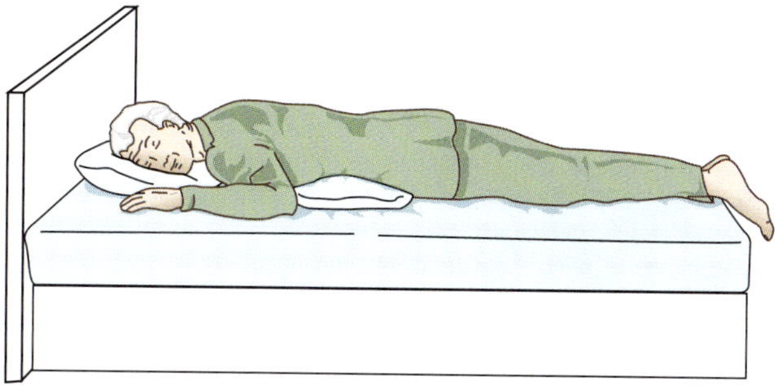

FIGURE 15-34C The patient may be moved down in bed so the feet hang over the end of the mattress.

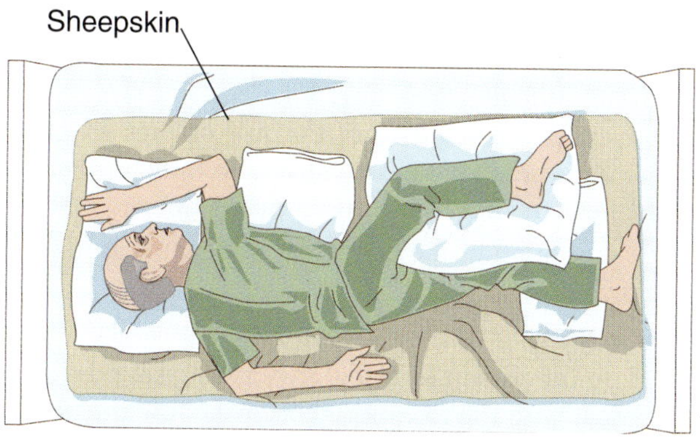

FIGURE 15-35 Semiprone position is a variation of prone.

5. Extend the right arm upward and toward the head of the bed. Place it on the head pillow with the fingers and palm against the bed.
6. Flex the upper arm on a pillow.
7. Lift up the sheepskin and place a foam block under the sheepskin above the iliac crest (hipbone).
8. Place another foam block under the sheepskin just below the iliac crest. You should be able to slide your hand between the hip and the bed.

SAFETY *Alert*

The semiprone and semisupine positions may be a source of confusion for some health care workers. These positions are not the same as the lateral positions. Patients in semiprone and semisupine positions are tilted at an angle so that pressure is not applied to the bony prominences, whereas the lateral position places pressure on many vital areas. The semiprone and semisupine positions are very comfortable and relieve pressure from all major pressure points on the patient's body.

Right Lateral Position (Figure 15-36). Reverse directions for left lateral position.

1. Start with the bed flat and the patient turned to the left side, with spine straight. Remember before turning to move the patient to the right side of the bed.
2. Place a pillow under the head so it extends 5 to 6 inches beyond the patient's face and down to the shoulders.
3. Position the right arm so the shoulder and elbow are flexed and the palm of the hand is facing up.
4. Place the left arm so it is extended or only slightly flexed and rest it on the hip or bring it forward and place it on a pillow. The patient's shoulder, elbow, and wrist should be at approximately the same height.
5. Place a pillow between the patient's legs, extending from above the knee to below the ankle. The patient's hip, knee, and ankle should be at approximately the same height.
6. A pillow may be placed behind the patient to help maintain the position.

Sims' Position (Figure 15-37). This is a variation of the lateral position with the patient on the left side, left leg extended and right leg flexed. This position is often used for rectal examinations and treatments and enemas.

1. Place a pillow under the patient's head as for lateral position.
2. Start with the bed flat and the patient moved and turned onto the left side.
3. Extend the patient's left arm and position it behind the patient's back.
4. Flex the right arm and bring it forward. Support the arm with a pillow.

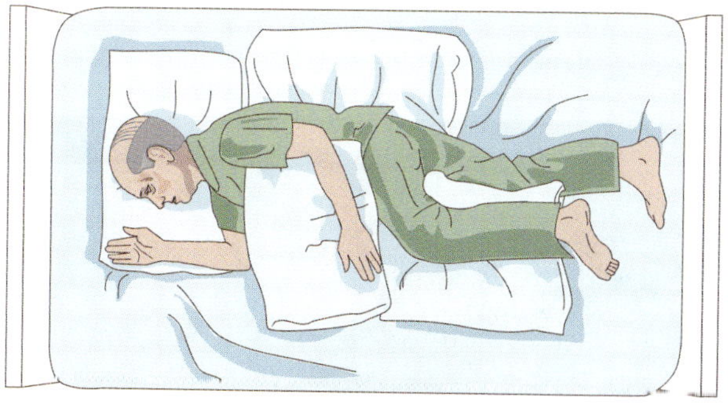

FIGURE 15-36 Right lateral position.

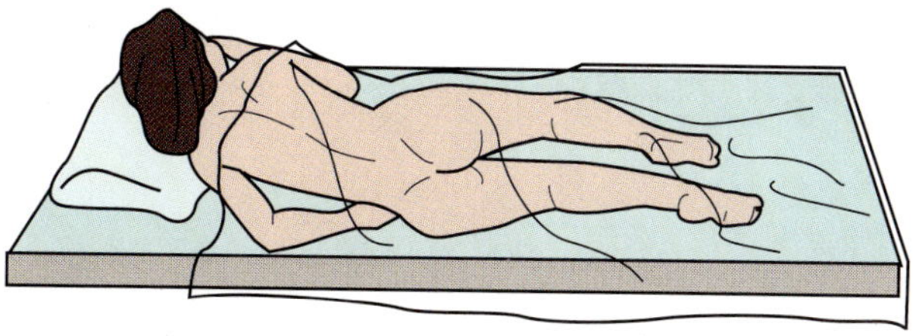

FIGURE 15-37 Sims' position.

Fowler's Position. This position, or a variation of it, is used for feeding patients in bed, for certain treatments and procedures, for the patient's comfort while visiting or watching television, and for those who have trouble breathing. This position increases pressure on the buttocks and increases the risk of skin breakdown and pressure ulcers. Because of this, patients should not be left in Fowler's position for prolonged periods. Check the care plan for instructions.

1. Start with the patient on the back, in the middle of the bed and in good alignment. The patient's hips should be at the place where the bed bends when the bed head is rolled up. Place the head of the bed at 30° for semi-Fowler's, 45° to 60° for Fowler's (Figure 15-38), and 90° for high Fowler's.
2. Place one or two pillows behind the patient's head to extend 4 to 5 inches below the patient's shoulders.
3. Flex elbows and place a pillow under each arm to prevent pull on the shoulders.
4. Place a pillow under each leg to extend from above the knee and to the ankle, to prevent pressure on heels.
5. Place a footboard or folded pillow to keep the feet in position, if necessary.

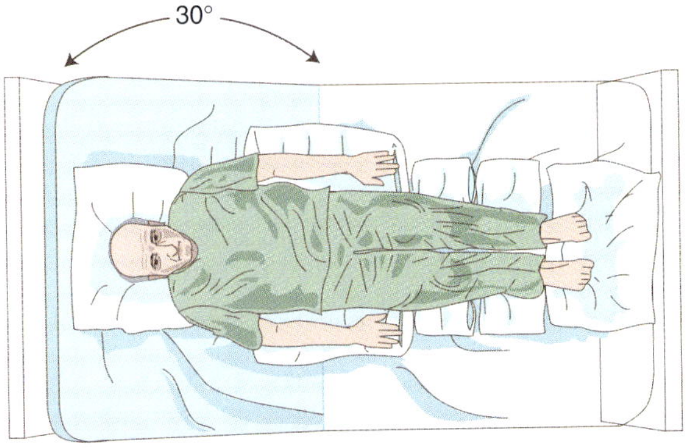

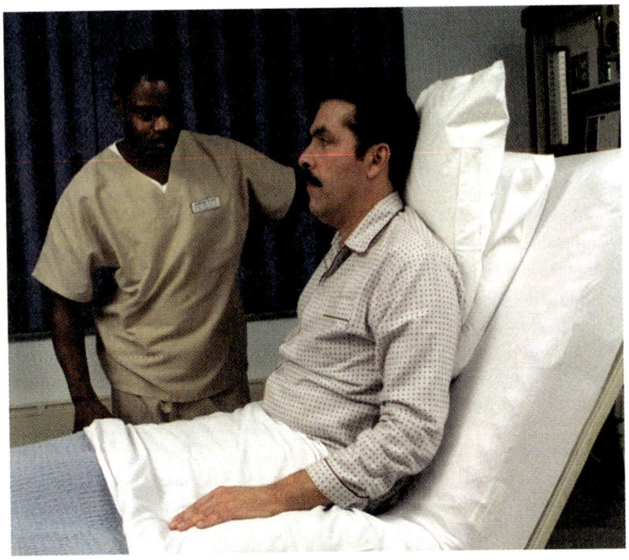

FIGURE 15-38 Fowler's position.

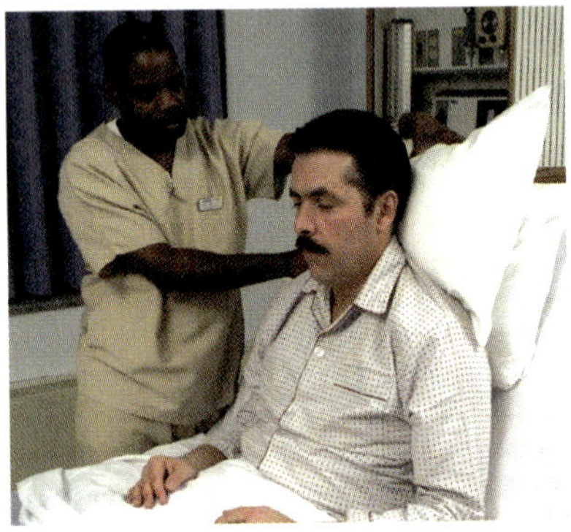

FIGURE 15-39 Orthopneic position.

Orthopneic Position (Figure 15-39). This is a variation of high Fowler's position and is used for patients who have difficulty breathing. Like Fowler's position, the orthopneic position increases the risk of pressure ulcers. Special skin care may be necessary. Check the care plan or ask the nurse manager for further instructions.

1. The position of the bed remains the same as high Fowler's.
2. Assist the patient to sit as upright as possible.
3. Have the patient lean slightly forward, supporting herself with the forearms. This makes the thorax larger, enabling the patient to inhale more air.
4. Place another pillow low behind the patient's back for support.

Sitting Position. Patients should be positioned in a comfortable, well-constructed chair, so that the head and spine are erect (Figure 15-40). The back and buttocks should be up against the chair back. The feet should be flat on the floor.

1. Pillows or postural supports may be needed to maintain the position.
2. A small pillow may be folded and placed at the small of the back to add comfort and support.
3. Do not permit the back of the patient's knees to rest against the chair.

SAFETY *Alert*

Patients can develop pressure ulcers when sitting in a chair. If the patient will be up in the chair for prolonged periods of time, make sure that the seat of the chair is padded. If the patient is able, remind him or her to push on the armrests and shift his or her weight every 15 minutes. Ambulate, stand, or reposition the patient in the chair at least every 2 hours to stimulate circulation and relieve pressure.

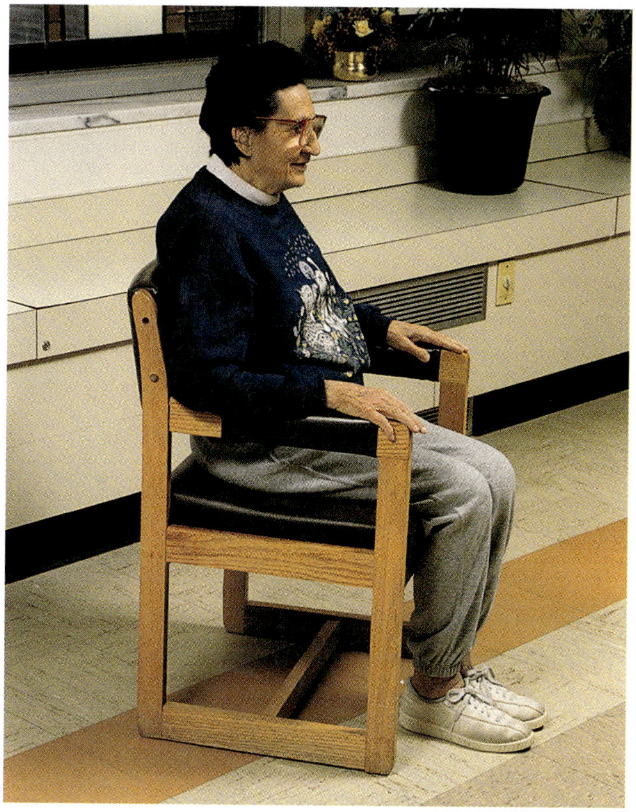

FIGURE 15-40 Maintaining good body alignment is important when patients are sitting in chairs.

Positioning Devices. Several types of devices, called orthoses, are used to maintain the position of an extremity. The correct use of these devices prevents contracture formation. Orthoses are also called **splints**. Figure 15-41 shows examples of orthoses for the upper extremities.

The physician may also order splints or orthoses for the lower extremities. A common type is called the *ankle foot orthosis (AFO)*. The AFO provides support for an unstable ankle and helps reduce extensor spasticity. The AFO is applied to the lower leg before the shoe is put on.

guidelines *for* The Use of Splints

- The splint must be applied correctly. Follow the manufacturer's directions for each splint.
- Follow the care plan for the patient's wearing schedule.
- Keep the extremity under the splint clean and dry.
- Keep the splint clean. If it becomes soiled, check with the nurse to see how it should be cleaned.
- Check the skin under the splint regularly for signs of redness, irritation, and skin breakdown.

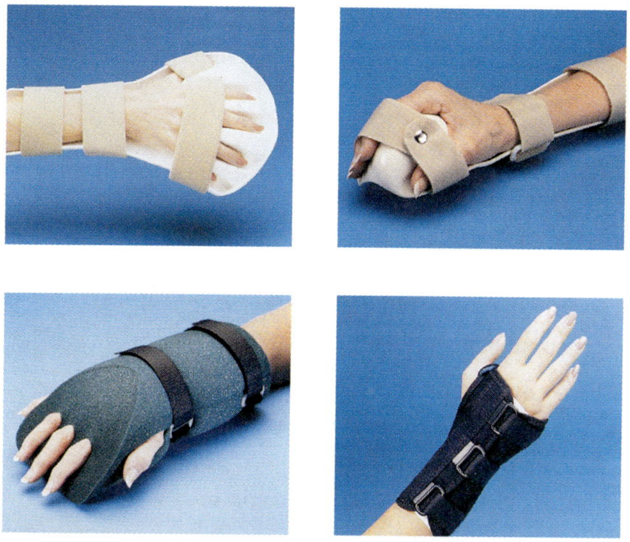

FIGURE 15-41 Several different orthoses are used to maintain good alignment of the hand, wrist, and fingers. *(Photos provided by Sammons Preston, Inc., a Bissell® HealthCare Company. Reprinted with permission.)*

REVIEW

A. Multiple Choice.

Select the one best answer for each of the following.

1. Patients may be at risk for incidents because they
   - **a.** ambulate in the hallway.
   - **b.** use a wheelchair for long distances.
   - **c.** keep one side rail up for turning independently when in bed.
   - **d.** receive certain medications affecting balance, coordination, and mental status.
2. Patient falls can be prevented by
   - **a.** encouraging the patient to remain in bed.
   - **b.** using restraints when the patient is up.
   - **c.** keeping the side rails up at all times.
   - **d.** caring for the patient's physical needs promptly.
3. Alternatives to restraints include
   - **a.** taking patients to the bathroom regularly.
   - **b.** giving medications to sedate the patient.

c. playing music throughout the day to distract the patient.
d. using side rails when in bed.

4. When restraints are used, they must be released
a. every 2 hours.
b. once each shift.
c. every hour.
d. every 4 hours.

5. When restraints are used on patients in bed,
a. there must be full side rails on the bed, in the raised position.
b. the bed should be elevated to the high position.
c. the restraints should be secured to the stationary part of the bed frame.
d. the electric bed adjustment switch should be removed to reduce the risk of injury.

6. Injuries caused by heat or cold are called
a. lacerations.
b. bruises.
c. thermal injuries.
d. aspiration.

7. Choking may be prevented by
a. giving the patient only fluids.
b. giving the patient finger foods.
c. using thickeners for liquids.
d. allowing only blended foods.

8. Beginning procedure actions include
a. handwashing.
b. raising side rails.
c. placing the call signal within reach.
d. opening the door.

9. Correct body alignment will
a. heal disease.
b. prevent infection.
c. help the body function more efficiently.
d. be harmful in certain circumstances.

10. Examples of supportive devices include
a. belts.
b. pillows.
c. side rails.
d. vests.

11. Supine position is
a. lying on the back.
b. lying on the abdomen.
c. lying on the side.
d. sitting in the chair.

12. A position used for patients who have trouble breathing is
a. orthopneic.
b. semiprone.
c. lateral.
d. supine.

13. Logrolling is a procedure performed for
a. persons who have had both legs amputated.
b. ambulatory patients.
c. all conscious patients.
d. patients who have had spinal surgery or spinal cord injury.

14. A trochanter roll is used to
a. maintain the hip in alignment.
b. maintain the feet in alignment.
c. support the patient's back.
d. prevent contractures of the hand.

15. Splints may be used to
a. maintain position of an extremity.
b. provide support for a fractured femur.
c. restrain the wrists.
d. prevent pressure ulcers.

B. True/False.

Mark the following true or false by circling T or F.

16. T F Restraints are attached to the side rails for security.
17. T F Restraints may be needed for some patients.
18. T F A physician's order is not necessary before applying restraints.
19. T F The position of bed patients should be changed at least every 2 hours.
20. T F The left Sims' position is often used for rectal treatments and enemas.
21. T F When turning a patient toward you, cross the patient's near leg over the leg that is farthest from you.
22. T F You must wash your hands before beginning and after completing every nursing assistant task.
23. T F After patient care, the bed should be left in the highest horizontal position.
24. T F Turning sheets make moving heavy patients an easier task.
25. T F You should always explain what you plan to do even if the patient seems not to hear or understand.

C. Matching.

Complete the following by matching Column I with Column II.

Column I

26. ____ supine

27. ____ prone

28. ____ orthopneic

29. ____ trochanter roll

30. ____ splint

31. ____ contracture

32. ____ supportive devices

33. ____ physical restraints

Column II

a. prevents external rotation of hip

b. joint deformity caused by shortening of the muscles

c. devices used to maintain patient's position

d. device used to maintain position of an extremity

e. position for patients with difficult breathing

f. lying on the back

g. lying on the abdomen

h. devices that inhibit movement

D. Nursing Assistant Challenge.

Sara Abrams is 76 years old, has Parkinson's disease, and is a resident in a long-term care facility. She is ambulatory, with a shuffling walk, and has tremors of her hands related to the Parkinson's. She is disoriented and frequently walks into other patients' rooms.

34. Discuss safety issues related to Ms. Abrams's condition.

35. Which of the Residents' Rights may be a special issue in this situation?

36. What steps can you take to meet Ms. Abrams's physical needs? Will doing so lower her risk of falling?

37. How can you incorporate exercise into her daily routine?

38. What types of activities might interest Ms. Abrams?

39. Are there are actions that can be taken to avoid restraints and falls?

EXPLORING THE WEB

Description	Location
Patient Safety	*http://www.patientsafety.com*
American Society for Healthcare Risk Management Hospital Connect	*http://www.hospitalconnect.com*
Before the Fall	*http://www.advancefornurses.com* (see past articles 6/24/02)
Developing Successful Strategies for Preventing Falls	*http://www.nursinghome.org*
National Center for Injury Prevention and Control	*http://www.cdc.gov/ncipc/pub-res/toolkit/toolkit.htm*
National Patient Safety Foundation	*http://www.ama-assn.org*
National Safety Council	*http://www.nsc.org*
Posey Corporation	*http://www.posey.com*
Restraint Reduction	*http://www.nursinghome.org*
The Right Steps (Orthoses)	*http://www.advancefornurses.com* (see past articles 9/25/00)
RN Plus Fall Prevention	*http://www.rnplus.com*
Skil-Care Corporation	*http://www.skil-care.com*
Untie the Elderly Newsletter	*http://www.ute.kendal.org*
Vail Beds	*http://www.vailbed.com*

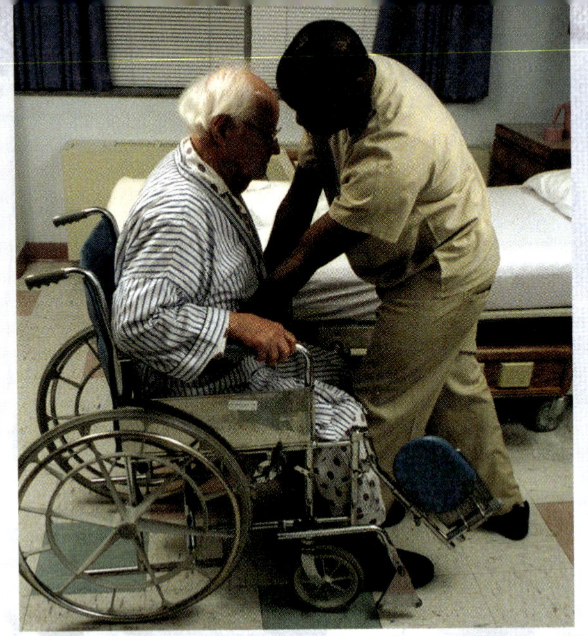

unit 16

The Patient's Mobility: Transfer Skills

objectives

After completing this unit, you will be able to:

- Spell and define terms.
- List the guidelines for safe transfers.
- Describe the difference between a standing transfer and a sitting transfer.
- Demonstrate correct application of a transfer belt.
- Demonstrate the following procedures:
  - Procedure 18 Applying a Transfer Belt
  - Procedure 19 Transferring the Patient from Bed to Chair—One Assistant
  - Procedure 20 Transferring the Patient from Bed to Chair—Two Assistants
  - Procedure 21 Transferring the Patient from Chair to Bed—One Assistant
  - Procedure 22 Transferring the Patient from Chair to Bed—Two Assistants
  - Procedure 23 Independent Transfer, Standby Assist
  - Procedure 24 Transferring the Patient from Bed to Stretcher
  - Procedure 25 Transferring the Patient from Stretcher to Bed
  - Procedure 26 Transferring the Patient with a Mechanical Lift
  - Procedure 27 Transferring the Patient onto and off the Toilet
  - Procedure 28 Transferring the Patient into and out of the Bathtub
  - Procedure 29 Transferring a Patient into and out of a Car

vocabulary

Learn the meaning and the correct spelling of the following words and phrases:

contraindication
full weight-bearing
gait belt
mechanical lift
nonweight-bearing
paralysis
paresis
partial weight-bearing
pivot
sitting transfer
standing transfer
transfer belt
weight-bearing

INTRODUCTION

As a nursing assistant, you will work with many patients who have impaired mobility. In the last unit you learned how to move and position patients in bed. In this unit you will learn how to transfer patients (to move them from one place to another). Patients transfer:

- Out of bed into a chair and back to bed from the chair
- Out of bed onto a stretcher and back to bed from the stretcher
- Onto and off of a toilet
- Into and out of a car
- Into and out of a bathtub or shower

Refer to Procedures 19 through 29 later in this unit.

TYPES OF TRANSFERS

There are basically two types of transfers. A **standing transfer** means the patient stands during the transfer with the help of one or two nursing assistants. A **sitting transfer** means the patient is sitting throughout the transfer, such as when a **mechanical lift** is used. A mechanical lift is a piece of equipment that is used to move dependent patients.

The nurse or the physical therapist determines which method is used to transfer a patient (Figure 16-1). It is important to follow instructions carefully to avoid injury. The method selected depends on:

1. The patient's physical condition. This takes into consideration:
   - **Paralysis** (inability to move) of any extremity
   - **Paresis**, which is weakness of an extremity
   - Absence of an extremity due to amputation
   - Recent hip surgery
2. The patient's strength, endurance, and balance. These abilities may be affected by:
   - Respiratory (lung) disease
   - Cardiac (heart) disease

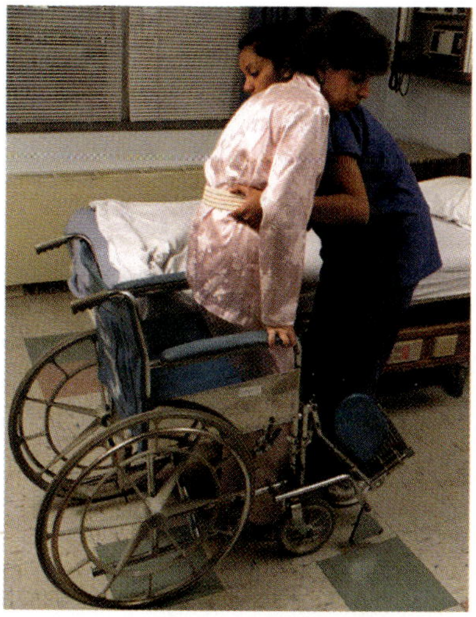

FIGURE 16-1 The nurse or physical therapist determines the method of transfer.

guidelines *for*

Safe Patient Transfers

Moving dependent patients can result in injury to you or the patient unless all safety measures are followed.

- Know the method of transfer that has been ordered by the nurse or physical therapist.
- Know the patient's capabilities.
- Use correct body mechanics.
- Place the bed in the lowest position before starting the standing transfer. Make sure the wheels on the bed and the transfer vehicle (wheelchair, stretcher) are locked before the move. It is helpful to elevate the head of the bed for bed-to-chair transfers.
- *Never allow patients to place their hands on your body during a transfer.* This is a dangerous practice. A patient who is disoriented or frightened can cause you to lose your balance. If this happens, the patient can pull you down, possibly injuring both of you.
- *Never place your hands under a patient's arms or shoulders.* This practice can cause the patient severe shoulder injury.
- Use a transfer belt for standing transfers unless it is contraindicated.
- Make sure the patient is wearing shoes with sturdy, nonslip soles and that clothing is not too loose or dragging on the floor.
- Be aware of any tubes, orthoses, or other items that must be dealt with during the transfer.
- Transfer the patient toward his strongest side if possible.
- Always explain to the patient what you are doing and how he can help.
- Test the patient's understanding and make sure she knows what you expect her to do during the transfer.
- Allow the patient to see the surface to which he is being transferred. Encourage the patient to keep his head up.
- Stand close to the patient during the transfer.
- If the patient has a weak or paralyzed leg, brace the knee of that leg with your knee or leg. If the patient has a paralyzed arm, be sure it is supported during the transfer to avoid dangling and pulling on the patient's shoulder.
- Give the patient only the assistance that she needs.
- Never have the patient use a footstool unless it is absolutely necessary.

- Neurological disease, such as multiple sclerosis or a stroke
- The ability to stand on one or both legs. This is called **weight-bearing**. For example, a patient may not be able to place full weight on a paralyzed leg. The physician may order the patient to be **non-weight-bearing** or only **partial weight-bearing** if the patient has had hip surgery. The ability to stand on both legs is called **full weight-bearing**. For a standing transfer, the patient must be able to stand and have at least partial weight-bearing on one leg.

3. The patient's mental condition. Can the patient understand and follow the instructions?
4. The patient's size. For example, transfer of a very tall or large person who cannot bear full weight would need two assistants or a mechanical lift.

In some situations you may be instructed to take the patient's pulse before and after she gets out of bed. If the patient has been inactive for a long time, the heart muscle may be deconditioned. Checking the pulse when the patient is active provides an evaluation of the heart's condition.

TRANSFER BELTS

A **transfer belt** is a webbed belt 1½ to 2 inches wide and about 54 to 60 inches long. It is an assistive and safety device used to transfer or ambulate patients who need help. (Refer to Procedure 18.) When it is used to assist a patient with ambulation, it is called a **gait belt**. Using a transfer belt avoids the need to grasp the patient around the rib cage or under the shoulders. Either of these methods can cause serious injury. It also allows you to have more control in directing the transfer. A transfer belt is not used to "lift" a patient. If the patient has no ability to bear weight, another method should be used for transferring.

OSHA Alert

Each year more than 12.8 million Americans consult their doctors about back problems. In fact, as many as 8 out of 10 individuals will suffer back pain during their lifetime. A transfer belt is an inexpensive item that helps protect you from injury and makes transfers safer and more secure for patients. Make the transfer belt a permanent part of your uniform. Wear it when you are on duty so it is readily available when needed to move a patient.

Contraindications (situations in which something is not indicated, inappropriate, or potentially dangerous) for use of the transfer belt include:

- Abdominal, back, or rib injuries, fractures, or recent surgery
- Abdominal pacemakers
- Advanced heart or lung disease
- Abdominal aneurysms
- Pregnancy
- Colostomy
- Gastrostomy tube or feeding tube

Medication pumps may be implanted under the skin of the abdomen in some patients. If the surgical site is well healed, it is probably safe to use the transfer belt. However, always follow the care plan or check with the nurse before using a transfer belt to move a patient with any type of implantable device.

PROCEDURE 18

APPLYING A TRANSFER BELT

1. Carry out beginning procedure actions.
2. Assemble equipment:
   - Transfer belt
3. Explain the procedure. Tell the patient that the belt is a safety device that will be removed as soon as the transfer is completed.
4. Apply the belt over the patient's clothing (Figure 16-2A). If the patient is undressed and being transferred from wheelchair to tub or shower chair, either leave the patient's shirt on, put the patient's robe on, or place a towel around the patient's waist and then apply the belt over the towel.

continues

PROCEDURE 18

continued

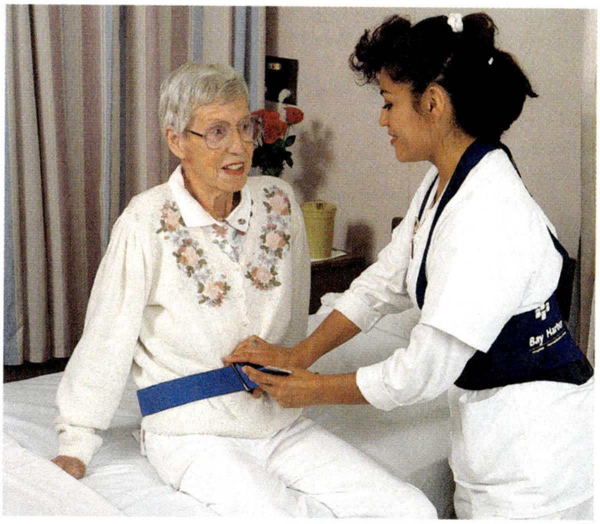

FIGURE 16-2A Always apply the transfer belt over clothing.

5. If the patient is going to transfer from bed to chair, the belt may be applied after the patient comes to a sitting position on the edge of the bed. If the patient has inadequate balance, the belt can be applied while the patient is still lying down in bed. You may need to readjust the belt after the patient sits up.
6. Keep the belt at the patient's waist level. Avoid placing it too high. Make sure the belt is right side out and is not twisted.
7. Buckle the belt in front by threading the belt end through the teeth side of the buckle first and then through both openings (Figure 16-2B). The buckle must be in front.
8. Check female patients to be sure the breasts are not under the belt.
9. The belt should be snug, so that it does not slide up, but not tight (Figure 16-2C). Check the fit of the belt by placing three fingers under it. There should be just enough space for your fingers to fit comfortably.
10. Before attempting to move the patient, be sure her feet are flat on the floor. If they are not, use the belt to assist the patient to the edge of the bed until her feet are resting firmly on the floor.
11. If you are transferring a patient into or out of a wheelchair, keep the footrests out of the way during the transfer. After the patient is seated, her legs should not dangle. The feet are supported on the floor or on the wheelchair footrests.
12. Teach the patient to assist by pushing off the bed or arms of the chair with her hands when you count to three.
13. Use an underhand grasp when holding the belt. For transfers, one hand should be on each side of the buckle in front.
14. Do not overuse the belt by pulling the patient up with force.
15. When the patient is standing, pivot to transfer.
16. The chair should be close enough so the patient can feel it with her hands after you pivot.
17. Remove the belt after the patient is safely moved.
18. Carry out procedure completion actions.

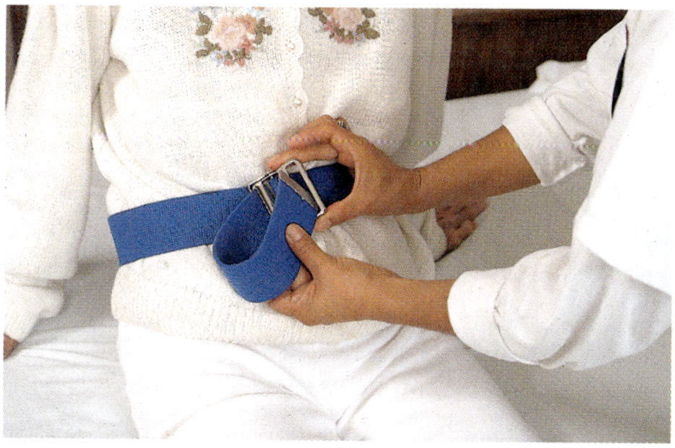

FIGURE 16-2B Thread the belt through the teeth side of the buckle first.

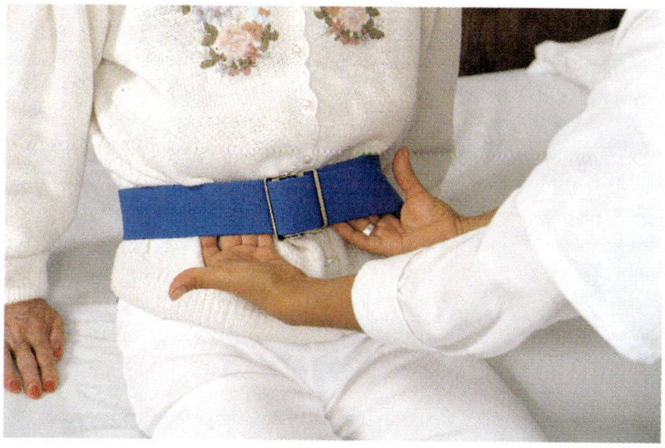

FIGURE 16-2C The belt should be snug but not tight.

PROCEDURE 19

TRANSFERRING THE PATIENT FROM BED TO CHAIR—ONE ASSISTANT

1. Carry out beginning procedure actions.
2. Assemble equipment:
   - Transfer belt
   - Chair for patient
   - Bath blanket
   - Robe or clothing
   - Shoes and socks
3. Place chair so the patient moves toward her strongest side. Set the chair parallel with the bed. Lock the wheelchair and raise or remove the footrests (Figure 16-3A). Cover the chair with a bath blanket, unless the patient is fully clothed.
4. Lower the bed to the lowest horizontal position and lock the bed wheels.

These instructions are for getting out of the right side (patient's right side) of the bed.

5. Stand against the right side of the bed with the side rail down. Ask the patient to slide toward the right side of the bed.
6. Have the patient roll over onto her right side, flexing the knees and bending the right arm so it can be used for propping the upper body. Bend the elbow of the left arm so this hand can be used to push off from the bed.

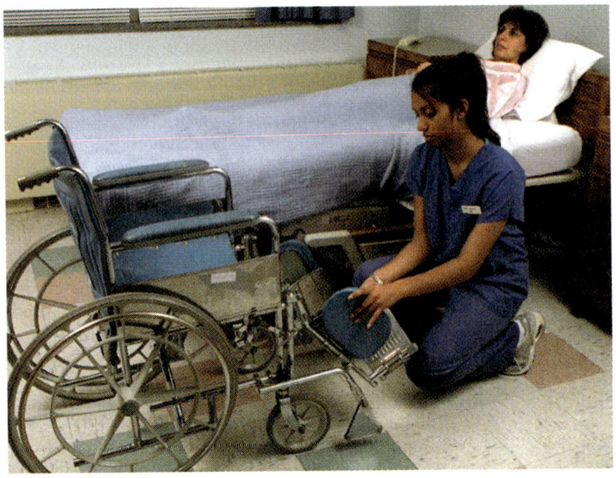

FIGURE 16-3A Lock the wheelchair and lift or remove the footrests before the patient transfers.

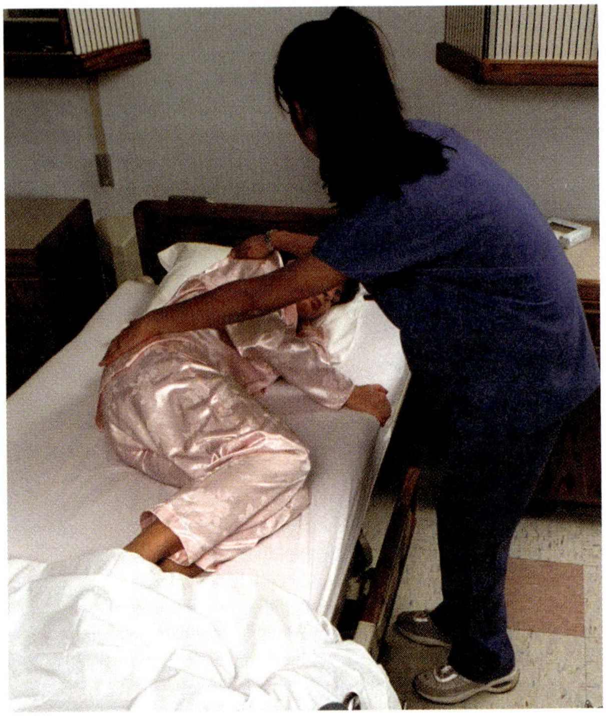

FIGURE 16-3B Instruct the patient to use her hands to push to the sitting position.

7. Instruct the patient to use the elbow of her right arm to raise the upper body and to push with the hand of the right arm so she comes to an upright position (Figure 16-3B).
8. Instruct the patient to let her legs slide off the bed at the same time.
9. If assistance is needed, place one arm under the shoulders (not the neck) and one arm over and around the knees (Figure 16-3C). Raise the patient's upper body at the same time you move the legs off the bed.
10. Give the patient time to adjust to sitting up and then apply the transfer belt. Assist to put on shoes and socks. (If the patient has problems with balance, the shoes and socks can be put on while the patient is lying down in bed.)
11. If the patient has a weak or paralyzed arm, do not let it hang or dangle during the transfer. Put it in

continues

PROCEDURE 19

continued

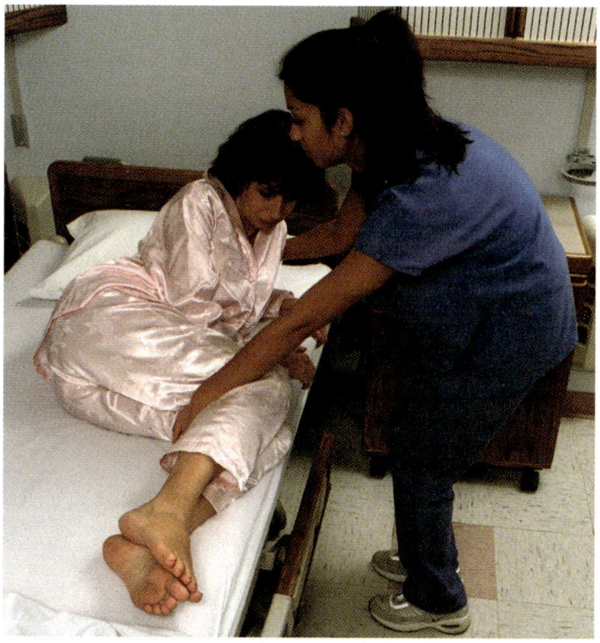

FIGURE 16-3C Place one arm under the patient's shoulders and one arm over and around the patient's knees.

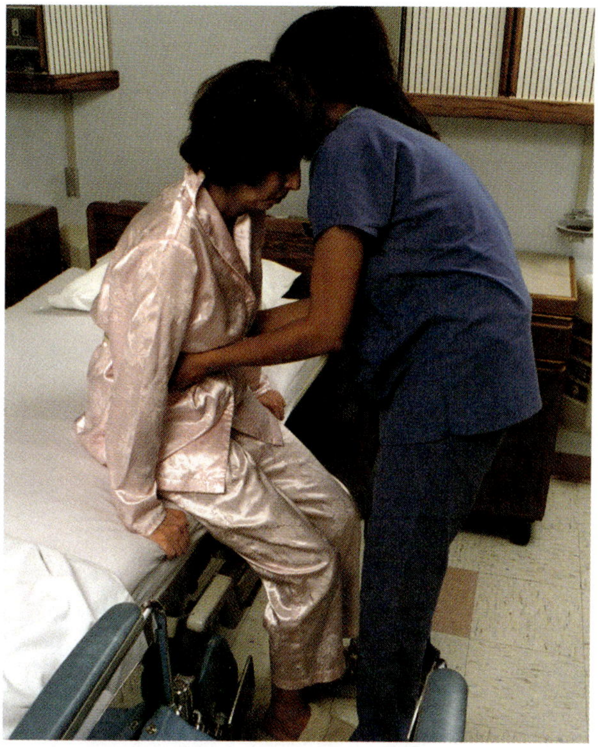

FIGURE 16-3D The stronger leg should be slightly back.

her pocket, or have her cradle it with her strong arm, or carefully tuck her weaker hand in the transfer belt or waist of the pants until she is again seated.

12. When the patient is ready to transfer:
    - Instruct her to move forward or closer to the edge of the mattress, to spread her knees, lean forward from the waist, and place her feet slightly back.
    - If one leg is weaker or should not bear weight, place this leg out in front with the strong leg slightly back (Figure 16-3D).
    - Remember to spread your feet apart and bend your knees and hips, keeping your back straight.
    - Hold the belt with an underhand grasp, one hand on each side of the front of the belt.
    - If the patient has a weaker leg, press your knee against her knee, or block the patient's foot with yours to prevent the weaker leg from sliding out from under her.
    - Tell the patient on the count of three to use her hands (if able) to press into the mattress, to straighten her elbows and knees, and to come to a standing position (Figure 16-3E).

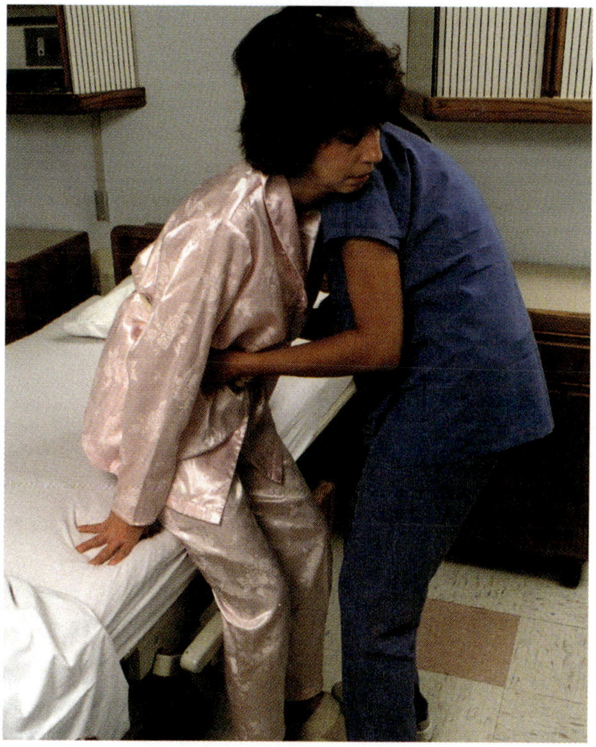

FIGURE 16-3E Tell the patient to straighten her elbows and knees to come to a standing position.

continues

PROCEDURE 19

continued

13. If patient cannot walk, have her **pivot** (turn the entire body as one unit) around to the front of the chair until the chair is touching the backs of her legs (Figure 16-3F).
14. Instruct the patient to place her hands on the arms of the chair (if able), to bend her knees, and to gently lower herself into the chair as you ease her downward (Figure 16-3G). Replace the footrests.
15. Position patient comfortably. Place the signal light within easy reach.
16. Straighten the bed and prepare it for the patient's return.
17. Carry out procedure completion actions.

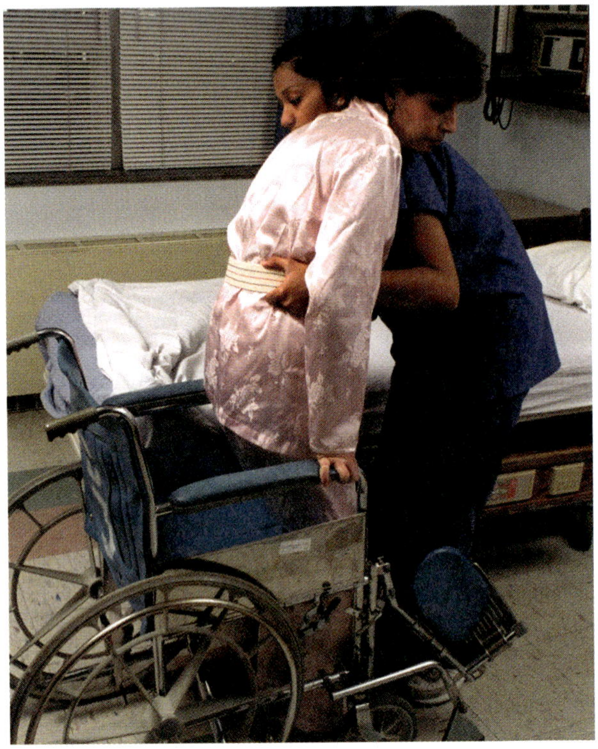

FIGURE 16-3F The patient pivots around to the wheelchair.

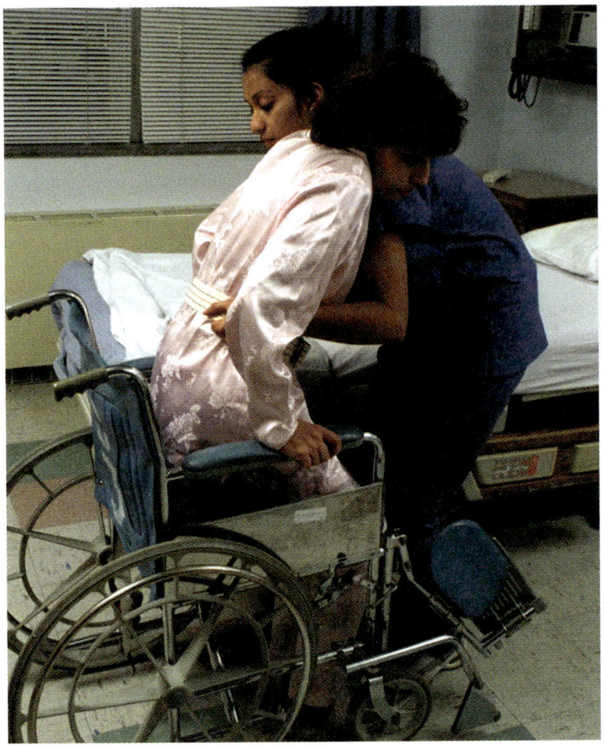

FIGURE 16-3G Tell the patient to bend her knees and lower herself into the chair.

SAFETY *Alert*

Remember to lock the brakes before transferring a patient into or out of a wheelchair. Turn the small front wheels so the large part faces forward. Lock the brakes any time the chair is parked. If you remove the wheelchair footrests during a transfer, remember to replace them.

PROCEDURE 20

TRANSFERRING THE PATIENT FROM BED TO CHAIR—TWO ASSISTANTS

Two people may be needed to transfer patients who are weak, disoriented, have limited weight-bearing ability, or are very large. Directions are given for transferring toward the patient's right side.

1. Follow steps 1 through 11 in Procedure 19.
2. The nursing assistants stand one on each side, facing the patient.
3. Each one places the hand closest to the patient through the belt, with an underhand grasp toward the front of the patient. The other hand of each assistant grasps the belt toward the back. Coordination of movement is necessary (Figure 16-4A).
4. The nursing assistant closest to the chair (on the patient's right side) stands in a position to step or pivot around smoothly to allow the patient access to the chair. This person stands with the left leg further back than the right leg.
5. The other nursing assistant uses the left knee to brace the patient's weaker left leg. This assistant's left leg is further back than the right leg.
6. Instruct the patient to bend forward and place the palms of the hands on the edge of the mattress to push off.
7. The patient's knees should be spread apart, with both feet back and the stronger foot slightly in back of the weaker foot.
8. The nursing assistants bend their knees and give a broad base of support.
9. On the count of three, the patient stands. Allow her to stand for a moment and bear weight. Tell her to keep her head up. Both nursing assistants help the patient pivot by slowly and smoothly pivoting their feet, legs, and hips to their left.
10. To sit, have the patient bend forward slightly, bend the knees, and lower onto the chair. At the same time, have her reach for the arms of the chair with both hands (Figure 16-4B).
11. Complete the procedure as instructed for a one-assistant transfer (Procedure 19).

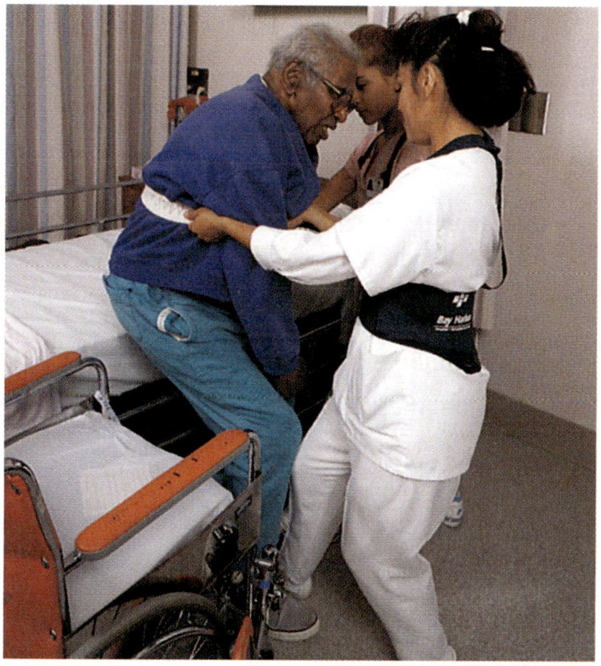

FIGURE 16-4A Coordination of movement is necessary.

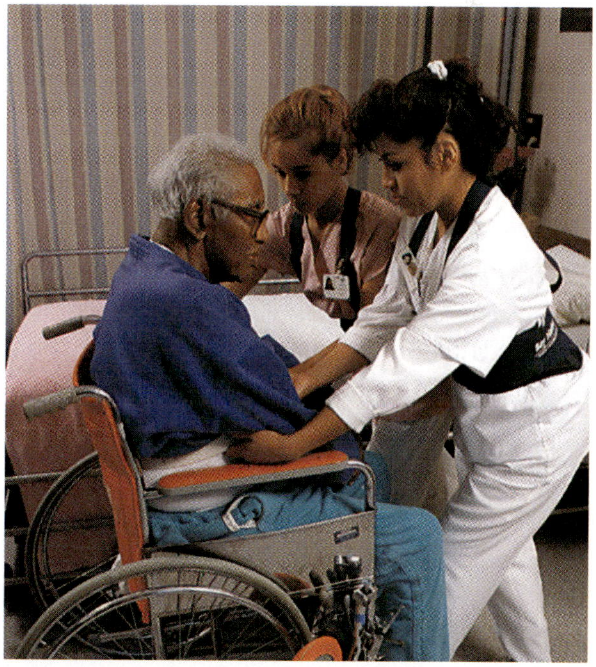

FIGURE 16-4B The patient reaches for the arms of the chair with both hands.

PROCEDURE 21

TRANSFERRING THE PATIENT FROM CHAIR TO BED—ONE ASSISTANT

1. Carry out beginning procedure actions.
2. Assemble equipment:
   - Transfer belt
3. Place chair so the patient moves toward his strongest side. Set chair parallel with bed.
4. Move the bed to the lowest horizontal position and lock the wheels. Fanfold top covers to foot of bed if necessary and raise the opposite side rail.
5. Lock the wheelchair and raise or remove the footrests.
6. Have the patient place both feet flat on the floor.
7. Place the transfer belt around the patient's waist.
8. Instruct the patient to move forward in the chair, to bend forward, and to spread his knees apart. Both feet should be back, with the stronger foot slightly in back of the weaker foot. Both of the patient's hands should be on the arms of the chair (Figure 16-5).

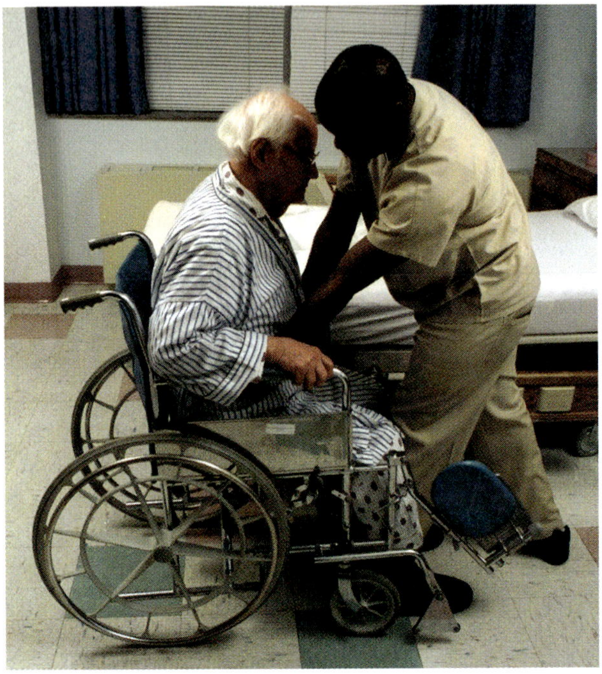

FIGURE 16-5 Instruct the patient to hold the chair arms with both hands.

9. Take hold of the transfer belt with an underhand grasp. Brace the patient's weaker leg with your knee or leg, as instructed in Procedure 19. Ask the patient to push off the chair on the count of three and to stand up as you provide the necessary assistance.
10. Allow the patient to remain standing for a time to stabilize position. Keep your grasp on the transfer belt and continue to brace the weak leg if necessary.
11. To complete the transfer, instruct the patient to step or pivot around to stand in front of the bed, facing away from it. Tell the patient to sit when the edge of the mattress is touching the back of his legs. To sit, have the patient bend forward slightly, bend his knees, and lower himself onto the mattress.
12. When the patient is safely in bed, remove the transfer belt.
13. Remove the patient's slippers and robe. Assist the patient to lie down. Position the patient as necessary. Draw top bedding over the patient. Fold the bath blanket (if used) from the wheelchair and return it to the bedside stand. Make sure the signal light is within reach.
14. Move the wheelchair out of the way.
15. Carry out procedure completion actions.

PROCEDURE 22

TRANSFERRING THE PATIENT FROM CHAIR TO BED—TWO ASSISTANTS

The directions given here are for moving the patient toward his left side.

1. Follow instructions 1 through 8 in Procedure 21.
2. Each nursing assistant places the hand closest to the patient through the belt with an underhand grasp in front of the patient; the other hand goes toward the back.
3. The nursing assistant closest to the bed (on the patient's left side) stands in a position to step or pivot around smoothly to allow the patient access to the bed. This person stands with the right leg further back than the left leg.
4. The other nursing assistant uses the left knee to brace the patient's weaker right leg. This person's right leg is further back than the left one (Figure 16-6A).
5. Ask the patient to push off the chair on the count of three and to stand up as you provide the necessary assistance.
6. Allow the patient to remain standing for a time to stabilize position. Keep your hands on the transfer belt and continue to brace the weak leg if necessary.
7. To complete the transfer, instruct the patient to step or pivot around to stand in front of the bed, facing away from it. Tell the patient to sit when the edge of the mattress is touching the back of his legs. To sit, have the patient bend forward slightly, bend his knees, and lower himself onto the mattress (Figure 16-6B).
8. When the patient is safely in bed, remove the transfer belt.
9. Remove the patient's slippers and robe. Assist the patient to lie down and position as necessary. Raise side rails if ordered. Draw top bedding over the patient. Fold the bath blanket (if used) from the wheelchair and return it to the bedside stand. Make sure the signal light is within reach.
10. Move the wheelchair out of the way.
11. Carry out procedure completion actions.

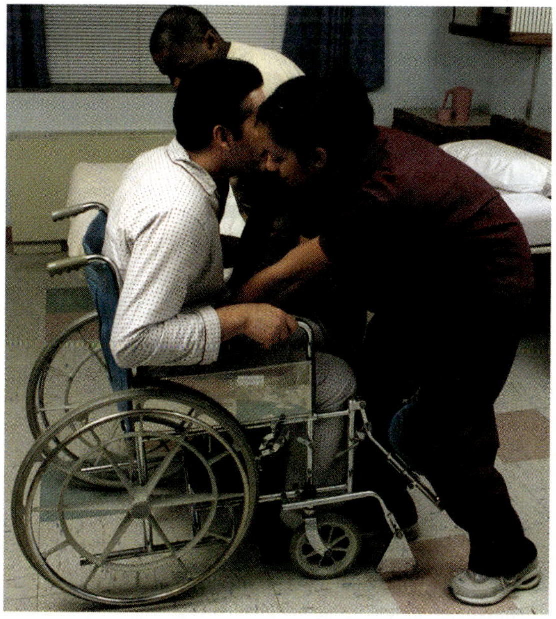

FIGURE 16-6A The nursing assistant uses the left knee to support the patient's weaker right leg.

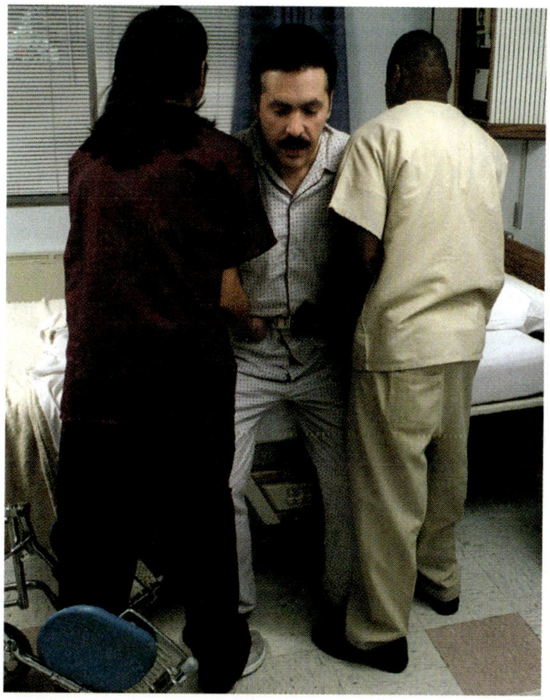

FIGURE 16-6B Tell the patient to bend forward, bend the knees, and lower himself onto the mattress.

PROCEDURE 23

INDEPENDENT TRANSFER, STANDBY ASSIST

This method is appropriate for the patient who has good balance and strength and can understand instructions. Put a transfer belt on the patient the first time this is attempted.

1. Follow the instructions for getting the patient to a sitting position on the side of the bed. (See Procedure 19.) For an independent transfer, the patient should be able to do this without help.
2. Have the patient place the strongest foot slightly in back of the other foot. The patient's knees should be spread slightly apart.
3. Instruct the patient to place the palms of the hands at the edge of the bed and to lean slightly forward.
4. Tell the patient to press the hands into the bed to push off, at the same time the legs straighten, to assume a standing position.
5. Once standing, have the patient reach for the far arm of the chair and then step or pivot to stand in front of the chair. Instruct the patient to sit when the edge of the seat is felt against the back of the legs.
6. Carry out procedure completion actions.

Reverse these directions when transferring from chair to bed.

STRETCHER TRANSFERS

This procedure is used to move a patient from her room to another room for surgery, treatments, or diagnostic tests. The procedure may be very frightening to the patient. Assure the patient that the procedure is safe.

Note: Procedures 24 and 25 are for moving an unconscious or semiconscious patient. For alert, fully awake patients, two people may be able to perform this procedure with one person against the stretcher and the other person on the opposite side of the bed. Instruct the patient how to help you.

PROCEDURE 24

TRANSFERRING THE PATIENT FROM BED TO STRETCHER

1. Carry out beginning procedure actions.
2. Assemble equipment:
   - Stretcher
   - Bath blanket
3. You will need three to four people for transferring an unconscious or comatose patient from bed to stretcher.
4. Lock the wheels of the bed. Raise the bed to a horizontal position equal to the height of the stretcher. Lower the side rails.
5. Place a bath blanket over the patient and fanfold top covers to the foot of the bed, out of the way.
6. Roll the turning sheet up against the patient on both sides. The sheet should be long enough to support the patient's head and shoulders during the move.
7. Position the stretcher close to the bed. Lock stretcher wheels.
8. Two or three people stand along the open side of the stretcher. The other person stands on the the open side of the bed. This assistant may need to get on the bed, on her knees, to avoid over-stretching her back.

Note: *Use an overhand grasp on the moving sheet to avoid wrist strain.*

continues

PROCEDURE 24

continued

- The assistant at the end of the bed grasps the moving sheet by placing one hand by the patient's legs and the other hand by the patient's hips.
- The middle assistant grasps the moving sheet by placing one hand by the patient's hips and the other hand by the patient's shoulders.
- The assistant at the head of the bed grasps the turning sheet by the patient's shoulder and head.
- On the count of three, all persons slide the moving sheet from bed to stretcher (Figure 16-7).

9. Center the patient on the stretcher in good body alignment. Secure the stretcher safety belt. Raise the side rails of the stretcher.
10. Transport the patient as directed.
11. Prepare the bed for the patient's return.
12. Carry out procedure completion actions.

SAFETY *Alert*

Patients on stretchers are not left alone.

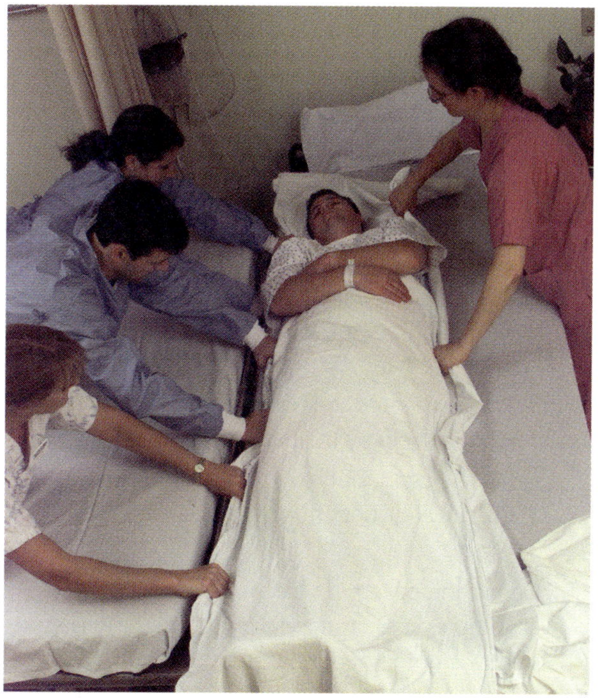

FIGURE 16-7 All persons slide the lifting sheet from bed to stretcher.

PROCEDURE 25

TRANSFERRING THE PATIENT FROM STRETCHER TO BED

1. Carry out beginning procedure actions.
2. Assemble equipment:
   - Stretcher
   - Bath blanket (patient should already be covered with one on the stretcher)
3. You will need three to four people for transferring an unconscious or comatose patient from stretcher to bed.
4. Lock the wheels of the bed. Raise the bed to a horizontal position equal to the height of the stretcher. Lower the side rails. Fanfold top covers to the foot of the bed, out of the way.
5. Place a bath blanket over the patient if necessary.
6. Roll the turning sheet up against the patient on both sides. The sheet should be long enough to support the patient's head and shoulders during the move.
7. Position the stretcher close to the bed. Lock the wheels and lower the side rails.

continues

PROCEDURE 25

continued

8. One person stands along the open side of the stretcher. The other two or three people stand on the open side of the bed. These assistants may need to get on the bed, on their knees, to avoid overstretching their backs.

   Note: *Use an overhand grasp on the moving sheet to avoid wrist strain.*

   - The assistant at the end of the bed grasps the moving sheet by placing one hand by the patient's legs and the other hand by the patient's hips.
   - The middle assistant grasps the moving sheet by placing one hand by the patient's hips and the other hand by the patient's shoulders.
   - The assistant at the head of the bed grasps the turning sheet by the patient's shoulder and head.
   - On the count of three, all persons slide the moving sheet from stretcher to bed (Figure 16-8).
9. Center the patient on the bed in good body alignment. Position the patient properly. Raise the side rails of the bed if ordered.
10. Carry out procedure completion actions.

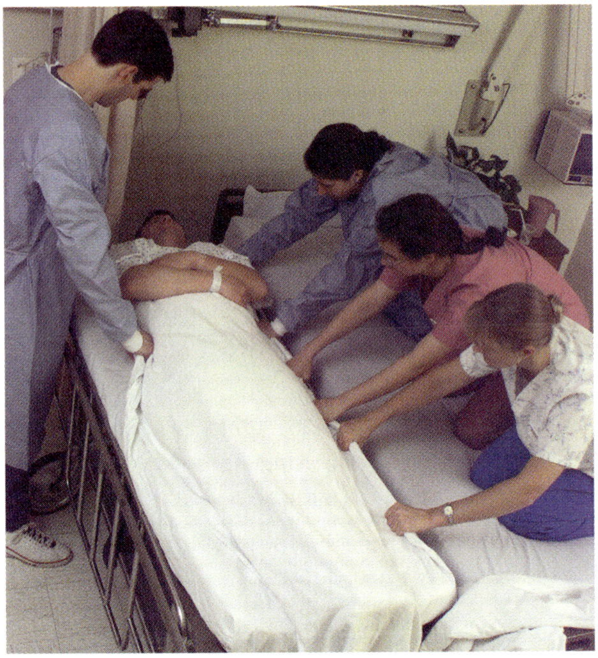

FIGURE 16-8 All persons slide the lifting sheet from stretcher to bed.

MOVING THE PATIENT WITH A MECHANICAL LIFT

The mechanical lift is used for moving heavy patients who have little or no ability to assist. Using a mechanical lift for transfers is safer for both the patient and the nursing assistant. Various types of seats are available so the patient can be moved in the sitting or supine position. Some mechanical lifts may be used to weigh bedfast patients.

Several types of mechanical lifts are available. Some are manually operated, others are electric. The most commonly used lift is the hydraulic lift. It is used when a patient is heavy, unable to assist, unbalanced, or has an amputation or other condition that makes transfer with a belt difficult or impossible. For safety reasons, the hydraulic lift should be operated by two or more nursing assistants. Never attempt to operate it alone. Some electric and battery-operated lifts can safely be used by one person. Know and follow your facility policy for use of the mechanical lift.

PROCEDURE 26

TRANSFERRING THE PATIENT WITH A MECHANICAL LIFT

This procedure is used for heavy patients who have little or no weight-bearing ability.

Note: *Check slings, chains, and straps for frayed areas or clasps that do not close properly. Check the hydraulic lift and the leg spreader to make sure they are both working. Do not use if there is oil on the floor or if equipment is defective. Report need for repair and obtain safe equipment.*

continues

PROCEDURE 26

continued

1. Carry out beginning procedure actions.
2. Assemble equipment:
   - Mechanical lift
   - Sling
   - Chair
3. Place a wheelchair or other chair parallel to the foot of the bed, facing the head. Lock the wheelchair.
4. Elevate the bed to a comfortable working height. Lock the bed wheels. Lower the nearest side rail. Roll the patient toward you.
5. Position the sling beneath the patient's body behind shoulder, thighs, and buttocks. Be sure the sling is smooth (Figure 16-9A).
6. Roll the patient back onto the sling and position properly (Figure 16-9B). If the sling has inserts for metal bars, insert them now.
7. Position lift frame over bed with base legs in maximum open position, and lock lift legs (Figure 16-9C).
8. Attach suspension straps or chains to the sling (Figure 16-9D). Check fasteners for security.

***Note:** Be sure that the correct end of the strap or chain is hooked to the correct place on the sling. Always hook straps or chains from inside to outside so the open part of the hook faces away from the patient.*

SAFETY *Alert*

Two people should carry out these procedures to ensure patient safety.

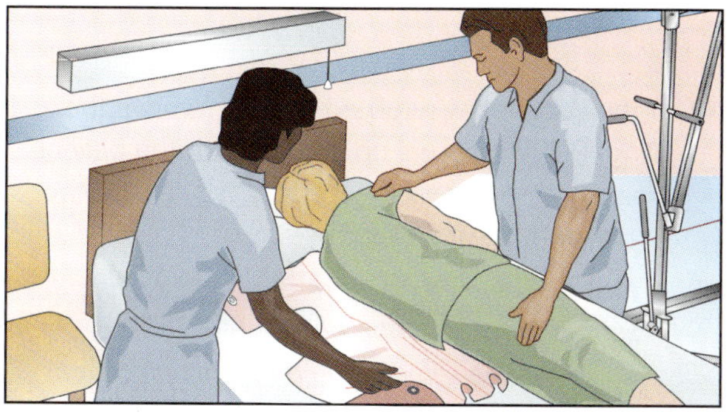

FIGURE 16-9A Position the sling under the patient.

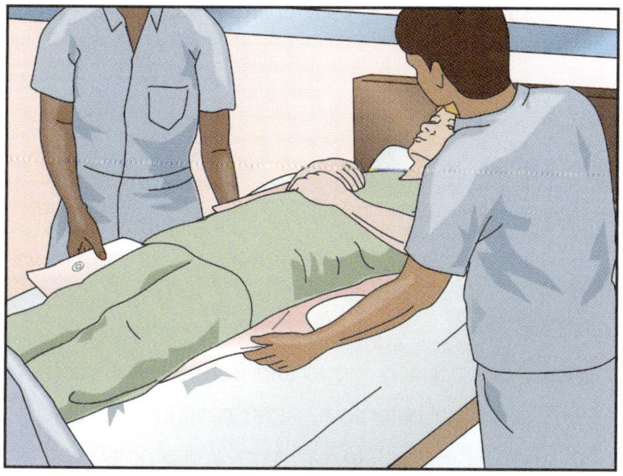

FIGURE 16-9B Roll the patient back onto the sling.

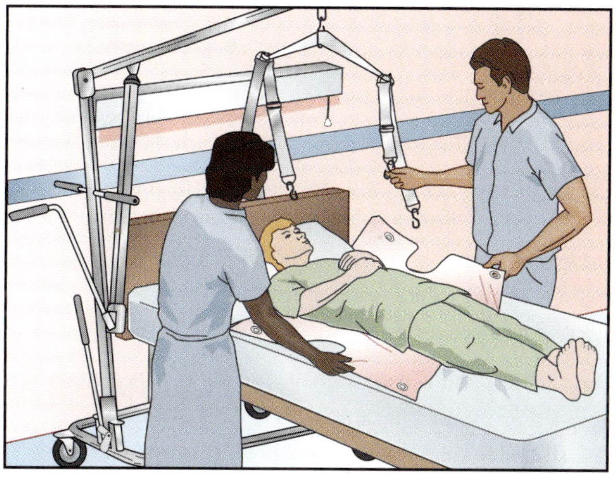

FIGURE 16-9C Position the lift frame over the bed.

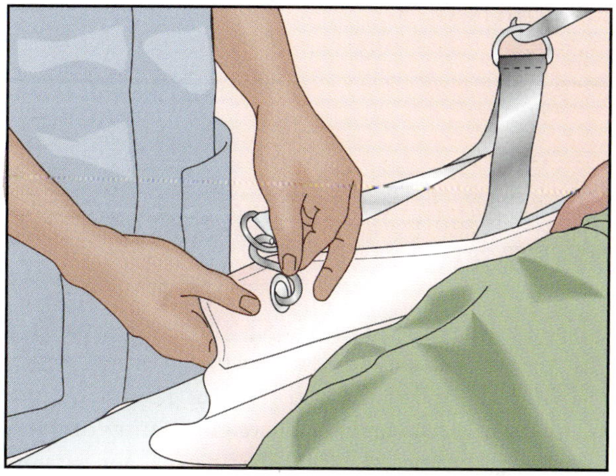

FIGURE 16-9D Attach the straps or chains to the sling.

continues

PROCEDURE 26

continued

9. Position the patient's crossed arms inside the straps.
10. Secure straps or chains if necessary.
11. One assistant operates the lift and the other assistant guides the movement of the patient. Lock the hydraulic mechanism, and slowly raise the boom of the lift until the patient is suspended over the bed. Talk to the patient while slowly lifting him free of the bed.
12. Guide the lift away from the bed.
13. Position the patient and lift over the chair or wheelchair (Figure 16-9E). Make sure that the wheels of the wheelchair are locked.
14. Slowly lower the patient into the chair or wheelchair. Pay attention to the position of the patient's feet and hands. One assistant stands behind the chair to pull and guide the patient's hips back into position.
15. Unhook the suspension straps or chains and remove the lift.
16. Position the footrests to support the feet.

Note: *Directions are reversed for moving patient from chair to bed. When raising the patient from the chair, monitor the position of the "S" hooks, which sometimes catch under the chair arms.*

17. If the patient is in a chair, the sling can remain underneath the patient so it is in position for transfer back to bed. If the sling has metal bars, remove them and make sure the sling is smooth and wrinkle-free. Make sure the signal light is within reach.

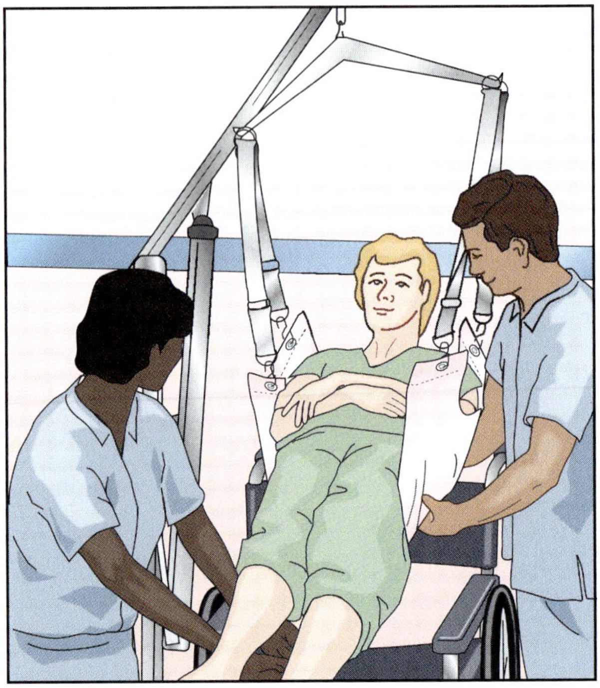

FIGURE 16-9E Position the lift frame over the chair.

18. If the patient has returned to bed, remove the sling. Pull top covers up and position the patient. Raise both side rails if necessary. Make sure the signal light is within reach.

Note: *The method for raising and lowering the lift and for moving the base legs varies for different types of equipment. Read the manufacturer's directions and practice using equipment before using it with patients.*

19. Carry out procedure completion actions.

TOILET TRANSFERS

The bladder is emptied much more efficiently if patients can use the toilet or commode rather than a urinal or bedpan. To use the toilet, the patient must possess transfer skills. Unless the patient has full weight-bearing on both legs and good balance, a wall rail is needed for support while transferring. (Refer to Procedure 27.) Towel racks are not safe for this purpose. Male patients may find it easier and safer to sit rather than stand while urinating.

SAFETY *Alert*

Many falls occur going to and from the bathroom, as well as in the bathroom. Assist patients with toileting regularly. Respond to call signals promptly. Do not leave the patient alone if you think doing so is unsafe.

PROCEDURE 27

TRANSFERRING THE PATIENT ONTO AND OFF THE TOILET

1. Carry out beginning procedure actions.
2. Assemble equipment:
   - Toilet tissue
   - Transfer belt
   - Disposable gloves
   - Commode if toilet is not available
3. Position the wheelchair at a right angle to the toilet or commode to face the wall rail. Lock the wheels. Raise or remove footrests.
4. Place a transfer belt around the patient's waist. Use an underhand grasp with one hand toward the patient's back and the other hand toward the patient's front.
5. Tell the patient to lean forward slightly, to place the strongest foot slightly behind the other foot, to bring herself to a standing position by pushing off from the wheelchair, and to grasp the wall rail with both hands (Figure 16-10A).
6. Have the patient pivot or step around until she feels the toilet against the back of her legs.
7. Slide the pants and underwear down over the patient's knees. You may need to keep one hand in the transfer belt and use the other hand to manipulate the patient's clothing (Figure 16-10B).
8. Assist the patient to a sitting position on the toilet and allow her time to eliminate.
9. When the patient is finished, put on the disposable gloves. Instruct the patient to stand and to reach for the wall rail. Use the toilet tissue to clean the patient if she was unable to do this herself. If the patient is steady, remove and dispose of your gloves. Then pull the patient's pants or underwear up.
10. If the sink is close enough, the patient can pivot or step to the sink to wash her hands before sitting down in the wheelchair. Otherwise, unlock the wheelchair, replace the footrests, and move the wheelchair to the sink so this step can be completed while the patient is seated.
11. Wash your hands.
12. Assist the patient to leave the bathroom. Make sure she is comfortable and has a signal light within reach.
13. Carry out procedure completion actions.

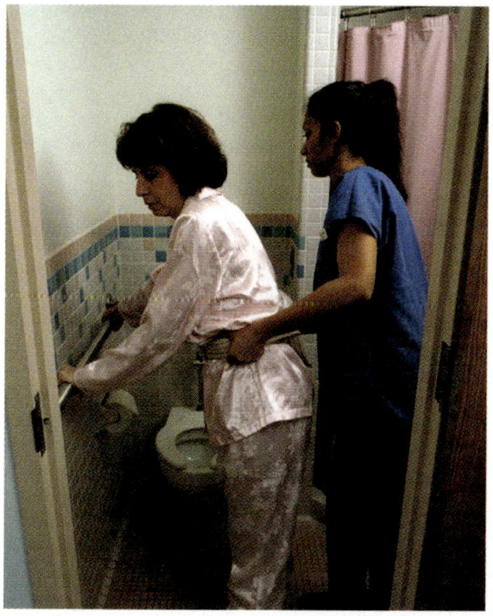

FIGURE 16-10A Tell the patient to grasp the wall rail with both hands.

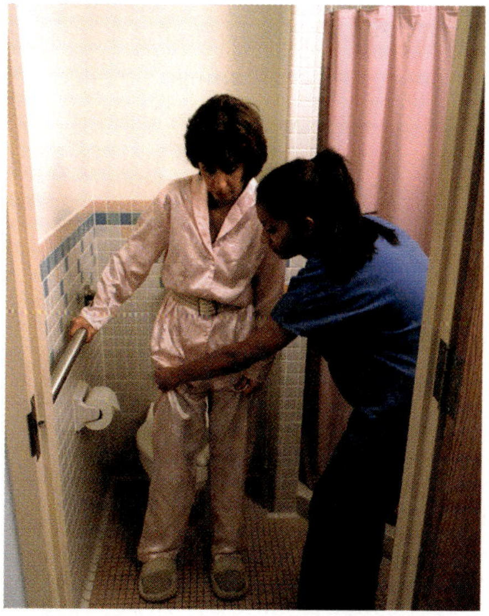

FIGURE 16-10B Keep one hand on the transfer belt and adjust the patient's clothing.

TUB TRANSFERS

In the institutional setting, a shower with chair or tub with hydraulic lift is available. If the patient is at home, a tub chair, rail on the wall beside the tub, and slip-proof mats in the tub are needed for safety. Add water to the tub after the patient has safely transferred, with cold water turned on first and off last. A hand-held shower attached to the faucet of the tub is safer and easier for self-bathing.

PROCEDURE 28

TRANSFERRING THE PATIENT INTO AND OUT OF THE BATHTUB

1. Carry out beginning procedure actions.
2. Assemble equipment:
   - Towels and washcloths
   - Soap
   - Hand-held shower if available
   - Tub chair
   - Slip-proof bath mats for floor and tub
   - Disposable gloves if necessary
   - Sturdy straight chair if necessary

Note: *If patient's wheelchair has a removable arm or side, remove it and place the wheelchair at the foot of the tub, facing the faucets.*

3. Place a sturdy chair beside the tub, facing the faucets, if wheelchair arm is not removable. (Use this in place of a wheelchair.)
4. Have the patient transfer from the wheelchair to the chair and then into the tub and onto the tub chair. Make sure the tub chair is even with the other chair.
5. Once the patient is seated in the chair beside the tub, instruct the patient to place the leg closest to the tub into the tub. If this is the weaker leg, the strong arm can be used to lift the leg over the side of the tub (Figure 16-11A).
6. Tell the patient to use the strongest arm to reach for the wall rail. Sliding across onto the tub chair, have the patient bring the other leg over the side of the tub (Figure 16-11B).

Note: *For this procedure, it is safer to have the weaker side toward the tub, if possible; that way the strong arm can be brought around to the wall rail.*

7. Proceed with the bath, giving assistance as needed or allowing the patient privacy to complete the bath, if possible. Stay within hearing distance.
8. When the patient is ready to get out of the tub, the strong side will be next to the outer chair. This allows the patient to get the strong leg out of the tub and to use the strong arm to move herself onto the chair. She then uses the strong arm to move her weaker leg out of the tub.
9. Assist the patient to dry and dress if necessary.
10. Carry out procedure completion actions.
11. Disinfect tub and tub chair.

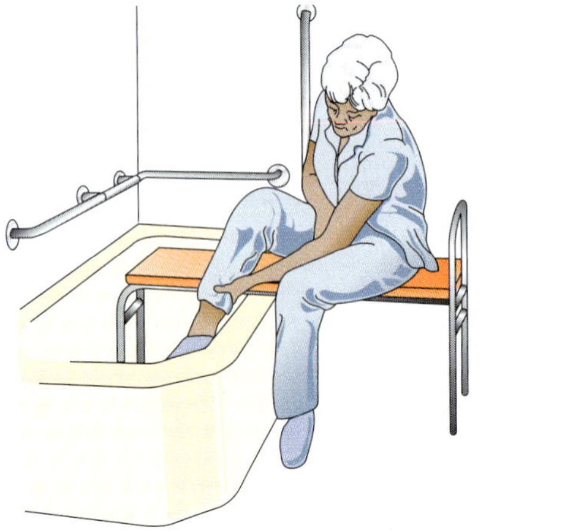

FIGURE 16-11A The patient uses the stronger arm to lift the weak leg over the edge of the tub.

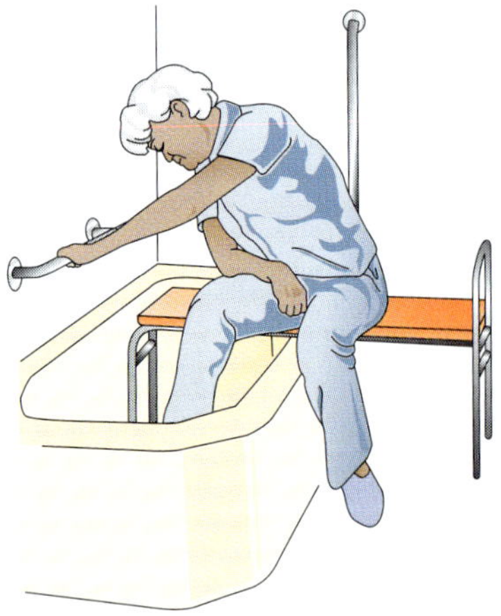

FIGURE 16-11B The patient brings the stronger leg over the side of the tub.

CAR TRANSFERS

You may need to assist a patient to transfer into a car when she is discharged from the facility. If you are working in the patient's home, you may need to be able to help the patient into and out of the car. A two-door car makes the transfer easier because the door is wider and gives more room for moving in and out of the car. With either a two-door or four-door car, the patient should always transfer onto the front seat. The front door is usually wider and opens wider.

PROCEDURE 29

TRANSFERRING A PATIENT INTO AND OUT OF A CAR

1. Carry out beginning procedure actions.
2. Assemble equipment:
   - Car
   - Wheelchair
   - Transfer belt
3. Place the wheelchair at a 45° angle to the car, with brakes set. Put transfer belt on the patient if necessary (Figure 16-12A). Have the patient come to a standing position in the usual manner.
4. If transferring to the stronger side, the dashboard and car door can be used for support (Figure 16-12B). If moving toward the weaker side, instruct the patient to use the strong arm and the door with the window open for support. Another person should hold the door for stability.
5. Tell the patient to pivot or step around so the side of the car seat is touching the back of the legs. After she sits down, have the patient raise one leg at a time into the car to face forward (Figure 16-12C). Assist with the seat belt.
6. To get the patient out of the car, reverse the procedure. Car seats are usually lower than other sitting surfaces and the patient may need help in getting to a standing position.
7. Carry out procedure completion actions.

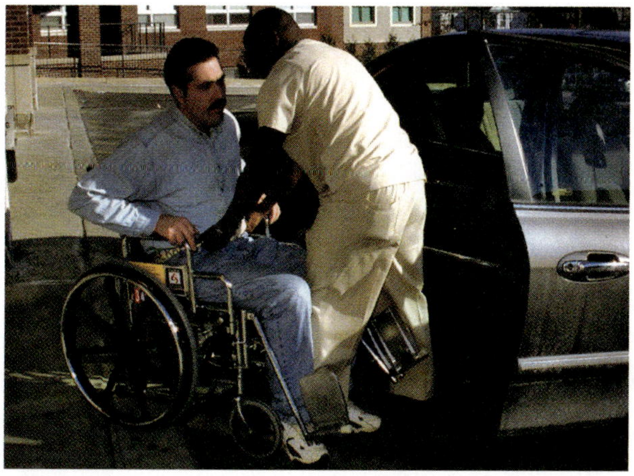

FIGURE 16-12A Apply the transfer belt and prepare to assist the patient to a standing position.

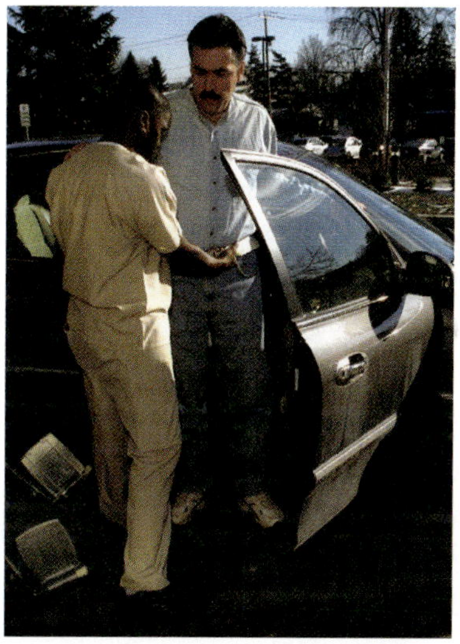

FIGURE 16-12B The dashboard and car door can be used for support.

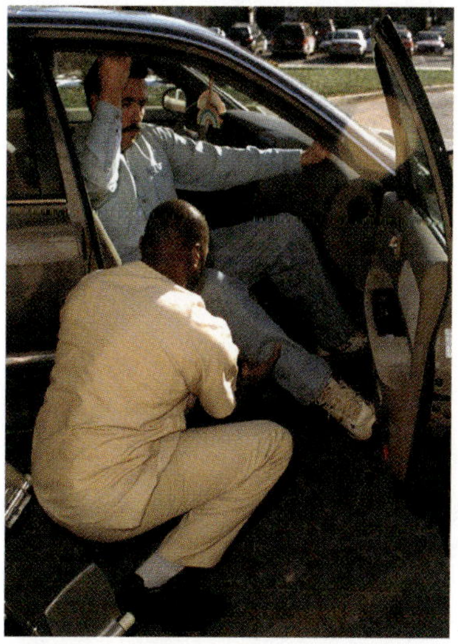

FIGURE 16-12C The patient lifts one leg at a time into the car.

REVIEW

A. Multiple Choice.

Select the one best answer for each of the following.

1. The method used for transferring a patient depends on
   a. the availability of two nursing assistants.
   b. the patient's personal preference.
   c. the patient's size, strength, endurance, and balance.
   d. where the patient is going.
2. A transfer belt should never be used on patients who
   a. have a long-term medication pump.
   b. have a colostomy.
   c. can stand on their feet.
   d. have an IV or catheter.
3. During a transfer, the patient should never
   a. be allowed to help in the move.
   b. place his hands on your body.
   c. wear shoes.
   d. be allowed to stand.
4. When transferring a patient, you should never place your hands under a patient's arms because the
   a. patient may not want you to stand so close.
   b. patient cannot see where she is going.
   c. patient's bones are fragile.
   d. patient may be ticklish.
5. Using a mechanical lift requires that
   a. there always be two persons to do the procedure.
   b. the patient be able to assist in the move.
   c. the patient be mentally alert.
   d. the patient weigh at least 300 pounds.

B. True/False.

Mark the following true or false by circling T or F.

6. T F During a transfer, the patient should place his or her hands on the nursing assistant's shoulders.
7. T F A transfer belt should always be used for standing transfers unless contraindicated.
8. T F Always transfer toward the patient's strongest side.
9. T F During a transfer, the nursing assistant should place his or her hands around the patient's trunk.
10. T F During a transfer, always explain to the patient how he or she can help.
11. T F Towel bars are not safe to use as grab bars.
12. T F Before using a mechanical lift, always check the slings and straps for frayed areas.
13. T F One person can safely transfer an unconscious patient from a stretcher to a bed.
14. T F When transferring a patient from a bed to a stretcher, raise the bed to the same horizontal height as the stretcher.
15. T F The unconscious patient should be secured with a safety belt during transport.

C. Nursing Assistant Challenge.

You are assigned to Mrs. McNeely, who is scheduled for surgery. She is alert and able to follow your directions. You know that when she returns from surgery she will be semiconscious from the medications and anesthesia. Consider the differences in procedures when she goes to surgery and when she returns to her room.

16. What instructions will you give Mrs. McNeely when she transfers from her bed to the surgical stretcher?
17. What will you need to do to transfer her back to bed after the surgery?

EXPLORING THE WEB

Description	Location
Ergonomics in Patient Transfers	*http://www.osha.gov/SLTC/hospital_etool/hazards/ergo/ergoequipment/ergoequip.html*
How to Use a Gait Belt	*http://www.medformation.com*
Lifting, Transferring, and Positioning Patients	*http://911papers.virtualave.net*
Policy for Gait Belt Use	*http://wdhfs.state.wy.us*
Transfer Procedures	*calder.med.miami.edu*

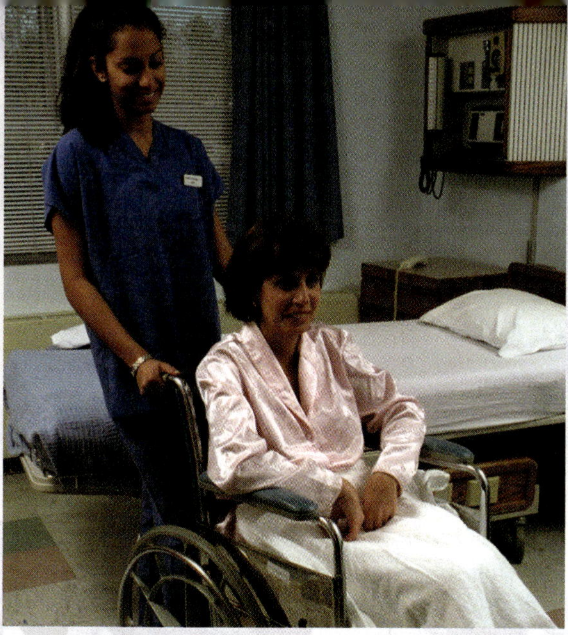

unit 17

The Patient's Mobility: Ambulation

objectives

After completing this unit, you will be able to:

- Spell and define terms.
- Describe the purpose of assistive devices used in ambulation.
- List safety measures for using assistive devices.
- Describe safety measures for using a wheelchair.
- Describe nursing assistant actions for
  - Ambulating a patient using a gait belt.
  - Propelling a patient in a wheelchair.
  - Positioning a patient in a wheelchair.
  - Transporting a patient on a stretcher
- Demonstrate the following procedures:
  - Procedure 30 Assisting the Patient to Walk with a Cane and Three-Point Gait
  - Procedure 31 Assisting the Patient to Walk with a Walker and Three-Point Gait
  - Procedure 32 Assisting the Falling Patient

vocabulary

Learn the meaning and the correct spelling of the following words and phrases:

ambulate	**gait**	**orthopedic**
assistive device	**gait training**	**prosthesis**

AMBULATION

The term **ambulate** means to walk. Some patients may not be able to walk because of a disease or injury. Patients who cannot walk may be able to self-propel their wheelchairs to increase their independence.

The term **gait** refers to the way in which a person walks. Many disorders can affect a person's gait, such as:

- A stroke—one side of the body is paralyzed (hemiplegia).
- Multiple sclerosis—one or both legs are weakened and balance may be disturbed.
- Huntington's disease—the patient has involuntary movements that disturb balance.
- Parkinson's disease—the patient has stiffness and slowness of movements, causing shuffling.
- Arthritis—pain and stiffness of joints.
- Amputation—the patient has a **prosthesis** (artificial limb).
- **Orthopedic** (bones and muscles) surgery.

Evaluation for Ambulation

Before initiating an ambulation program, the nurse or physical therapist (Figure 17-1) will evaluate the patient's:

- Tolerance to movement in bed
- Ability to participate in active (as opposed to passive) exercise
- Ability to safely transfer with minimal assistance
- Ability to stand and bear weight
- Strength, endurance, and balance
- Mental state, to determine if the patient can follow directions
- Ability to walk alone (whether the assistance of a person or equipment is needed)

Normal Gait Pattern

There are two phases to a normal gait (walking). The leg is on the floor during the first phase and the leg is brought forward during the second phase. Walking begins with the ankle in *dorsiflexion* (toes pulled toward shin) and the heel striking the floor first (Figure 17-2), rolling onto the ball of the foot. The patient must be able to stand straight on this leg while bringing the other leg forward. The arms normally swing slightly during walking. Each arm moves in the same direction as the opposite leg. To walk safely, the patient must have adequate joint motion in the hips and knees and strength in the muscles of the hips, buttocks, and legs. The physical therapist may work with the patient on exercises to promote movement and strength before the patient starts walking.

Gait Training

The physical therapist may work with the patient on **gait training** (teaching the patient to walk). The therapist will teach the patient how to:

- Walk correctly
- Walk on different surfaces, such as linoleum floors, carpet, grass, gravel, etc.
- Go up and down stairs (Figure 17-3)
- Get in and out of a chair
- Use an assistive device if one is ordered

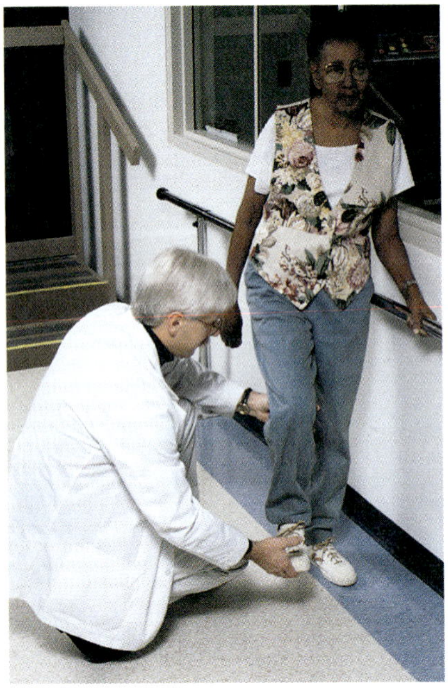

FIGURE 17-1 The physical therapist evaluates the patient's ability to ambulate and need for assistive devices.

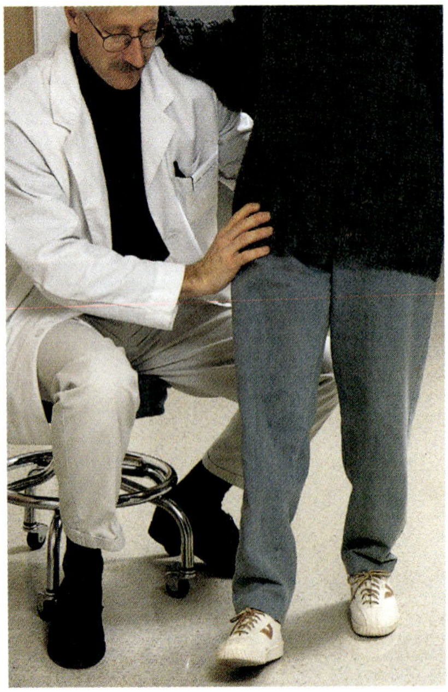

FIGURE 17-2 Walking begins with the ankle in dorsiflexion and the heel striking the floor first.

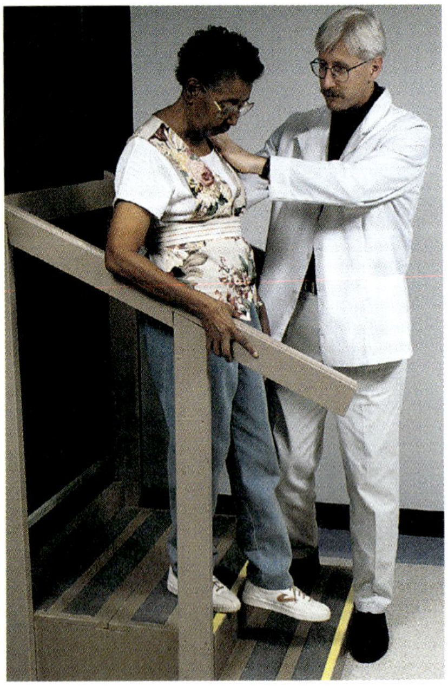

FIGURE 17-3 The physical therapist teaches the patient how to walk on stairs.

guidelines *for*

Safe Ambulation

- Encourage independent patients to use the hand rail when walking.
- Always stand on the patient's affected side when walking with her.
- Always use a gait belt (transfer belt) if the patient needs assistance with ambulation. Grasp the belt in the back with an underhand grip (Figure 17-4). Place your other hand on the patient's shoulder if balance is unsteady.
- Make sure the patient is wearing sturdy shoes with nonslip soles and that laces are tied. Clothing should not be too loose or drag on the floor.
- Check floor for clutter or puddles that could cause a fall.
- If you are unsure of the patient's endurance or balance, ask another nursing assistant to follow behind you with the wheelchair. If the patient becomes weak, dizzy, or tired, she can sit in the wheelchair.
- Check rubber tips on bottoms of canes, crutches, and walkers, and also check the rubber handgrips (Figure 17-5). These should be replaced if the ridges are cracked, loose, or worn down. If the ridges are filled with debris, use alcohol and cotton swabs to clean them. Replace the handgrip if it is loose or cracked.
- Check screws, nuts, and bolts for tightness. Do not use any device that appears unsafe. Report the problem to the appropriate person.
- Practice good body mechanics for both yourself and the patient.

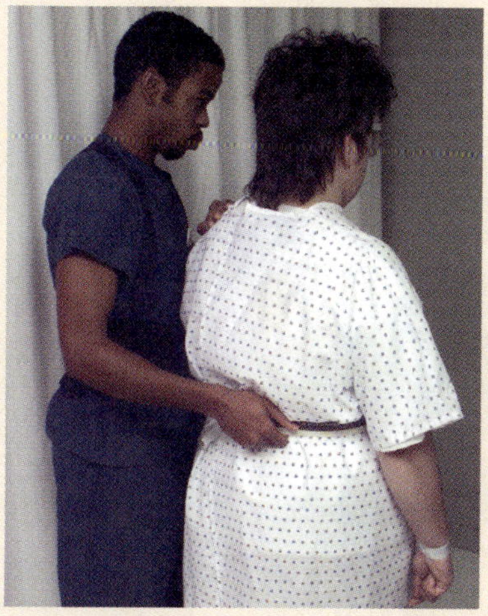

FIGURE 17-4 Hold the gait belt in back, using an underhand grip.

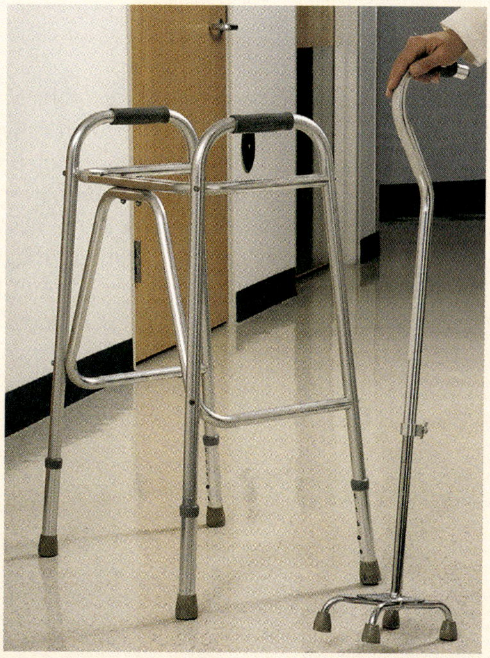

FIGURE 17-5 Check the rubber tips and handgrips.

- Teach the patient to practice safety.
- Position your body so it moves with the patient's body. You should not interfere with the patient's movement. Match the patient's stride.
- Encourage the patient to stand upright and erect when walking.
- Encourage the patient to take large, even steps. Teach him or her to maintain a wide base of support. The distance between the feet should be equal to the patient's shoulder width.
- Allow adequate time for ambulation. Avoid making the patient feel rushed.
- Allow the patient time to rest, if necessary.
- Provide only the amount of assistance needed.
- If the patient is not motivated, place a chair ahead of him or her. Tell the patient the goal is to walk to the chair.
- Stop ambulation immediately if the patient shows signs of illness, pain, extreme fatigue, shortness of breath, dizziness, sweating, or anxiety. Notify the nurse.
- Never leave the patient standing unattended. When you are through, leave the patient safely sitting in a chair.

ASSISTIVE DEVICES

An **assistive device** is often prescribed. These devices include:

- Crutches
- Canes
- Walkers

An assistive device can help compensate for problems the patient has with walking. A walker or crutches may be ordered if the patient has only partial weight-bearing on one leg. Canes are usually ordered for persons who have problems with balance. There are several types of crutches, canes, and walkers. Each device is selected according to the needs of the patient and the cause of the problem. The nurse or physical therapist will adjust the device to fit the patient. The gait used with the device is determined by the patient's abilities, the cause of the impairment, and the type of assistive device being used. The nurse or physical therapist will select the appropriate gait. You should know the gaits that have been chosen. When you walk with the patient, you can then help make sure the patient is using the device correctly.

Use of Crutches

Standard crutches (Figure 17-6) are seldom recommended for older adults. They can be cumbersome to handle and require considerable balance and two strong arms. Metal forearm crutches may be used by patients who have weakness of both legs. These crutches are also called Lofstrand crutches or Canadian crutches. The cuff of the crutch encloses the forearm so the patient can release that hand without dropping the crutch (Figure 17-7).

Forearm crutches with platforms permit weight-bearing on the forearms, providing stability. During use, the elbows are at a constant 90° angle to the shoulder (Figure 17-8). The patient may need assistance in attaching the arm straps of

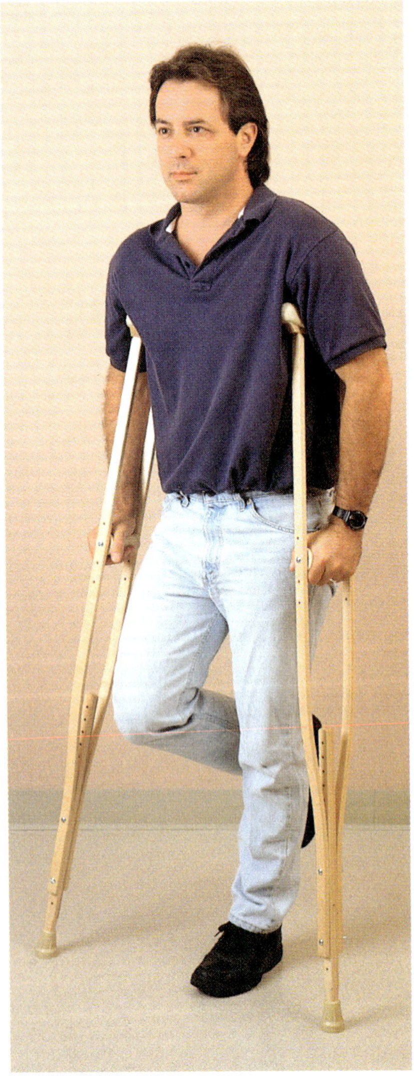

FIGURE 17-6 Standard crutches are not usually appropriate for elderly patients.

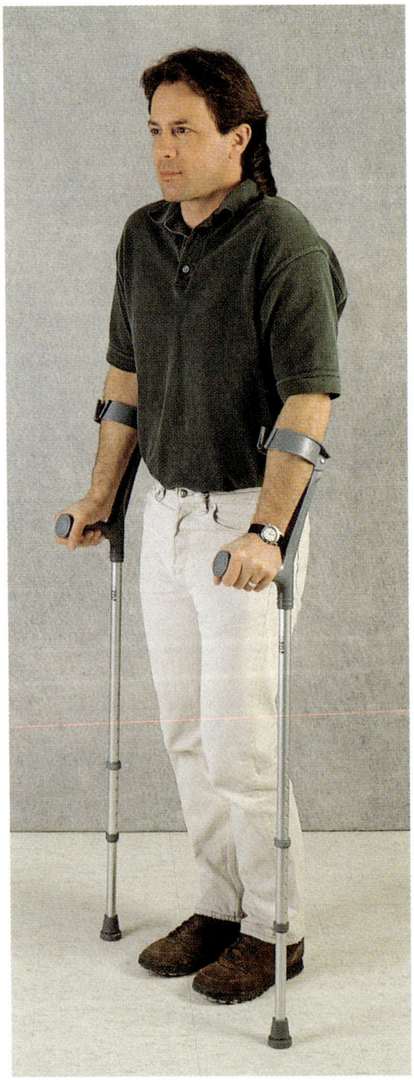

FIGURE 17-7 Forearm crutches can be released to free the hand without dropping the crutch.

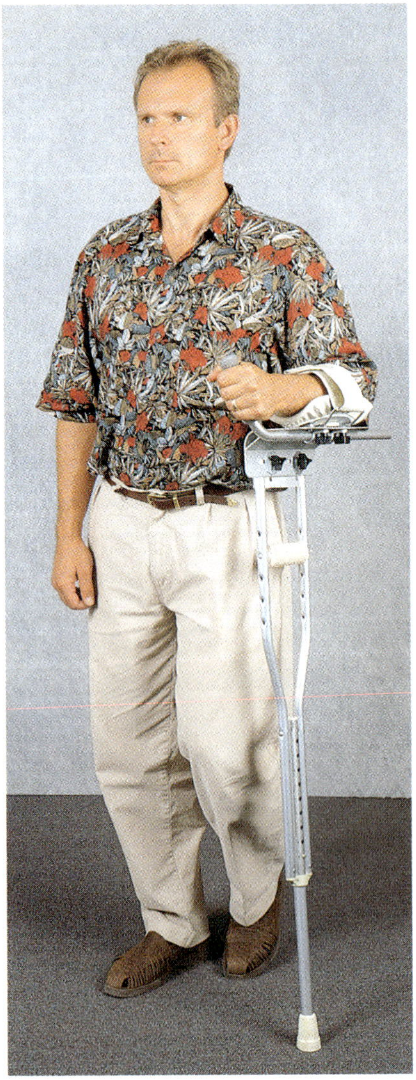

FIGURE 17-8 Forearm crutches with platforms permit weight-bearing on the forearms to provide stability.

SAFETY *Alert*

Occasionally, you will observe a patient using an assistive ambulation device incorrectly. For example, a patient may carry a walker, or use the walker to hold onto when rising from a chair. Assistive ambulation devices are designed to be used for ambulation, not transfers. Using them for other purposes may be unsafe. Inform the nurse. He or she will arrange for a therapist to evaluate the patient for appropriate ways of meeting her ambulation and transfer needs.

the platforms. If you care for patients with crutches, you will be taught the gaits the patients are to use.

Use of Canes

Quad canes and tripod canes provide a wide base of support. Pyramid canes are four-pronged devices with a broad base, and are narrower at the top. Single-prong canes with T-handles or J-handles have straight handles with a handgrip and are easier to hold than half-circle handled canes. For proper fit, the elbow is flexed 30° when the hands are on the handgrip, and the patient's wrist is even with the hip joint. Canes are recommended for aiding balance rather than for providing support. (Refer to Procedure 30.) The cane is always held by the arm on the *strong* side of the body. The patient will be taught to use either a two-point gait or a three-point gait with a cane.

PROCEDURE 30

ASSISTING THE PATIENT TO WALK WITH A CANE AND THREE-POINT GAIT

1. Carry out beginning procedure actions.
2. Assemble equipment:
   - Cane as ordered
   - Gait belt
3. Make sure the patient has on sturdy shoes with nonslip soles. Check clothing to be sure it does not hang down over shoes.
4. Place the bed in the lowest horizontal position with brakes locked. Assist the patient to sit on the edge of the bed. Place a gait belt on the patient and assist the patient to a standing position. Stand on the patient's affected side. Place your closest hand in the gait belt, using an underhand grip.
5. Instruct the patient to hold the cane on her stronger side, with the tip about 4 inches to the side of the stronger foot. Her weight should be distributed evenly between her feet and the cane (Figure 17-9A).

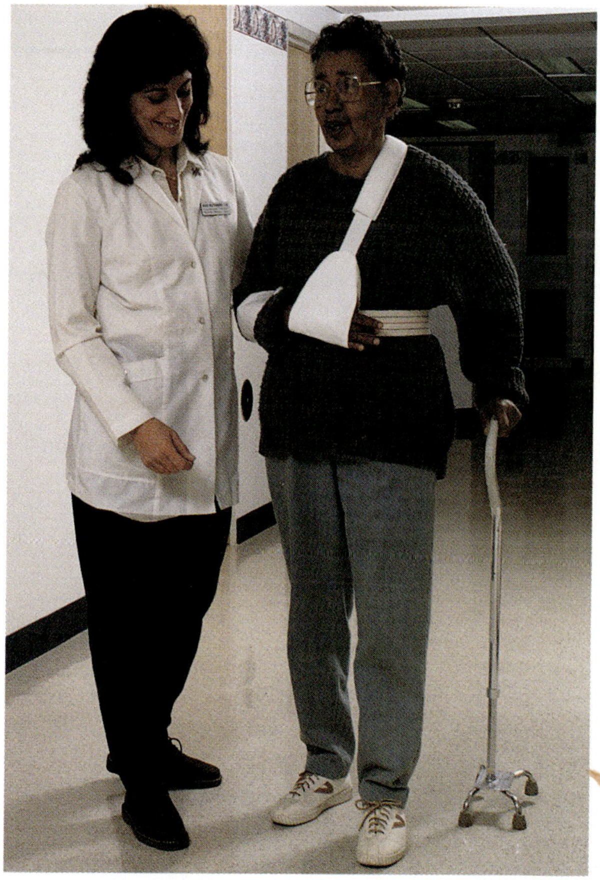

FIGURE 17-9A The patient holds the cane on the strong side of the body. The patient's weight should be distributed evenly between her feet and the cane before she starts to walk.

continues

PROCEDURE 30

continued

6. Tell the patient to shift her body weight to the strong leg and advance the cane about 4 inches so she is supporting her weight on the strong leg and the cane. Move the weak leg forward so it is even with the cane (Figure 17-9B).
7. The patient then shifts her weight to the weak leg and the cane, moving the strong leg forward, ahead of the cane. This pattern is repeated while the patient is walking.
8. Note the patient's endurance, balance, and strength while walking. Stop immediately if the patient has trouble and help her to the closest chair. Call the nurse.
9. Assist the patient to sit in the chair or to lie down in bed. Remove the gait belt. Store the cane in an appropriate area.
10. Document the distance the patient ambulated and her tolerance of the procedure.
11. Carry out procedure completion actions.

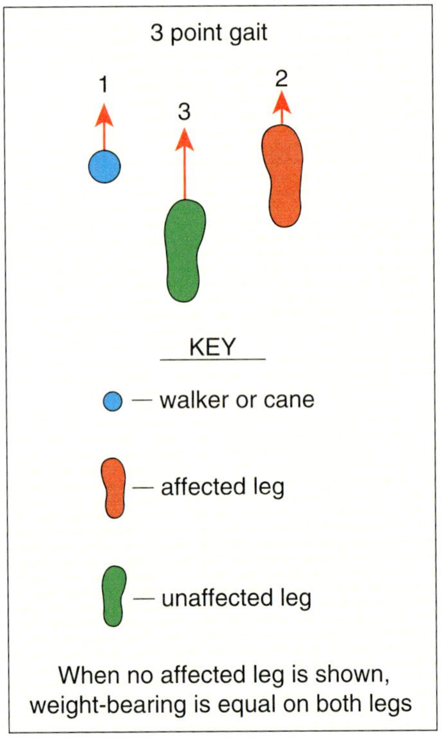

FIGURE 17-9B Three-point gait.

Two-Point Gait with Cane. The steps for this procedure are as follows:

1. Follow steps 1 through 5 in Procedure 30.
2. Tell the patient to move the cane and weaker leg forward at the same time, while his weight is on the stronger leg (Figure 17-10).
3. He then shifts his weight to the weak leg and cane, and moves the stronger leg forward.
4. This pattern is repeated while the patient is walking.
5. Repeat steps 8 through 11 in Procedure 30.

Use of Walkers

Walkers also come in a variety of styles. Walkers are recommended for individuals who have general weakness of both legs, partial weight bearing on one leg, or mild balance problems. The patient needs strength in both arms to pick up the walker. The walker should be wide enough to allow the patient to walk into it. For proper fit, the elbow is flexed 30° when the hands are on the handgrip, and the top of the walker reaches the hip joint. Most walkers are adjustable. The nurse or physical therapist will make any necessary changes. There are many additional features available from most manufacturers.

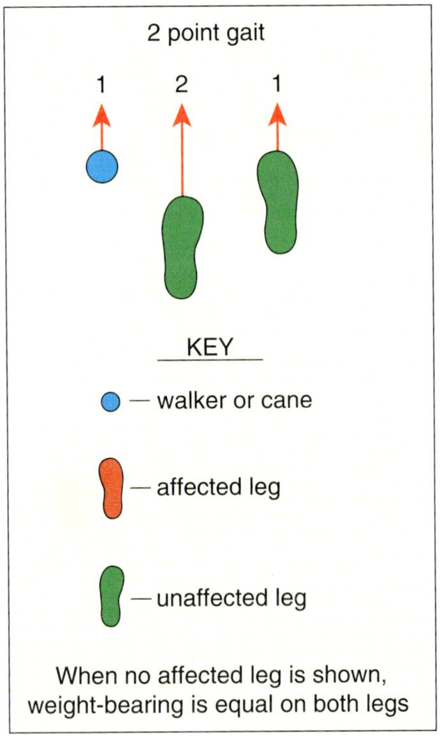

FIGURE 17-10 Two-point gait.

PROCEDURE 31

ASSISTING THE PATIENT TO WALK WITH A WALKER AND THREE-POINT GAIT

1. Carry out beginning procedure actions.
2. Assemble equipment:
   - Walker as ordered
   - Gait belt
3. Make sure the patient has on sturdy shoes with nonslip soles. Check clothing to be sure it does not hang down over shoes.
4. Place a gait belt on the patient and assist the patient to a standing position. Place the walker in front of the patient and have her grasp the walker with both hands. Stand on the patient's affected side. Place your closest hand in the gait belt, using an underhand grip (Figure 17-11).

Note: *The walker is not a transfer device and should not be used to help the patient stand up. The patient grasps the walker after she is standing. To sit, the patient releases her grip on the walker while still standing, and then places her hands on the arms of the chair before sitting.*

5. Instruct the patient to stand with her weight evenly distributed between the walker and both legs, with the walker in front of her.
6. Have the patient shift her weight to the strong leg as she lifts and moves the walker 6 to 8 inches ahead. All four legs of the walker should strike the floor at the same time.
7. The patient then brings her weak foot forward into the walker.
8. Now have her bring her strong foot forward even with the weak foot.
9. This process is repeated while the patient is walking.
10. Note the patient's endurance, balance, and strength while walking. Stop immediately if the patient has trouble and help her to the closest chair. Call the nurse.
11. Assist the patient to sit in the chair or to lie down in bed. Remove the gait belt. Store the walker in an appropriate area.
12. Document the distance the patient ambulated and her tolerance of the procedure.
13. Carry out procedure completion actions.

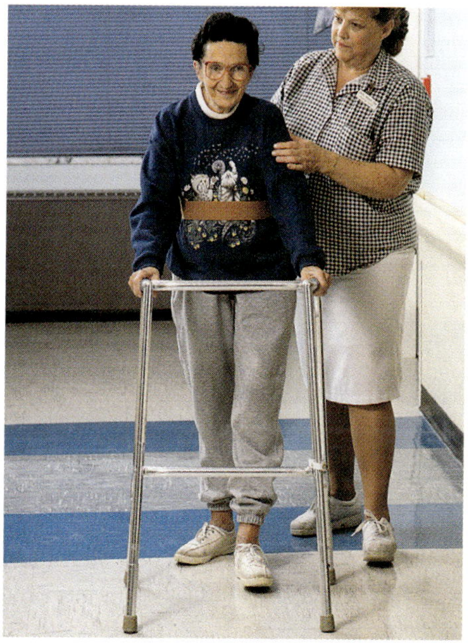

FIGURE 17-11 Stand on the patient's affected side while she grasps the walker with both hands.

Two-Point Gait with Walker. The steps for this procedure are as follows:

1. Complete steps 1 through 5 in Procedure 31.
2. Have the patient shift his weight to the strong leg as he lifts and moves the walker and the weak leg 6 to 8 inches ahead.
3. Now have him shift his weight to the weaker leg and the walker (with most of the weight on the walker).
4. He then moves his strong leg 6 to 8 inches ahead.
5. This process is repeated while the patient is walking.
6. Note the patient's endurance, balance, and strength while walking. Stop immediately if the patient has trouble and help him to the closest chair. Call the nurse.
7. Assist the patient to sit in the chair or to lie down in bed. Remove the gait belt. Store the cane in an appropriate area.
8. Document the distance the patient ambulated and his tolerance of the procedure.
9. Carry out procedure completion actions.

THE FALLING PATIENT

If a patient starts to fall, you must protect both yourself and the patient. If the patient has started to fall, do not try to hold her upright. This will strain your back and may injure the patient. *If a patient does fall, call the nurse to assess the patient for injuries before she is moved.*

SAFETY Alert

If you find a patient on the floor, remain in the room and call for help. Leave the patient on the floor. Provide any emergency measures that you are qualified to provide. If the nurse suspects a fracture, he or she will instruct you on how to return the patient to bed. Rolling him or her onto a sheet or blanket will make the transfer less traumatic. After proper emergency treatment and positioning on the sheet, the patient is lifted back to bed.

SAFETY Alert

Fall prevention is a major concern in health care facilities. Patients with a previous history of falls are always at higher risk than other patients. Other risk factors include advancing age, muscle weakness, gait and balance problems, neurological and musculoskeletal disorders, use of psychoactive medication, dementia, lower extremity disability or foot problems, and visual impairment. Environmental risk factors include slippery surfaces, uneven floors, loose rugs, poor lighting, unstable furniture, and objects on the floor.

Some elderly individuals have basic trust issues, particularly if the caregiver is young. They have their own way of doing things and believe they know best. The caregiver's way may be safest, but to gain compliance, avoid telling the individual that he or she is wrong. Rather, try to incorporate the patient's method into a safer way of accomplishing the task.

PROCEDURE 32

ASSISTING THE FALLING PATIENT

1. Keep your back straight, bend from the hips and knees, and maintain a broad base of support as you assist the falling patient. Maintain your grasp on the transfer belt.
2. Ease the patient to the floor, protecting her head.
3. As you ease the patient to the floor, bend your knees and go down with the patient (Figure 17-12).
4. Call for help.
5. Assist in returning the patient to bed or chair.
6. Carry out procedure completion actions.

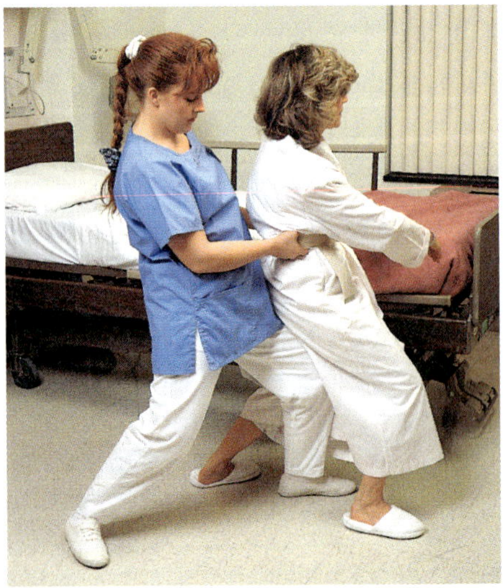

FIGURE 17-12 Ease the falling patient to the floor; bend your knees and go down with the patient.

USE OF WHEELCHAIRS

Many individuals who are unable to ambulate can gain some independence with the use of a wheelchair. A wheelchair should fit the person who is using it. Correct fit and body alignment will prevent contractures (Figure 17-13). If the chair fits correctly, there will be:

- About 4 inches between the top of the back upholstery and the patient's axillae.
- Armrests that support the arms without pushing the shoulders up or forcing them to hang.
- Two to 3 inches clearance between the front edge of the seat and the back of the patient's knee.
- Enough space between the patient's hip and the chair to slide your hand between the patient's hips on each side and the side of the wheelchair; the right amount of space avoids internal or external rotation of hips.
- Two inches between the bottom of the footrests and the floor.
- 90° angles between the feet and the legs, whether they are on the footrests or on the floor (when the footrests have been removed).

If the wheelchair does not fit the patient, check with the nurse or physical therapist to see how you can use pads or other devices to adapt the chair to the patient.

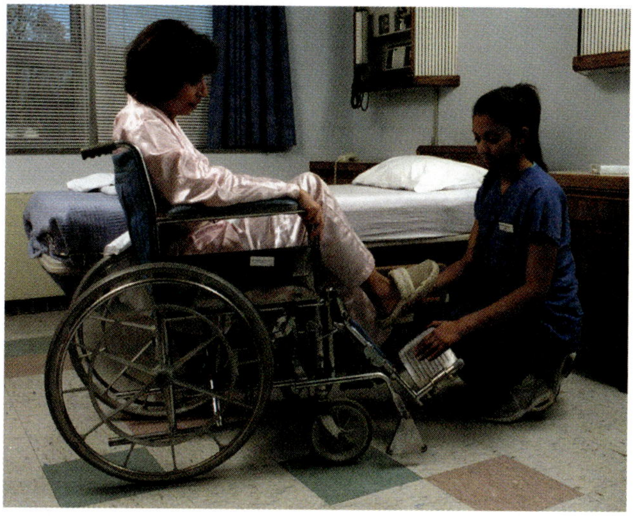

FIGURE 17-13 The wheelchair should fit the patient.

SAFETY *Alert*

There is no "one size fits all" wheelchair. Patients may have difficulty propelling a wheelchair that does not fit properly. A chair that does not fit correctly increases discomfort. Positioning problems are common. Patients may lean to the side, slide forward, or sit slumped in the chair. The risk of skin breakdown is increased. Positioning aids may be necessary. Sometimes unnecessary restraints are used to correct positioning problems. For many patients, a properly fit wheelchair solves the problem! If you suspect that the patient's problems are due to a wheelchair of the wrong size, inform the nurse.

guidelines *for*

Wheelchair Safety

- Check the wheelchair to see that brakes are working and wheels are securely attached. If the patient needs footrests, make sure they are in place. Replace the arm of wheelchair if it was removed during transfer.
- The small, front caster wheels of the chair provide the ability to move in all directions. The large part of the wheel faces back when the chair is moving. When the chair is parked, position the large part of the front wheel facing forward. This changes the center of gravity in the chair. Positioning the wheels to face forward prevents tipping if the patient leans forward. It helps stabilize the chair if the patient picks up an item from the floor. To reposition the wheels, back the chair up, then move it forward.
- Keep the wheelchair locked when not moving.
- Apply brakes and lift footrests out of the way when the patient is getting in or out of the wheelchair.
- Instruct the patient not to try to pick up an object off the floor. If there is satisfactory trunk stability and balance, the patient may be taught to do so, but instruct the patient to:
  - avoid shifting weight in the direction of the reach
  - not move forward in the seat
  - not reach down between the knees

The safest method is to position the chair alongside the object with casters in forward position, lock the chair, and reach only as far as the arm will extend.

continues

guidelines *continued*

- Check the patient's body alignment while in the wheelchair and reposition the patient when necessary.
- Prevent bath blankets, lap robes, or clothing from getting caught in wheels.
- Observe the patient's affected arm. A paralyzed arm may fall over the side of the wheelchair and become caught in the wheel.
- Guide the wheelchair from behind, grasping both handgrips (Figure 17-14).
- Approach corners slowly and look before you go around them.
- Take care when approaching swinging doors. Prop the door open to propel the chair through the door. If this is not possible, back through swinging doors.
- Back the wheelchair over the threshold in a doorway.
- Always back into doorways and elevators when transporting a patient by wheelchair (Figure 17-15).
- When leaving an elevator, push the stop button and ask others to step out. Turn the wheelchair around and back it out the door.
- When transporting a patient in a wheelchair down a ramp or incline, walk backward, slowly pulling the chair. Periodically look over your shoulder, as you would when backing up in a car, to make sure that the path is clear.
- When parking a wheelchair, avoid blocking a doorway. Apply the brakes.

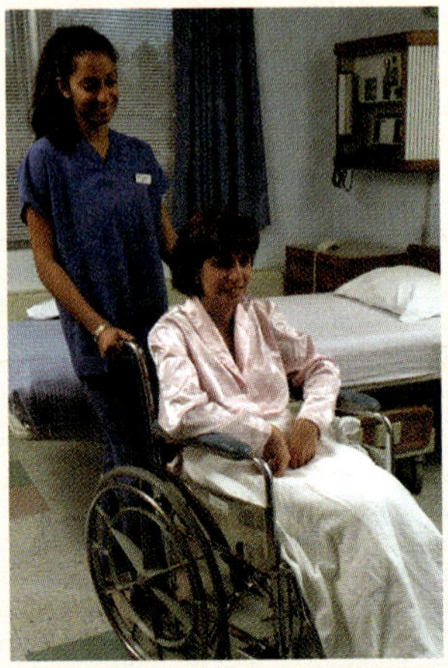

FIGURE 17-14 Guide the wheelchair from behind, grasping both handgrips.

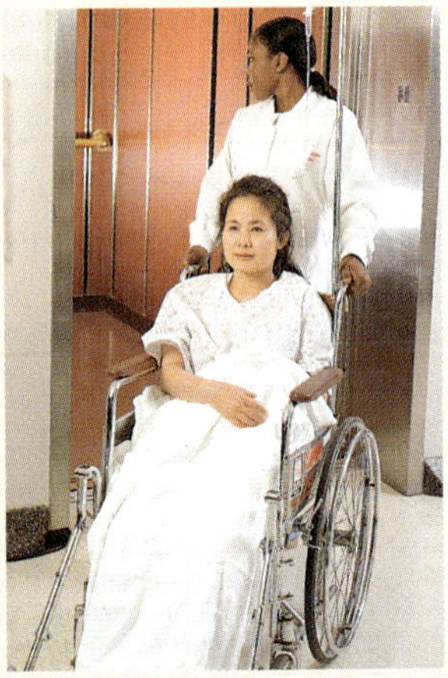

FIGURE 17-15 Always back into doorways and elevators when transporting a patient in a wheelchair.

POSITIONING THE DEPENDENT PATIENT IN A WHEELCHAIR

The dependent person may slide down in the wheelchair, requiring assistance to regain body alignment. Several procedures can be used to correct the dependent patient's position in the wheelchair. Lock the drive wheels and position the caster wheels in the forward position before repositioning the patient.

1. Stand in front of the patient; make sure that the feet are in alignment and the arms are on the armrests. Help the patient lean forward and push with the hands and legs as you push against the patient's knees (Figure 17-16).
2. For an alternate method, place a soft towel or small sheet under the patient's buttocks and use this as a pull sheet to move the patient up in the chair. This requires two people (Figure 17-17).

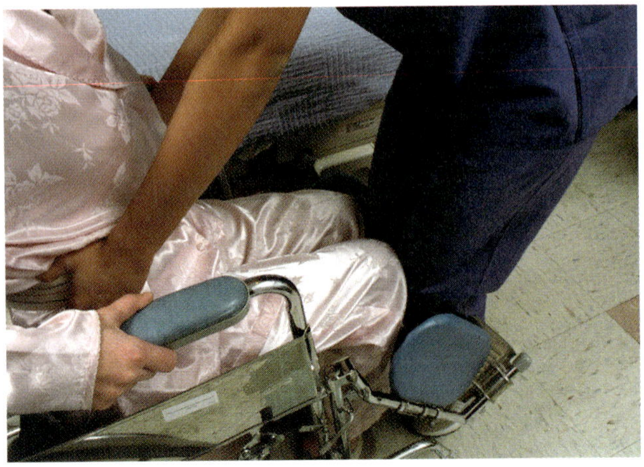

FIGURE 17-16 Push against the patient's knees as she pushes with her hands and legs.

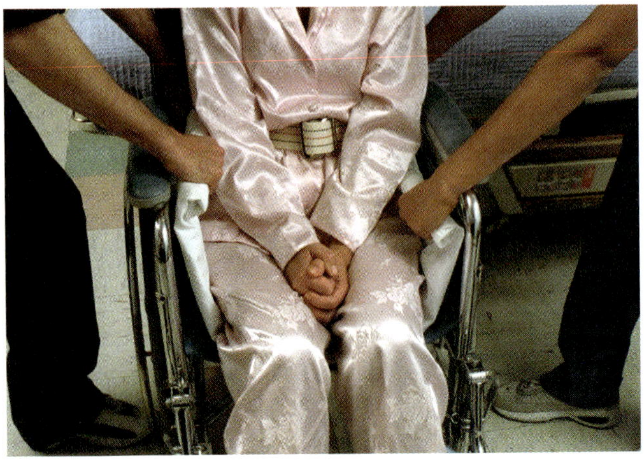

FIGURE 17-17 A draw (lift) sheet may be used to correct the patient's body alignment.

3. This method also requires two people. Place the transfer belt around the patient's waist. One assistant stands in back of the wheelchair and grasps the transfer belt with one hand on each side of the patient. The other one stands in front of the patient and places her hands and arms under the patient's knees. On the count of three, this assistant supports the lower extremities while the other one moves the patient back in the chair (Figure 17-18). This is not recommended for a heavy patient.
4. This method also requires two people. Stand in back of the wheelchair and have another assistant in front of the patient. Both assistants work with knees and hips bent and backs straight. Lean forward with your head over the patient's shoulder. Instruct the patient to fold the arms. Place your arms around the patient's trunk. Grasp the patient's right wrist with your left hand and grasp the patient's left wrist with your right hand. The other assistant encircles the patient's knees with hands and arms. On the count of three, both assistants lift and move the patient up (Figure 17-19).
5. One person can do this procedure. The patient needs to be oriented and able to follow directions. Stand in front of the patient. Flex your knees and hips and keep your back straight. Position your feet, one on each side of the patient's feet. Brace your knees against the patient's knees. Have the patient lean forward. Lean forward over the patient's right shoulder with the patient's head under your right arm. Encircle your arms around the patient's trunk. The patient's arms are folded together (Figure 17-20). Rock the patient forward and on the count of three, when the patient's weight is over the legs, push against the patient's knees to move back in the chair.

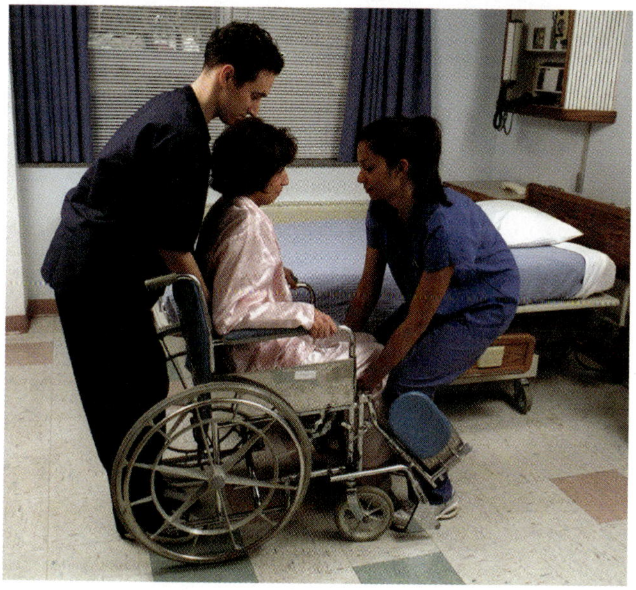

FIGURE 17-18 One assistant supports the lower extremities while the other uses the transfer belt to move the patient back in the chair.

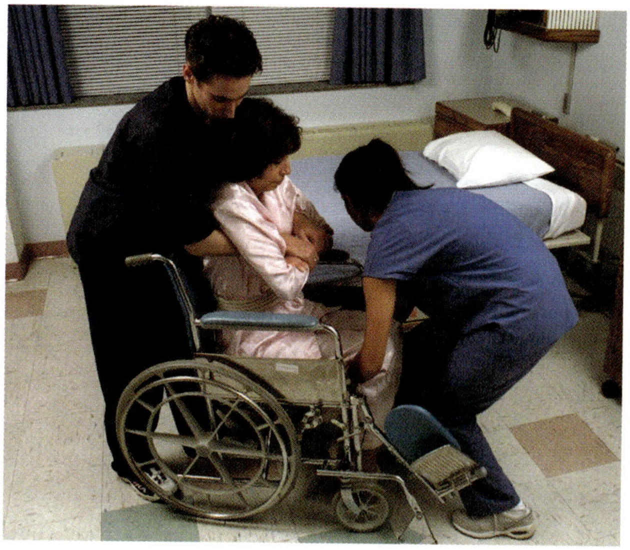

FIGURE 17-19 One assistant encircles the patient's legs with her hands and arms.

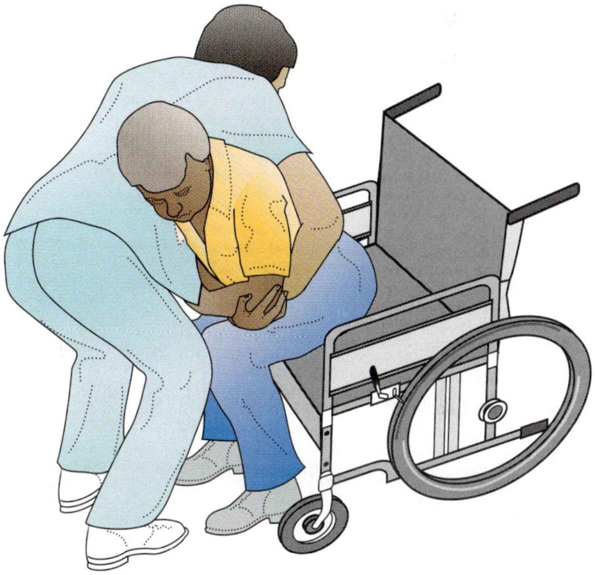

FIGURE 17-20 Put your arms around the patient's trunk.

If the patient can bear weight, it is easier and more beneficial to assist the patient to stand and then sit back down, getting the hips to the back of the chair. Wedge cushions placed in the wheelchair will prevent the patient from sliding forward.

WHEELCHAIR ACTIVITY

Pressure over the buttocks is dramatically increased when the patient is sitting. Teach the patient (and provide assistance if necessary) to periodically relieve the pressure by shifting weight every 15 minutes. *Be sure wheelchair is locked before beginning any activities involving patient movement in the chair.*

Wheelchair Push-ups

1. Teach the patient to place one hand on each armrest, keeping both elbows bent.
2. Then have patient lean forward slightly, pushing on the armrests and straightening the elbows while lifting the buttocks off the seat of the wheelchair. Have the patient hold this position to the count of five if possible (Figure 17-21).

Leaning

If the patient cannot do push-ups, teach her to place the hands on the armrests or thighs and lean forward slightly, and then to each side to relieve pressure on the buttocks (Figure 17-22). Monitor patients who have balance problems, to avoid falling out of the chair.

Other Preventive Measures

Place a folded bath blanket in the seat of the chair if the patient is wearing a hospital gown, so the skin does not contact the vinyl chair seat. Use pressure-relieving pads in the seat of the chair if the patient will be up for a prolonged period of time. Use pillows, pads, or other props to maintain the patient in good body alignment. Patients should always sit upright, without leaning to either side.

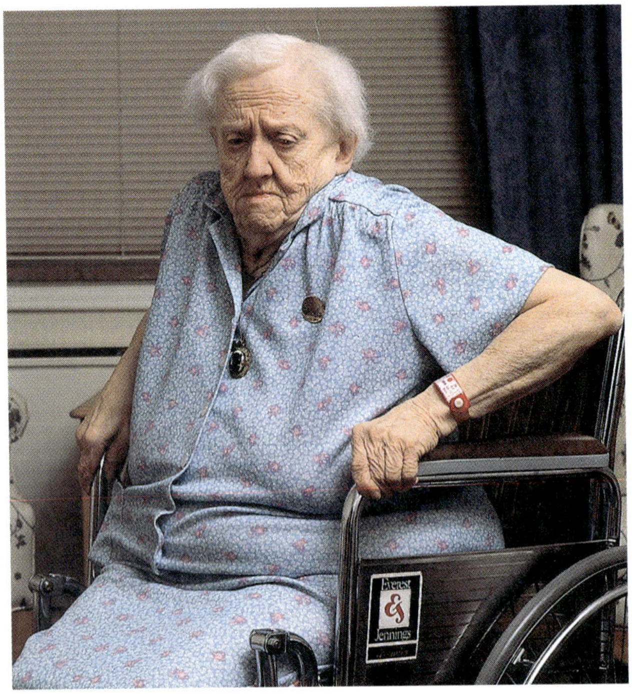

FIGURE 17-21 Wheelchair push-ups can relieve pressure on the buttocks, preventing pressure ulcers.

TRANSPORTING A PATIENT BY STRETCHER

Before moving a patient on a stretcher, make sure that the side rails are up and all safety belts are fastened. Push the stretcher by standing at the patient's head. Moving the stretcher in this manner enables you to use good body mechanics and see potential hazards. Approach corners slowly and look before you go around them. Take care when approaching swinging doors. Prop the door open to propel the stretcher through the door. If this is not possible, back through swinging doors.

When entering an elevator, push the stop button to lock the doors open. Back the stretcher into the elevator by walking backward and pulling the head end of the stretcher. Stand by the patient's head while the elevator is in motion. When the elevator stops, push the stop button to lock the door open. Push the stretcher out so the feet exit the elevator first. If the threshold is uneven, go to the foot end of the stretcher and pull it out of the elevator. After the stretcher is safely out of the elevator, unlock the door mechanism.

When transporting a stretcher down a ramp or incline, walk backward, slowly guiding the stretcher from the head end. Periodically look over your shoulder to make sure that the path is clear.

When parking a stretcher, avoid blocking a doorway. Never leave a patient who is on a stretcher unattended or unsupervised.

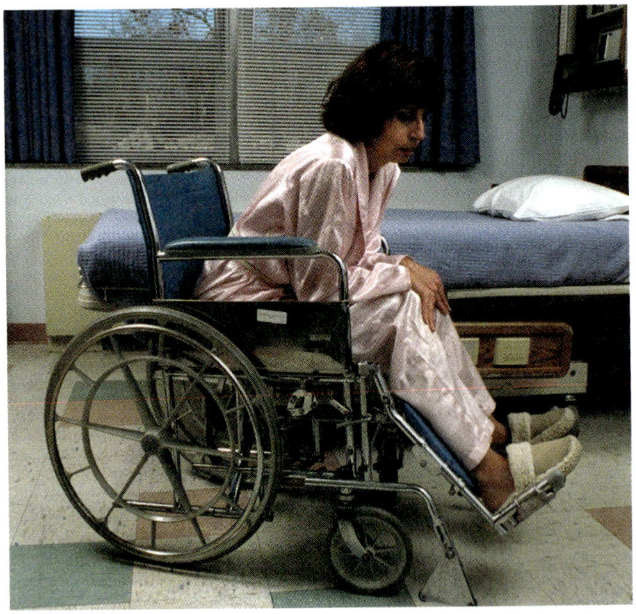

FIGURE 17-22 The patient can lean forward slightly to relieve pressure.

REVIEW

A. Multiple Choice.

Select the one best answer for each of the following.

1. When ambulating a patient with a weak right side, you should stand
- **a.** in back of the patient.
- **b.** on the patient's right side.
- **c.** on the patient's left side.
- **d.** in front of the patient.

2. When ambulating the patient, you should hold the gait belt with
- **a.** an overhand grasp in back of the patient.
- **b.** an underhand grasp in back of the patient.
- **c.** one hand on each side of the patient.
- **d.** one hand in front of the patient.

3. Before helping a patient to walk with a cane or walker, you should check the
- **a.** distance between the patient's feet.
- **b.** screws and bolts for tightness.
- **c.** height of the wheelchair.
- **d.** length of each step.

4. The cane is always held
- **a.** on the patient's weaker side.
- **b.** on the patient's stronger side.
- **c.** in the dominant hand.
- **d.** in the nondominant hand.

5. When using a two-point gait with a cane, the patient will
- **a.** place the strong foot forward, then the cane, then the weaker foot.
- **b.** place the strong foot and cane forward at the same time and then the weaker foot.
- **c.** place the weaker foot and cane forward at the same time and then the stronger foot.
- **d.** place the weaker foot forward, then the stronger foot, and then the cane.

6. If a patient starts to fall, you should
- **a.** try to hold the patient upright to prevent a fall.
- **b.** let go of the patient immediately, to avoid back strain.
- **c.** ease the patient to the floor.
- **d.** leave the patient and go for help.

7. When using a walker, the walker is set down so that
- **a.** the front legs strike the floor first and then the back legs.
- **b.** the back legs strike the floor first and then the front legs.
- **c.** all four legs strike the floor at the same time.
- **d.** how the walker is set down depends on the patient's problem.

8. When transporting a patient in a wheelchair, always
- **a.** stay to the right in corridors.
- **b.** guide the wheelchair from the front going down ramps.
- **c.** push the patient into an elevator frontwards.
- **d.** position the patient's feet at a 45° angle.

9. Conditions that can affect a patient's gait include
- **a.** diseases such as Parkinson's disease.
- **b.** having a catheter.
- **c.** having hand surgery.
- **d.** transferring independently.

10. Assistive devices are usually selected by the
- **a.** nursing assistant.
- **b.** physician.
- **c.** physical therapist.
- **d.** family.

B. True/False.

Mark the following true or false by circling T or F.

11. T F Always back in as you move a patient in a wheelchair into an elevator.

12. T F When transporting a patient in a wheelchair, always walk on the left of the corridor.

13. T F A wheelchair should always be locked unless the patient is being moved.

14. T F A cane is held in the patient's weaker hand.

15. T F When using a walker, the front two tips of the walker should strike the floor first and then the back two tips should strike the floor.

16. T F When assisting a patient to ambulate, you need to use a gait belt only if the patient is using an assistive device.

17. T F To relieve pressure on the buttocks, the patient should be taught how to do wheelchair push-ups or how to lean to relieve pressure.

18. T F To pick an article up from the floor, the patient should lean forward and reach down between the knees.

19. T F A cane is used for patients who are unable to bear weight on one leg.

20. T F The patient needs to be able to use both hands to manipulate a walker.

C. Nursing Assistant Challenge.

Mr. Santozi is 76 years old and has had right hip surgery. His physician does not want him to bear full weight on the affected leg. He uses a walker to assist his ambulation. He has been taught to use a three-point gait. When you help him out of bed, he reaches for the walker to help pull himself up from the bed. As you watch him walk down the hall, you note that he is setting the walker down by the front legs first and then the back legs. When he walks, he pushes the walker and his strong leg ahead at the same time. What errors is Mr. Santozi making, and how can you help him?

EXPLORING THE WEB

Description	Location
Ambulating with a Gait Belt	*http://www.gc.maricopa.edu*
Ambulation Training	*http://sandiego.networkofcare.org*
Articles on Falls and Risk	*http://www.amda.com*
Assisted Walking	*http://www.ohsah.bc.ca*
Preventing Falls and Fractures	*http://www.crouse.org*
Safety Procedures	*http://www.texashste.com*
Strategies for Improving Resident Mobility	*http://www.nursinghome.org*
Merry Walker	*http://www.merrywalker.com*
Making Health Care Safer	*http://www.ahrq.gov/clinic/ptsafety/spotlight.htm*
Procedure for Ambulation Aids	*http://www-nmcp.med.navy.mil/nursing/procman/ambulationaids.doc*

section 6

Measuring and Recording Vital Signs, Height, and Weight

UNIT 18
Body Temperature

UNIT 19
Pulse and Respiration

UNIT 20
Blood Pressure

UNIT 21
Measuring Height and Weight

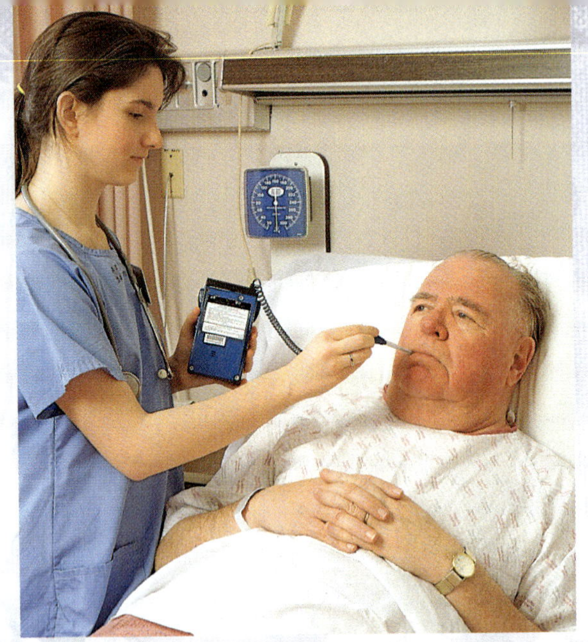

unit 18

Body Temperature

objectives

After completing this unit, you will be able to:

- Spell and define terms.
- Name and identify the three types of clinical thermometers and tell their uses.
- Read a thermometer.
- Identify the range of normal values.
- Demonstrate the following procedures:
  - Procedure 33 Measuring an Oral Temperature (Glass Thermometer)
  - Procedure 34 Measuring Temperature Using a Sheath-Covered Thermometer
  - Procedure 35 Measuring a Rectal Temperature (Glass Thermometer)
  - Procedure 36 Measuring an Axillary or Groin Temperature (Glass Thermometer)
  - Procedure 37 Measuring an Oral Temperature (Electronic Thermometer)
  - Procedure 38 Measuring a Rectal Temperature (Electronic Thermometer)
  - Procedure 39 Measuring an Axillary Temperature (Electronic Thermometer)
  - Procedure 40 Measuring a Tympanic Temperature
  - Procedure 41 Cleaning Glass Thermometers

vocabulary

Learn the meaning and the correct spelling of the following words and phrases:

body core	digital thermometer	flagged	tympanic thermometer
body shell	electronic thermometer	metabolism	vital signs
Celsius scale	Fahrenheit scale	probe	
clinical thermometer			

INTRODUCTION

Measurement of body temperature is a common nursing assistant task. Body temperature is one of the **vital** (living) **signs**. The patient's other vital signs include the pulse, respiration, and blood pressure. Although they are not part of the vital signs, the height and weight of the patient are also commonly measured.

Specific equipment is used to determine or measure these values. They must be accurately measured because they tell us a great deal about the patient's condition. Do not tell the patient the results. This is not your responsibility. Tell the patient you will ask the nurse to discuss the results with him. Although they are usually determined as a combined procedure, each vital sign is discussed in a separate unit. Measurement of height and weight is discussed in Unit 21.

Many facilities use electronic equipment that automatically registers the four vital signs simultaneously.

TEMPERATURE VALUES

Temperature values may be expressed in either of two scales. They are the:

- **Fahrenheit scale**, which is indicated by an *F*.
- **Celsius scale** (centigrade scale), which is indicated by a *C*.

A small ° before either capital letter indicates degrees or levels of temperature.

A formula can be used to convert temperature readings from Celsius to Fahrenheit and from Fahrenheit to Celsius. See Table 18-1 for some important equivalents. Figure 18-1 compares the markings of the Fahrenheit and Celsius thermometers.

DEFINITION OF BODY TEMPERATURE

Temperature is the measurement of body heat. It is the balance between heat produced and heat lost.

TABLE 18-1 COMPARISON OF FAHRENHEIT AND CELSIUS TEMPERATURE SCALES

	Celsius (C)	Fahrenheit (F)
Freezing	0°	32°
Body temperature	37°	98.6°
Pasteurization	63°	145°
Boiling	100°	212°
Sterilizing (Autoclave)	121°	250°

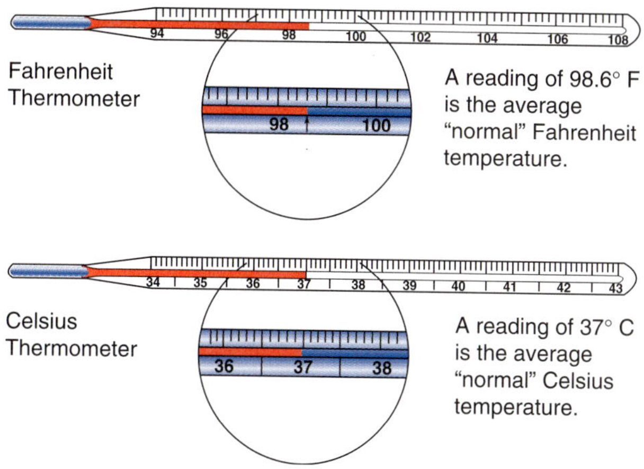

FIGURE 18-1 Fahrenheit and Celsius thermometers.

Body temperature is:

- Fairly constant. There is a daily variation of 1 to 3°F. Body temperature is lowest in the morning. It is higher in the afternoon and evening.
- Lower the closer to the body surface it is measured. The temperature at the center of the body (**body core**) is much higher than the temperature at the surface of the body.
- Different in the same person when determined from different body areas (Table 18-2). It is important to know the "normal" temperature for an individual, because the normal may vary from person to person.
- Less stable in children. Table 18-3 shows average temperatures in infants and children.
- Affected by
  - illness
  - external temperature/environment
  - medication
  - age
  - infection
  - time of day
  - exercise
  - emotions
  - pregnancy

TABLE 18-2 TEMPERATURE VARIATIONS IN THE SAME PERSON

	Oral	Axillary	Rectal
Average Temperature	98.6°F	97.6°F	99.6°F
Range	97.6–99.6°F (36.5–37.5°C)	96.6–98.6°F (36–37°C)	98.6–100.6°F (37–38.1°C)

TABLE 18-3 AVERAGE TEMPERATURES IN INFANTS AND CHILDREN

Age	Temperature
3 months	99.4°F
6 months	99.5°F
1 year	99.7°F
3 years	99.0°F
5 years	98.6°F
9 years	98.0°F

- menstrual cycle
- crying
- hydration

Excessive body temperature puts stress on vital body organs.

TEMPERATURE CONTROL

Activities to control and regulate body temperature are managed by special cells in the brain.

- Heat is produced by chemical reactions (**metabolism**) in the body core and muscular contractions. For this reason, rectal temperature is highest.
- Blood carries the heat to the skin (**body shell**). The heat is lost from the skin to the outside.
- Heat loss is largely controlled by regulating the amount of blood reaching the skin and through perspiration.
- Average oral temperature range is 96.8°F (36°C) to 100.4°F (38°C). Average temperature is 98.6°F (37°C).

MEASURING BODY TEMPERATURE

Temperature is usually measured in one of four body areas:

- mouth (oral)—most common.
- ear (aural or tympanic)—takes the least amount of time.
- rectal—most accurate of commonly used sites (mouth, rectal, axillary); rectal temperature registers 1°F higher than oral.
- axillary or groin—least accurate; measures temperature under the arm or at the groin. (This method is used only when the patient's condition does not permit the use of oral, aural, or rectal sites.) An axillary or groin temperature registers 1°F (or 0.6°C) lower than oral temperature.

The patient's condition determines which is the best site for measuring the temperature. The site used most often is the mouth. It is not, however, always the best or safest site to use. In some situations, it is wiser to use the rectal site.

For example, if the patient is a child or irrational, a glass thermometer in the mouth could result in injury. Patients with respiratory problems, those who breathe through the mouth, or those who are very weak or unconscious may not be able to keep an oral thermometer in their mouths for a long enough time to ensure an accurate recording. In these situations, the best choice is the aural site, because the care provider holds the tympanic thermometer in the ear. The reading registers within seconds, so the tympanic thermometer is a good choice for restless patients as well. If the tympanic thermometer is not available, the rectal site might be used. Use a rectal thermometer inserted in the anus for the proper time. Be sure to hold the rectal thermometer in place to avoid possible injury.

CLINICAL THERMOMETERS

A patient's temperature is determined by using a **clinical thermometer**. There are several types of clinical thermometers.

The Glass Clinical Thermometer

The glass clinical thermometer is a slender glass tube containing liquid; the liquid expands when exposed to heat and moves up or down the tube. Three types of glass clinical thermometers are in general use (Figure 18-2). They are the oral, security, and rectal thermometers. They differ mainly in the size and shape of the bulb. The bulb is the end that is inserted into the patient. When only the security or stubby type is in use, the rectal thermometers are marked with a red dot at the end of the stem.

Thermometers containing mercury have been used for many years. However, recently the trend in health care has been to avoid the use of products containing mercury, because the mercury can be very toxic to humans and wildlife, if the product is broken. This is true even if mercury exposure occurs in very small amounts.

A mercury thermometer is a small glass tube containing

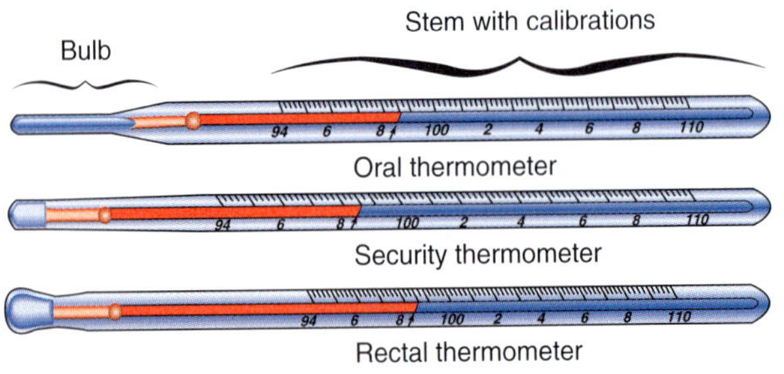

FIGURE 18-2 Clinical thermometers (from top to bottom): oral, security, rectal.

liquid mercury, a silvery-white substance that registers body heat. Alternative products are now being used in many glass thermometers because of mercury's potential for toxicity. Some thermometers contain a red or blue liquid. These are alcohol thermometers and contain no mercury. Another, less common thermometer contains galinstan, a substance similar to mercury in appearance. These thermometers are mercury-free, however, and are generally marked as such.

Mercury can be toxic in small amounts, particularly if it vaporizes and is inhaled. Even small mercury spills must be cleaned up properly to prevent contamination and illness. If you accidentally break a thermometer or other medical device containing mercury, follow your facility policies and procedures for cleaning the spill.

Electronic Thermometer

The **electronic thermometer** (Figure 18-3) is used in many hospitals. One unit can serve many patients because the nursing assistant simply changes the disposable sheath that fits over the probe.

- The electronic thermometer is battery-operated. It registers the temperature on the viewing screen in a few seconds.
- The portion called the **probe** is inserted into the patient.
- The probes are colored red for rectal use and blue for oral or axillary use.
- The probe is covered by a plastic sheath before use. The plastic sheath stays on during use. It is discarded after use.

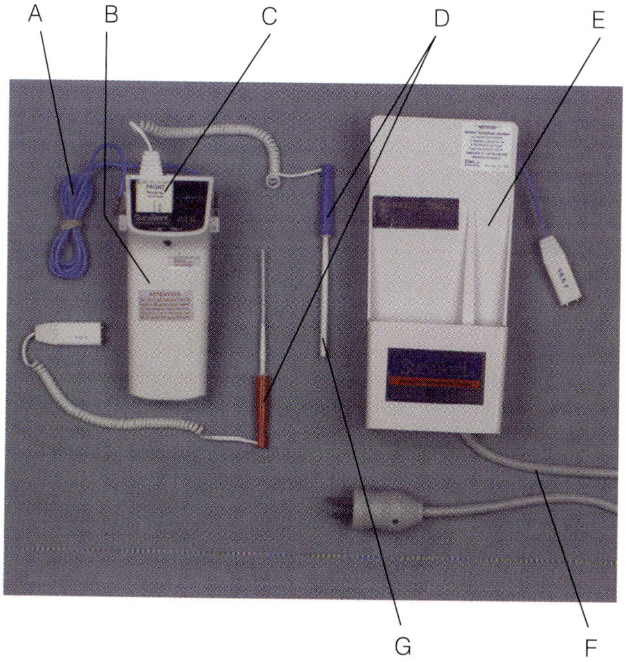

FIGURE 18-3 An electronic thermometer. The temperature is registered in large, easy-to-read numerals. The disposable protective sheath (probe cover) is placed over the probe tip. The probe is inserted in the patient's mouth in the usual manner. (A) Plastic cord goes around the nursing assistant's neck when carrying the thermometer. (B) Thermometer (C) Box of disposable probe covers (D) Probe (Blue = oral, Red = rectal) (E) Charging unit (F) Probe cord (G) Disposable probe cover.

Digital Thermometer

Digital thermometers are hand-held and have a probe that is inserted into the patient's mouth or rectum (Figure 18-4). Sheaths are used to cover the oral or rectal probe before use and are discarded after use. The unit is battery-operated. After the sheath-covered probe is inserted, the temperature can be read within 20 to 60 seconds. The temperature is shown as a digital (number) display.

Disposable Oral Thermometers

Plastic or paper thermometers are used for oral temperatures in some facilities. They are used once and discarded. They have dots on them. The dots change color from brown to blue, according to the patient's temperature.

> **SAFETY Alert**
>
> The disposable thermometer is made of rigid plastic. Remove the thermometer from the patient's mouth slowly. Pulling the thermometer out rapidly from between closed lips can cause tears of the lips and mucous membranes in the mouth.

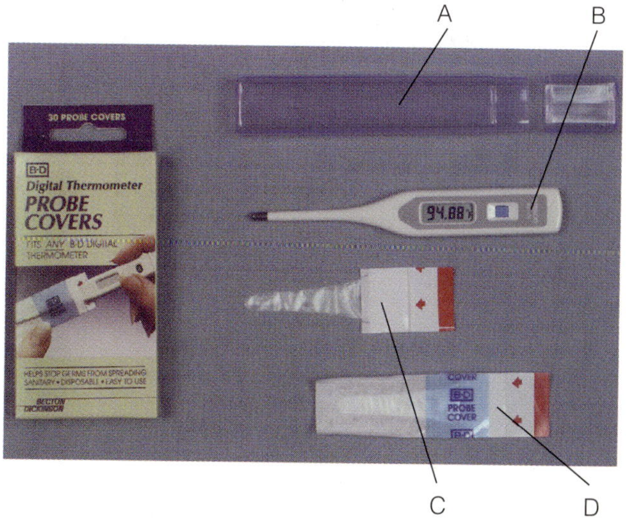

FIGURE 18-4 Digital thermometer (A) Carrying case (B) Digital thermometer (C) Probe cover less backing (D) Probe cover with backing.

Tympanic Thermometer

The **tympanic thermometer** is an instrument that measures the temperature from blood vessels in the tympanic membrane (ear drum) in the ear (Figure 18-5). The temperature reading obtained is close to the core body temperature. To obtain an accurate reading, the probe must be placed solidly into the ear canal. The instrument has a built-in converter that provides the equivalent temperature in rectal or oral values (in both the Fahrenheit and Celsius systems). The type of temperature reading (mode) is selected by the user. The disposable speculum is inserted into the ear canal, gently sealing the canal. The instrument is activated, usually by pressing a button, and within a few seconds it registers the temperature of the blood flowing through the vessels in the eardrum.

Using the Glass Thermometer

The glass thermometer is a long, cylindrical, calibrated tube that contains a column of heat-sensitive liquid (Figure 18-6).

- Starting with 94°F (34°C), each long line indicates a one-degree elevation in temperature.
- Only every other degree is marked with a number.
- In between each long line are four shorter lines.
- Each shorter line equals two-tenths (2/10 or 0.2) of 1 degree.

The liquid (the solid color line shown in Figure 18-6) in the bulb of the thermometer rises in the hollow center of the stem as heat is registered. To read the thermometer:

- Hold it at eye level.
- Find the solid column in the center.
- Look along the sharper edge between the numbers and lines.

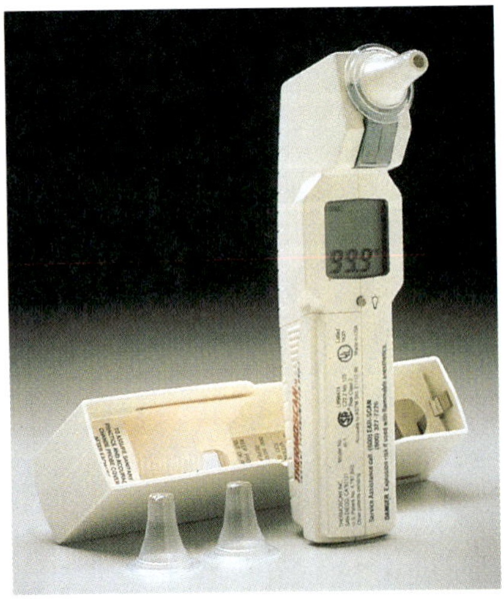

FIGURE 18-5 Cordless, hand-held tympanic thermometer that measures the temperature of the tympanic membrane in the ear. The window on the handset indicates the digital temperature reading. *(Courtesy of Thermoscan® Inc., San Diego, CA.)*

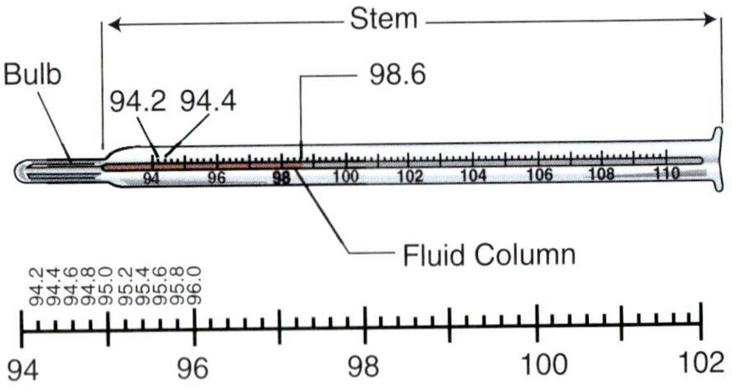

FIGURE 18-6 Reading a thermometer. This thermometer reads 98.6°F. Most Fahrenheit thermometers have an arrow indicating 98.6°F.

- Read at the point at which the liquid ends.
- If it falls between two lines, read it to the closest line.

Some glass thermometers come individually prepackaged for patient use. The patient receives it as part of the admission package.

Using the Electronic Thermometer

Battery-operated electronic thermometers are commonly used. The temperature registers in large numbers on the screen. The probe is placed into the patient. The probe stem is colored blue for oral or axillary use and red for rectal use. A new, disposable probe cover is used for each patient. Following use, the cover is discarded. The temperature registers in about 30 seconds.

Using the Tympanic Thermometer

Many facilities use tympanic thermometers. The temperature is taken by measuring the heat given off by the tympanic membrane (in the ear). This method has several advantages:

- Tympanic thermometers are accurate and easy to use.

SAFETY *Alert*

If you accidentally break a mercury thermometer, apply gloves and eye protection. Your facility may also require use of a mask to prevent inhalation. Pick up broken glass and other debris and place in a puncture-resistant container. Follow facility policies for picking up mercury. Use an index card to consolidate the droplets, then seal them in a plastic bag or covered container. Small droplets can be picked up with adhesive tape or wet paper towels. Seal the container and affix a label identifying the material as "mercury spill debris."

guidelines *for* Using an Oral or Rectal Thermometer

Oral Thermometer

1. Do not use if the patient is:
   - uncooperative
   - restless
   - unconscious
   - chilled
   - confused or disoriented
   - coughing
   - an infant or child under the age of 6
   - unable to breathe through the nose
   - recovering from oral surgery
   - irrational
   - very weak
   - receiving oxygen (except nasal prongs)
   - on seizure precautions
2. An oral temperature reading could be false on denture wearers.
3. To measure an oral temperature accurately, wait 15 minutes if patients have been smoking, eating, or drinking, then take the temperature.

Rectal Thermometer

1. Do not use if the patient has:
   - diarrhea
   - fecal impaction
   - combative behavior
   - rectal bleeding
   - hemorrhoids
   - had rectal surgery or rectal or colonic disease
   - recently had a heart attack
   - recently had prostate surgery
   - a colostomy
2. Always hold a rectal thermometer in place the entire time.

- The temperature registers in a few seconds. Because of this, taking the temperature of an agitated patient is safer and faster.
- Temperatures that cannot be taken orally can be taken by the tympanic method, eliminating the need to take rectal or axillary temperatures.

guidelines *for* The Safe Use of a Glass Thermometer

- Make sure the thermometer is clean.
- Wear disposable gloves when measuring oral and rectal temperatures.
- Check glass thermometers for chips.
- Shake the thermometer down before use. Shake away from the patient and hard objects.
- Cover the thermometer with a disposable plastic sheath.
- Do not leave the patient alone with a thermometer in place.
- Allow a glass thermometer to register for at least 3 minutes for oral temperature, 3 minutes for rectal temperature, and 10 minutes for axillary temperature. Each facility may have it's own guidelines. Be sure to follow your facilities guidelines.
- Hold rectal and axillary thermometers in place.
- When using a rectal thermometer, lubricate the bulb end of the thermometer before inserting it into the rectum.
- After removing the thermometer and before reading it, wipe the thermometer from end to tip with an alcohol wipe or cotton ball.
- Do not touch a bulb end or disposable sheath that has been in patient's mouth (oral thermometer) or anus (rectal thermometer).
- Discard the sheath according to facility policy after use.
- Clean and disinfect the thermometer after use.

- The tympanic thermometer allows you to select a core, oral, or rectal mode. This means the reading will correlate with the mode selected. Choose the mode according to your facility's policy.
- Wait for 15 minutes to take the temperature if the patient has been outdoors or if the patient has been lying on the ear you will use.

The tympanic temperature is the fastest and most convenient method, but it can also give inaccurate readings if the user's technique is not precise. To ensure an accurate reading, insert the probe tip into the ear as far as it will go. Next, rotate the probe handle until it is aligned with the jaw, like speaking on the telephone. Quickly press the "scan" button. Using this method will help ensure accurate temperature readings.

PROCEDURE 33

MEASURING AN ORAL TEMPERATURE (GLASS THERMOMETER)

1. Carry out beginning procedure actions.
2. Assemble the following equipment on a tray:
   - Gloves (standard precautions)
   - Container with clean thermometers
   - Container for used thermometers
   - Cotton balls
   - Container for soiled tissues
   - Container with tissues
   - Pad and pencil
   - Watch with second hand
3. Have the patient rest in a comfortable position in a bed or chair. Put on gloves.
4. Remove the thermometer from the container by holding the stem end. Rinse the thermometer with cold water and wipe with tissue from stem to bulb end if the thermometer has been in disinfectant. Check to be sure the thermometer is intact. Read the center column. It should register below 96°F. If necessary, shake it down. (To shake down (Figure 18-7A), move away from tables and other hard objects. Grasp the stem tightly between your thumb and fingers. Shake down with a downward motion.) If used in your facility, place the thermometer in a disposable plastic cover sheath.
5. Ask the patient if he or she has had anything to eat or drink or has smoked within the last 15 minutes. Wait 15 minutes before taking an oral temperature if the answer is yes.
6. Insert the bulb end of the thermometer under the patient's tongue, toward the side of the mouth (Figure 18-7B). Tell the patient to hold the thermometer gently with lips closed for 3 minutes.
7. Remove the thermometer, holding it by the stem. Wipe from stem end toward bulb end (Figure 18-7C).
8. Discard tissue in the proper container.
9. Read the thermometer and record the temperature on a pad (Figure 18-7D).
10. Place the thermometer in the container for used thermometers. If the thermometer is to be reused for this patient:
    - Wash it twice in cold water and soap with two separate cotton balls, wiping from stem to bulb.
    - Rinse and dry it.
    - Return it to the individual disinfectant-filled holder.

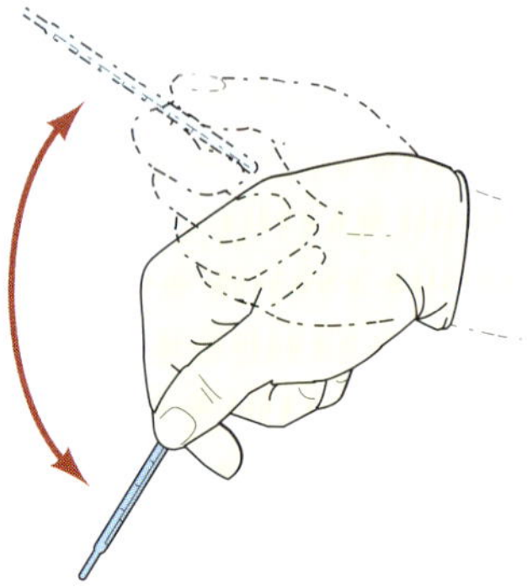

FIGURE 18-7A Shake the liquid down in the column by holding the thermometer by the stem and snapping the wrist. Check the reading. Repeat until the reading is below 96°F.

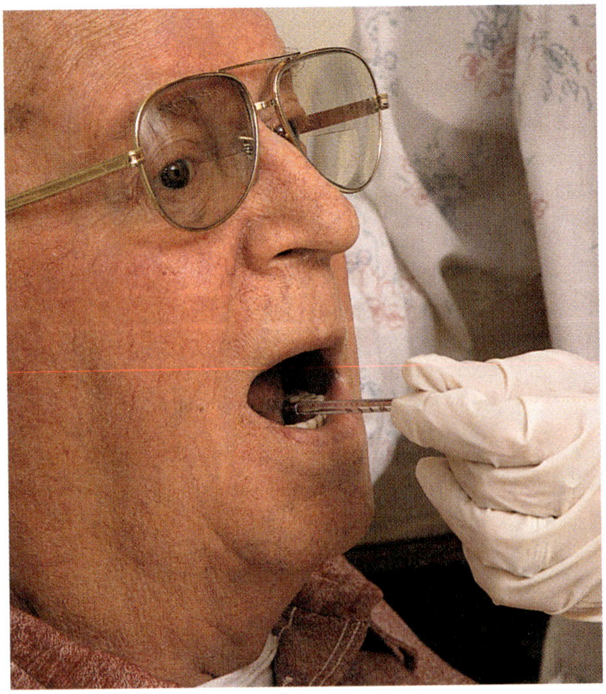

FIGURE 18-7B The bulb end of the thermometer is inserted under the tongue, left 3 minutes, then removed.

continues

PROCEDURE 33

continued

- Remove gloves and discard according to facility policy.

11. Carry out procedure completion actions.

12. Report any unusual variations to the nurse at once.

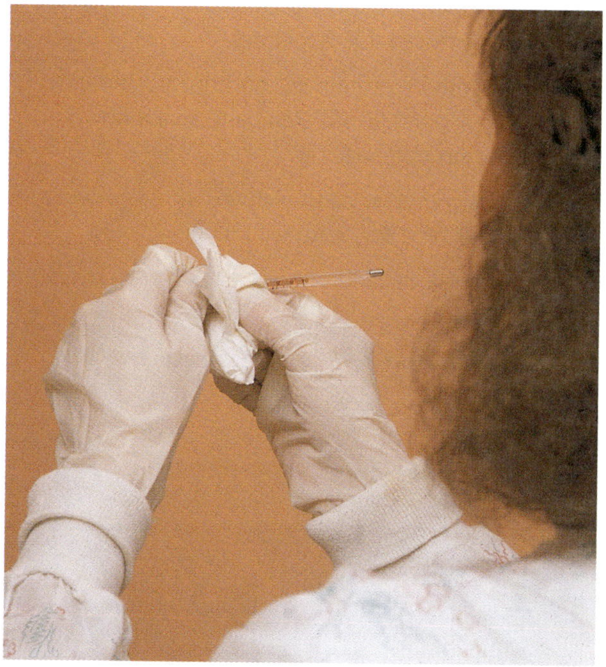

FIGURE 18-7C Wipe the thermometer after removing it from the patient's mouth or discard the disposable sheath. Always wipe from the stem to the bulb. Do not touch the bulb.

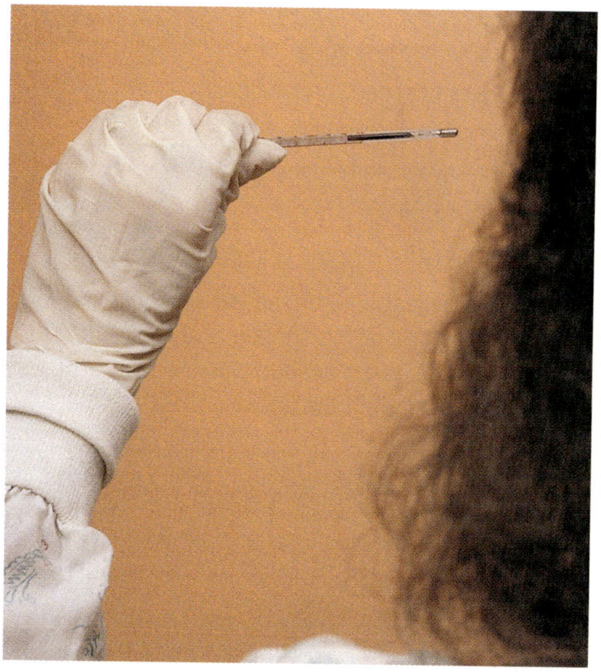

FIGURE 18-7D Hold the thermometer at eye level. Locate the column of liquid in the center and read to the next closest line.

guidelines *for*

Using a Tympanic (Ear) Thermometer

- Make sure the thermometer lens is clean and that there is no dirt or debris on the lens at the end of the probe tip.
- Use each probe cover only once. Make sure the cover is on snugly, without ripples.
- Store the thermometer out of the path of any cold air flow. If the thermometer is in a cold area, allow it to warm up before use, or it may read low.
- Make sure the patient is not directly in the path of cold air or being fanned. This action cools the ears, which can cause a low temperature reading.
- If the patient is lying on one ear, use the opposite ear.
- If the patient has a hearing aid, use the opposite ear or remove the aid and wait 15 minutes.
- The tympanic thermometer can be set to oral, core, or rectal mode. In most cases, oral is appropriate. The mode will be shown in the LCD readout screen. If the screen says "CAL," the thermometer is in the unadjusted mode, which is used only for calibration and other bench work.
- Insert the probe tip into the ear as far as possible, then rotate the handle to the correct position in alignment with the jaw.

PROCEDURE 34

MEASURING TEMPERATURE USING A SHEATH-COVERED THERMOMETER

1. Carry out beginning procedure actions.
2. Assemble needed equipment:
   - Gloves (standard precautions)
   - Clinical thermometer
   - Protective sheath (unopened package)
   - Pad and pencil
3. Have the patient rest in a comfortable position.
4. Ask the patient if he or she has had anything to eat or drink or has smoked within the last 15 minutes. Wait 15 minutes before taking an oral temperature if the answer is yes.
5. Apply gloves.
6. Shake the thermometer down to below 96°F.
7. Holding the thermometer in one hand, insert it into the marked end of a protective sheath wrapper (Figure 18-8A).
8. Holding onto the sheath tab on the stem end of the thermometer, peel back the paper cover to expose the plastic sheath (Figure 18-8B).
9. Hold the paper wrapper in one hand (Figure 18-8C). Twist on the paper wrapper to break the seal with the tab and remove the paper wrapper, leaving the plastic sheath on the thermometer (Figure 18-8D).
10. Keeping the protective sheath over the thermometer, insert the bulb end of the thermometer under the patient's tongue, toward the side of the mouth.
11. Tell the patient to hold the thermometer gently, with lips closed, for 3 minutes.
12. Remove the thermometer and discard the used sheath (Figure 18-8E). Read and shake down. Record on notepad.
13. The thermometer can be stored in the patient's bedside stand for reuse with a new sheath.
14. Remove gloves and discard according to facility policy.
15. Carry out procedure completion actions.
16. Report any unusual variations to the nurse at once.

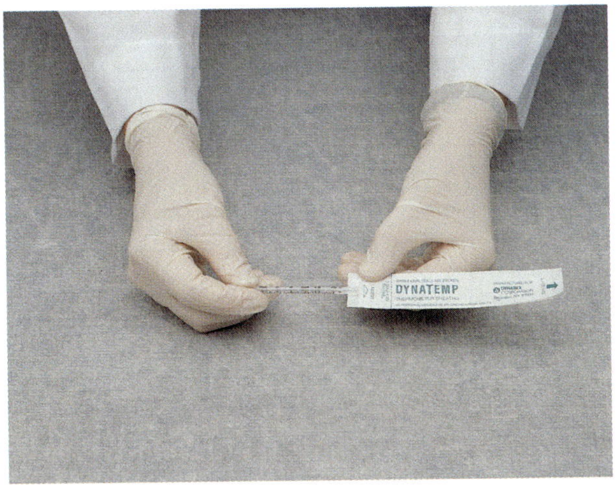

FIGURE 18-8A Inserting a thermometer into a disposable thermometer sheath.

continues

Cleaning Glass Thermometers

Glass thermometers are reusable. Therefore, they must be cleaned and disinfected between uses. If each patient has an individual thermometer kept in solution at the bedside, you must clean and disinfect it after each use. If a general supply of thermometers is used to determine routine temperature, they too must be disinfected before reuse.

Each used thermometer must be carefully washed with soapy, cold, running water to remove saliva or other body secretions. It must be rinsed to remove the soap and then carefully dried before disinfecting.

PROCEDURE 34

continued

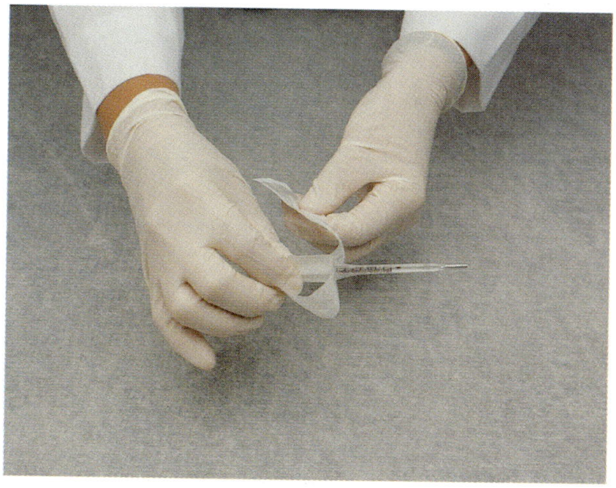

FIGURE 18-8B To remove the sheath, peel back the outer paper wrapper to expose the inner plastic sheath.

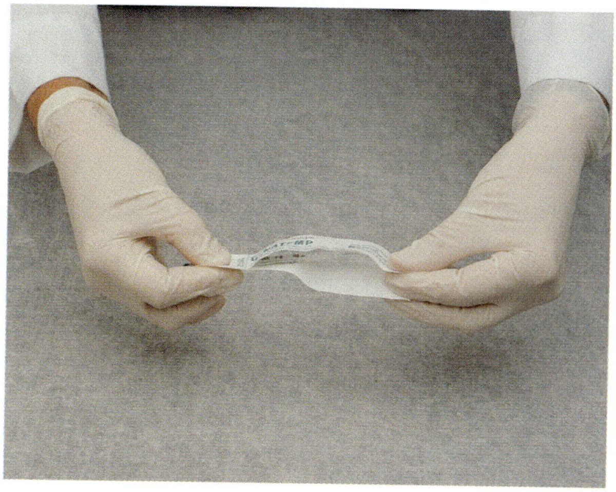

FIGURE 18-8C Grasp the outer paper wrapper.

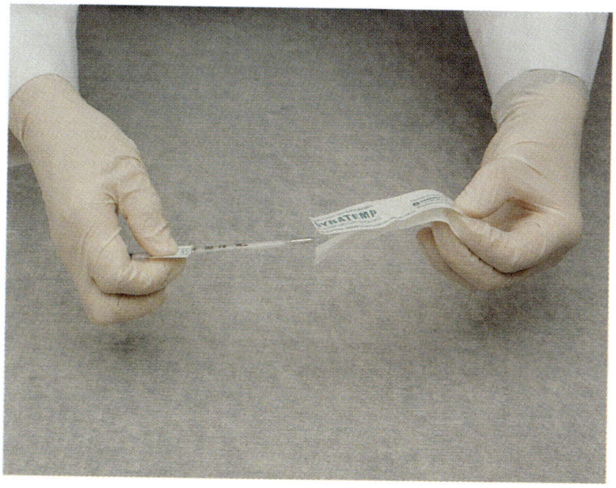

FIGURE 18-8D Holding onto the paper tab with one hand, twist and remove the outer paper wrapper.

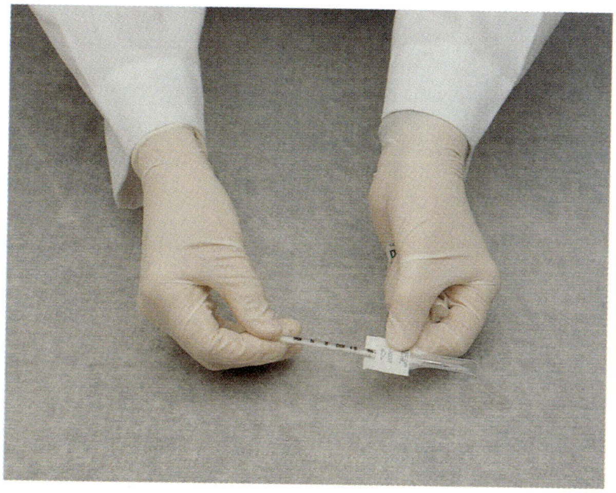

FIGURE 18-8E The sheath-covered thermometer is inserted into the patient's mouth. After the temperature is taken, the sheath is removed and discarded in the biohazard trash container.

Remember that glass breaks very easily, so be careful when washing and drying thermometers. Check each one for chips before putting it into disinfectant and before using a thermometer with a patient.

Documentation

In many facilities, temperatures are recorded on a temperature clipboard. They are then transferred to the individual patient charts. Changes in readings may be **flagged** (specially noted) by placing a circle around the reading or a star beside it. Make sure to report any changes from previous temperature readings directly to the nurse. Your accurate observations, reporting, and documentation contribute to the nurses' evaluation and assessment of the patient.

PROCEDURE 35

MEASURING A RECTAL TEMPERATURE (GLASS THERMOMETER)

1. Carry out beginning procedure actions.
2. Assemble equipment on a tray:
   - Container with clean rectal thermometer
   - Container for used thermometers
   - Container for soiled tissues
   - Lubricant
   - Container with tissues
   - Pad and pencil
   - Watch with second hand
   - Gloves (standard precautions)
3. Put up opposite side rail. Lower backrest of bed. Ask the patient to turn to the left side, if possible. Assist the patient if necessary.
4. Place a small amount of lubricant on a tissue.
5. Put gloves on. Remove the thermometer from the container by holding the stem end. Read the liquid column. Be sure it registers below 96°F. Check the condition of the thermometer.
6. Apply a small amount of lubricant to the bulb with a tissue.
7. Fold the top bedclothes back to expose the patient's anal area.
8. (Refer to Figure 18-9.) Separate the buttocks with one hand. Insert the thermometer gently into the rectum 1 inch. Hold in place. Adjust the bedclothes for privacy as soon as the thermometer is inserted.
9. The thermometer should remain inserted for 3 minutes, or according to facility policy. Hold the thermometer in place for the full time.

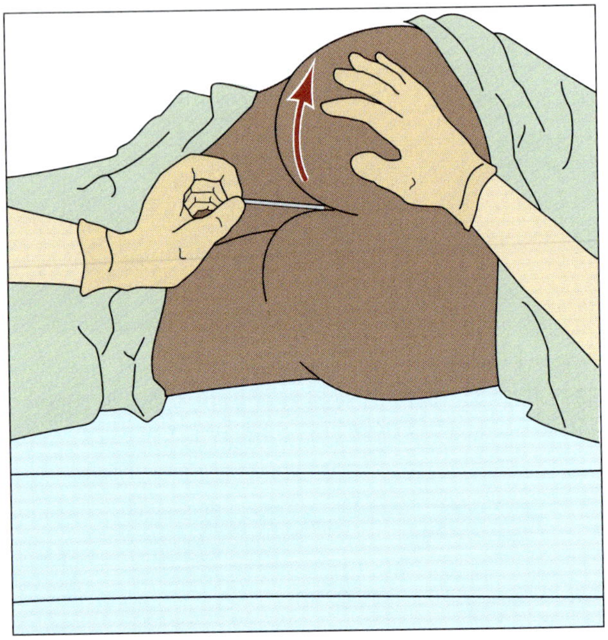

FIGURE 18-9 The rectal thermometer is lubricated and then inserted 1 inch into the rectum.

SAFETY Alert

Always hold the rectal thermometer in place. Never leave the patient unattended during the rectal temperature procedure.

10. Remove the thermometer, holding it by the stem. Wipe from stem toward bulb end.
11. Discard tissue in the proper container.
12. Read the thermometer. Record the reading on a pad.
13. Wipe the lubricant from the patient. Discard tissue.
14. Place the thermometer in the container for used thermometers. If the thermometer is to be reused for this patient:
    a. Wash it in cold water and soap.
    b. Rinse and dry it.
    c. Return it to the individual disinfectant-filled holder.
15. Remove gloves and discard according to facility policy.
16. Lower the opposite side rail.
17. Carry out procedure completion actions.

Note: *Remember, when a rectal temperature is recorded, you must add (R) after the reading.*

PROCEDURE 36

MEASURING AN AXILLARY OR GROIN TEMPERATURE (GLASS THERMOMETER)

1. Carry out beginning procedure actions.

Note: Use disposable gloves if there may be contact with open lesions, wet linens, or body fluids.

2. Assemble equipment on a tray:
   - Gloves
   - Container with clean oral thermometers
   - Container for used thermometers
   - Container for soiled tissues
   - Container with tissues
   - Disposable sheath, if used
   - Pad and pencil
   - Watch with a second hand
3. Shake the thermometer down to below 96°F. Cover the thermometer with a disposable sheath, if used.
4. Wipe the area dry and place the thermometer. Put on gloves if the groin area is used for temperature measurement.
   a. The patient's arm is held close to the body if an axillary site is used (Figure 18-10).
   b. The thermometer must be in the fold against the body if the groin site is used.
   c. Hold the thermometer in place for 10 minutes.
   d. Remove, wipe (or discard sheath, if used), and read the thermometer. Note the reading on a pad.
   e. Shake the thermometer down.
   f. Clean and replace as with an oral thermometer if the thermometer is to be reused.

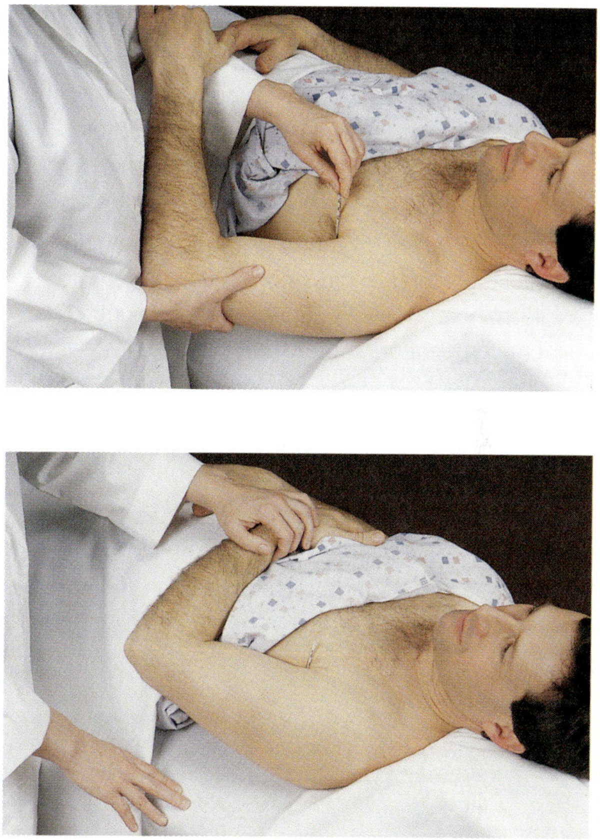

FIGURE 18-10 Hold the thermometer in place.

5. If the groin area was used, remove gloves and discard according to facility policy.
6. Carry out procedure completion actions.

Note: Remember, when an axillary temperature is recorded, you must add (AX) after the reading.

SAFETY *Alert*

Remember that the axillary method of taking a temperature is the least accurate method. Use it only when other methods are impractical or unavailable. Hold the glass thermometer in place for a full 10 minutes. Do not leave the bedside during this procedure.

PROCEDURE 37

MEASURING AN ORAL TEMPERATURE (ELECTRONIC THERMOMETER)

1. Carry out beginning procedure actions.
2. Obtain an electronic thermometer, disposable probe covers, and gloves, if this is your facility policy. (Gloves are not necessary with an *oral temperature* using this type of thermometer. Know and follow your facility policy.)
3. Ask the patient if he or she has had anything to eat or drink or has smoked within the last 15 minutes. Wait 15 minutes before taking an oral temperature if the answer is yes.
4. Cover the probe (blue) with a protective sheath.
5. Insert the covered probe under the patient's tongue toward the side of the mouth (Figure 18-11).
6. Hold the probe in position. Ask the patient to close the mouth and breathe through the nose.
7. When a buzzer signals that the temperature has been determined, remove the probe from the patient's mouth.
8. Discard the sheath in the appropriate container (Figure 18-12). Do not touch the sheath. Remove gloves, if used, and discard according to facility policy.
9. Return the probe to its proper position.
10. Record the temperature on your pad.
11. Return the thermometer unit to the charger.
12. Carry out procedure completion actions.

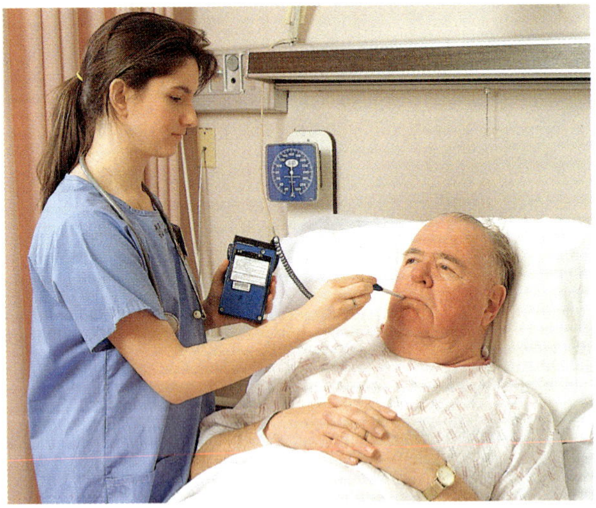

FIGURE 18-11 The thermometer probe is placed to one side of the patient's mouth and positioned under the tongue.

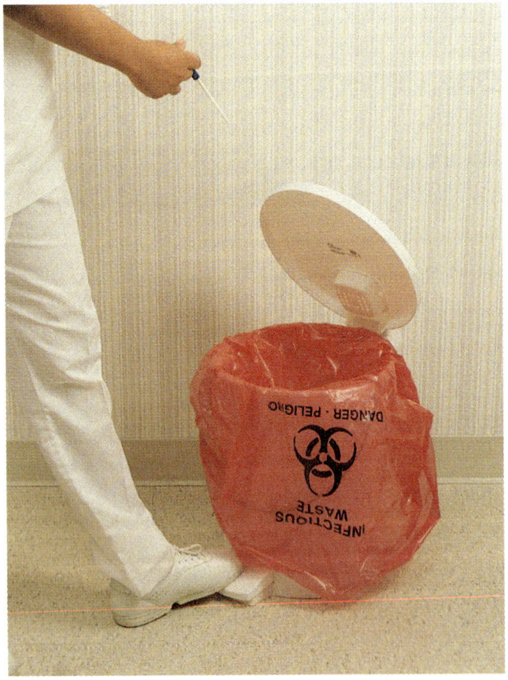

FIGURE 18-12 Once the temperature has been taken, the sheath is discarded.

PROCEDURE 38

MEASURING A RECTAL TEMPERATURE (ELECTRONIC THERMOMETER)

1. Carry out beginning procedure actions.
2. Assemble equipment on a tray:
   - Gloves
   - Electronic thermometer with rectal (red) probe
   - Probe cover
   - Lubricant
3. Lower the backrest of the bed. Ask the patient to turn on his side. Assist the patient if necessary.
4. Put on gloves. Place a small amount of lubricant on the tip of the sheath (Figure 18-13).
5. Fold the top bedclothes back to expose the patient's anal area.
6. Separate the buttocks with one hand. Insert the sheath-covered probe about 1 inch into the rectum, or as recommended by thermometer manufacturer. Hold in place. Replace the bedclothes for privacy as soon as the thermometer is inserted.
7. Read the temperature when registered on the digital display.

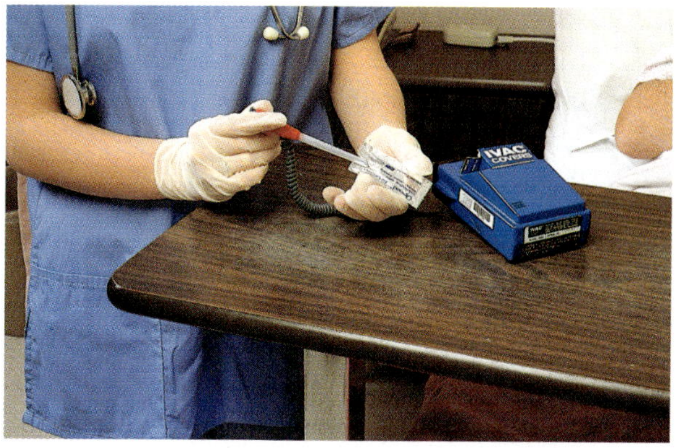

FIGURE 18-13 Remove the thermometer and apply a small amount of lubricant on the tip of the sheath.

8. Remove the probe and discard the sheath. Wipe lubricant from the patient. Discard tissue. Return probe to its proper position.
9. Remove gloves and dispose of according to facility policy.
10. Record the temperature on your pad.
11. Return the thermometer unit to the charger.
12. Carry out procedure completion actions.

PROCEDURE 39

MEASURING AN AXILLARY TEMPERATURE (ELECTRONIC THERMOMETER)

1. Carry out beginning procedure actions.

Note: *Use disposable gloves if there may be contact with open lesions, wet linens, or body fluids.*

2. Equipment needed: same as for oral temperature measurement using an electronic thermometer. (See Procedure 37.)
3. Wipe the axillary area dry and put the covered probe in place. Keep the patient's arm close to the body. Hold the probe in place until the temperature shows on the digital display and the buzzer signals that it has been recorded.
4. Remove the thermometer probe. Dispose of the sheath. Return the probe to its proper position.
5. Record the temperature on your pad.
6. Return the thermometer unit to the charger.
7. Carry out procedure completion actions.

PROCEDURE 40

MEASURING A TYMPANIC TEMPERATURE

1. Carry out beginning procedure actions.
2. Assemble equipment:
   - Disposable gloves if there may be contact with blood or body fluids, open lesions, or wet linens
   - Tympanic thermometer
   - Probe covers
3. Place a clean probe cover on the probe.
4. Select the appropriate mode on the thermometer.
5. Check the lens to make sure it is clean and intact (Figure 18-14A).
6. Put on disposable gloves if you may have contact with blood or body fluids, open lesions, or wet linens.
7. Position the patient so you have access to the ear you will be using.
8. Gently pull the ear pinna back and up (Figure 18-14B). This straightens the ear canal so the thermometer can be placed for an accurate reading. Note: When this thermometer is used for children under age 3, pull the pinna down and back. In children over age 3, pull the pinna up and back. This straightens the ear canal, enabling the sensor to detect heat in the eardrum. When the probe is positioned correctly, the probe tip will point at the midpoint between the eyebrow and sideburn on the opposite side of the face.
9. Place the probe in the patient's ear, aiming it toward the tympanic membrane. Insert the probe until it seals the ear canal (Figure 18-14C). Do not apply pressure.
10. Rotate the probe handle slightly until it is aligned with the jaw, as though the patient were speaking on the telephone.

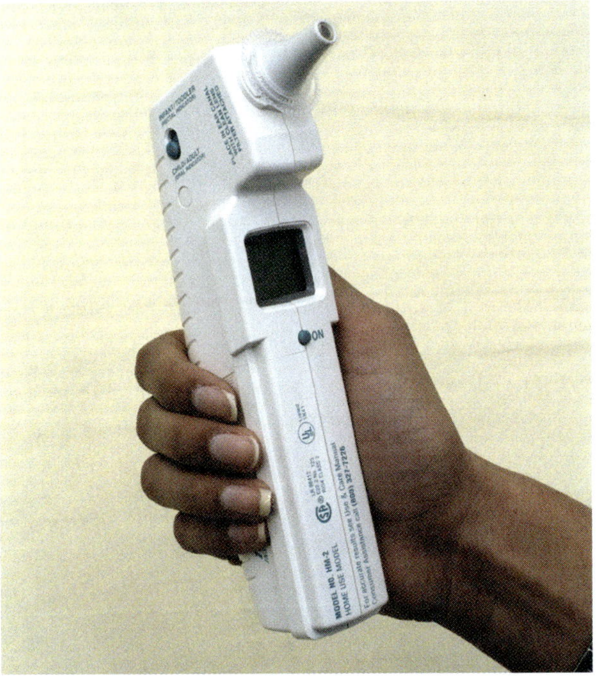

FIGURE 18-14A Check the lens of the tympanic thermometer to make sure it is clean and intact.

11. Quickly press the activation button (Figure 18-14D). Leave the thermometer in the ear for the time recommended by the manufacturer.
12. When you have a reading, remove the probe from the patient's ear and dispose of the cover. See Table 18-4 for normal ranges of tympanic temperatures by age group.
13. Record the temperature on your pad.
14. Return the thermometer unit to the charger.
15. Carry out procedure completion actions.

TABLE 18-4 NORMAL RANGES FOR TYMPANIC TEMPERATURES

Years of Age	Fahrenheit	Celsius
0–2	97.5–100.4°F	36.4–38.0°C
3–10	97.0–100.0°F	36.1–37.8°C
11–65	96.6–99.7°F	35.9–37.6°C
>65	96.4–99.5°F	35.8–37.5°C

continues

PROCEDURE 40

continued

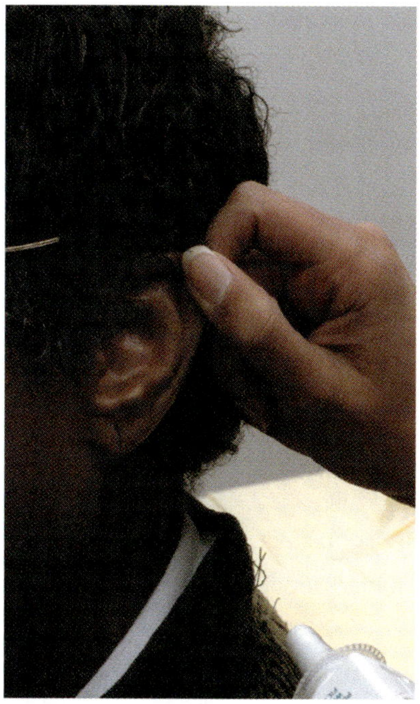

FIGURE 18-14B Gently pull the ear pinna back and up.

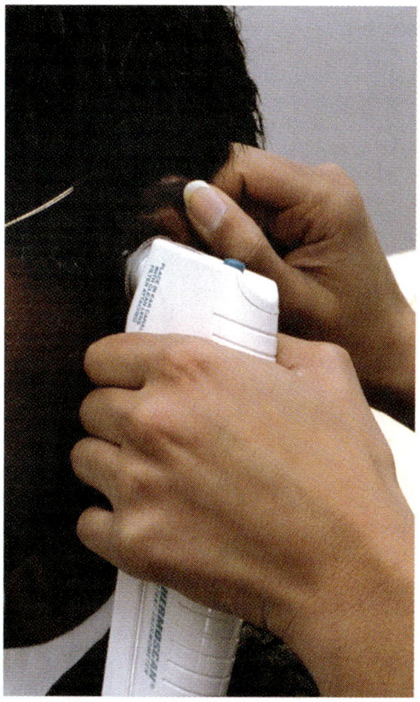

FIGURE 18-14C Place the covered probe in the patient's ear, aiming it toward the tympanic membrane. Insert the probe until it seals the ear canal.

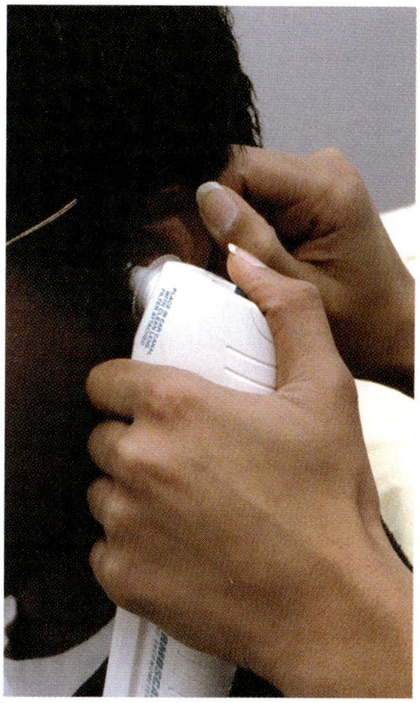

FIGURE 18-14D Press the activation button and leave the thermometer in the ear for the time recommended by the manufacturer.

PROCEDURE 41

CLEANING GLASS THERMOMETERS

1. Wash your hands.
2. Assemble equipment on a tray:
   - Towel
   - Label
   - Washcloth
   - Soiled thermometers in container of soapy water
   - Wash basin
   - Container for clean thermometers
   - Liquid soap
   - Container of cotton balls
   - Facility-approved disinfectant
   - Disposable gloves
3. Take tray of equipment to soiled utility room.
4. Place a towel on the sink side.
5. Wash and dry the container and cover for clean thermometers. Place on the towel with the cover top up.
6. Place gauze in the bottom of the container.
7. Place a clean wash basin in the sink. Line the bottom of the basin with a washcloth. (This is done to reduce the risk of breakage if you accidentally drop a thermometer.) Fill the basin one-third full with cool water. Apply gloves.
8. Slowly turn on the cold water faucet.

continues

PROCEDURE 41

continued

9. Moisten a sponge/cotton ball and apply soap.
10. Pick up one thermometer at a time, holding it by the stem.
    a. Using a circular motion, cleanse the thermometer from stem to bulb.
    b. Discard cotton ball.
    c. Carefully rinse the thermometer.
    d. Using a circular motion and a new, dry cotton ball for each, dry each thermometer.
    e. Check thermometers for chips and shake down to 96°F (21°C) or below before placing them in the clean container (Figure 18-15A).
    f. Fill the clean container half full with disinfectant (Figure 18-15B).
    g. Empty the water from the dirty container.
11. Shut off the faucet. Squeeze out the washcloth and put it into the laundry. Shut the basin drain and add hot water and soap.
12. Wash, rinse, and dry the dirty thermometer container and wash basin.
13. Remove gloves and discard according to facility policy.
14. Add disinfectant, if necessary, so that each thermometer is completely covered by it.
15. Place a cover on the container. Place a label with the date, time, and your initials on the container. Remember that disinfectants take time to be effective.
16. Place towel in laundry. Dispose of used sponges or cotton balls in trash.
17. Leave area neat and tidy.
18. After disinfecting:
    a. Remove label. Remove thermometers.
    b. Empty disinfectant.
    c. Wash and dry container.
    d. Place 4 × 4 folded sponge on the bottom of the container.
19. Rinse and dry thermometers.
20. Place dry, clean thermometers on a sponge in the container and cover (Figure 18-15C).
21. Store according to facility policy in clean area.
22. Wash your hands and report completion of task to the nurse.

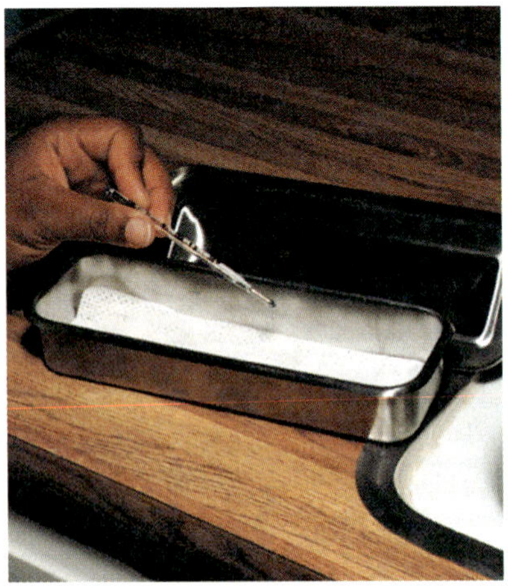

FIGURE 18-15A Place in a clean container that has folded gauze on the bottom to prevent breakage of thermometers.

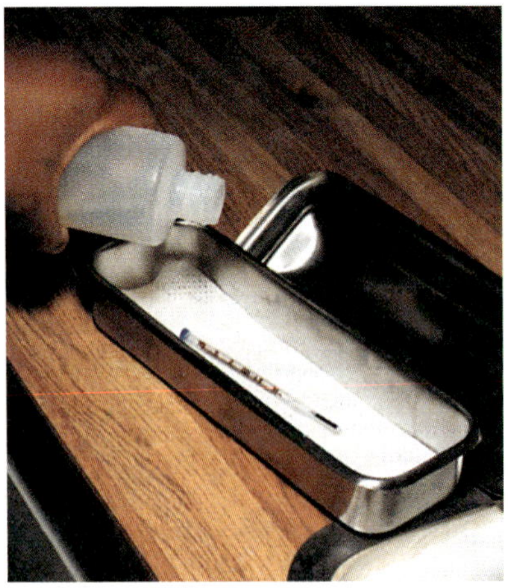

FIGURE 18-15B Add disinfectant solution, being sure to cover the entire thermometer.

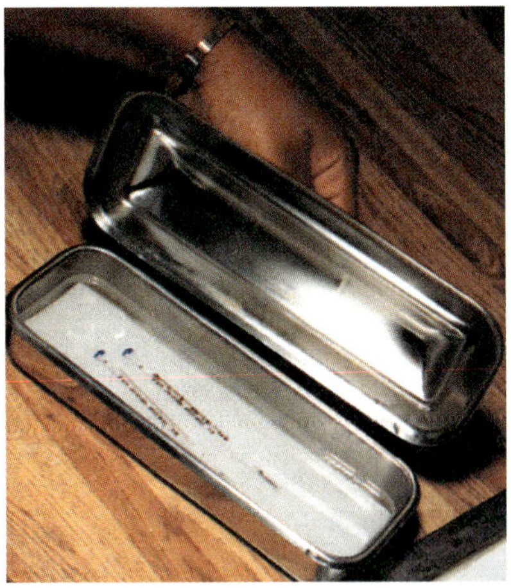

FIGURE 18-15C Allow thermometers to soak for the required time, then remove and rinse well before storing in a clean, dry container.

REVIEW

A. True/False.

Mark the following true or false by circling T or F.

1. T F When charting an axillary temperature, always print AX after the reading.

2. T F Readings taken with a plastic thermometer may not be entirely accurate.

3. T F Temperature is the measurement of body heat.

4. T F The most common method of measuring the temperature of a cooperative adult is by mouth.

5. T F To measure a rectal temperature, the patient is best positioned on her back.

6. T F 96.8°F is an average oral temperature.

7. T F Only temperature variations of more than 5°F should be reported to the nurse.

8. T F Clinical thermometers can be identified by the shapes of their bulbs.

9. T F The probe of an electronic thermometer is covered with a red sheath for rectal use.

10. T F The axillary temperature of a patient will register approximately one degree higher than his oral temperature.

11. T F The tympanic temperature reading is the most accurate.

12. T F A freezing temperature registered in Celsius readings would be 32°.

13. T F It would be unsafe to use glass oral thermometers with children.

14. T F If safely placed, rectal thermometers need not be held.

15. T F Wait 5 minutes after the patient has taken hot liquids to measure an oral temperature.

16. T F When washing used glass thermometers, always wash them in hot, soapy water.

17. T F Always wipe the axillary area before placing a thermometer.

18. T F When using an electronic thermometer, you should not allow your fingers to touch the probe sheath.

19. T F All rectal thermometers should be lubricated before insertion.

20. T F The oral thermometer should remain in place for one minute.

21. T F The liquid column in a glass oral thermometer should register below 96°F at the beginning of the procedure.

22. T F There may be times when a temperature has to be measured in the groin area.

23. T F Each long line on the stem of a clinical thermometer indicates an increase of 2 degrees of temperature.

24. T F Each short line on the stem of the clinical thermometer indicates a 0.2-degree increase in temperature.

25. T F Measuring the temperature in the groin area gives the most accurate indication of body temperature.

B. Completion.

Complete the statements by choosing the correct words from the following list.

Fahrenheit	less
higher	temperature
pulse	tympanic

26. Vital signs include ______ , ______ , respiration, and blood pressure.

27. A normal temperature reading of 98.6° would be in the ______ scale.

28. A ______ thermometer is used to measure the temperature in the ear.

29. A 3-month-old child might be expected to have a slightly ______ temperature normally than a child who is 9 years old.

30. Temperature is ______ stable in children than in adults.

C. Nursing Assistant Challenge.

31. Mrs. LeJune is having difficulty breathing and is very restless. The nurse instructs you to measure her temperature. What type of thermometer would you choose if all were available?

a. Glass oral thermometer
b. Glass rectal thermometer
c. Electronic oral thermometer
d. Tympanic thermometer

32. You are about to measure a rectal temperature with a glass thermometer. You find a small chip in the glass. What should you do?

a. Use the thermometer, because it is just a small chip.
b. Throw the thermometer in the wastepaper basket.
c. Break the thermometer in half so no one else will use it.
d. Replace it with another thermometer.

33. You are assigned to measure your patient's rectal temperature using a glass thermometer. How long should you hold the thermometer in place?
a. 3 minutes
b. 10 minutes
c. 15 minutes
d. 20 minutes

EXPLORING THE WEB

Description	Location
Assessment	*http://www.delmarhealthcare.com/olcs/white/pnotes.asp* (see Chapter 25)
Measuring vital signs	*http://www.delmarhealthcare.com/olcs/delaune/ppt/DeLaunechapter%2027.ppt*
Temperature regulation	*http://phy025.lubb.ttuhsc.edu*
Accuracy of Core Temperature Measurement with the IVAC® CORE·CHECK™ Tympanic Thermometer System	*http://www.alarismed.com*
Accuracy of the CORE·CHECK® Tympanic Thermometer for Pediatric Core Temperature Measurement	*http://www.alarismed.com*
The Facts About Tympanic Thermometers and Cross Contamination	*http://www.alarismed.com*
Going Green (resource kit for eliminating mercury in health care)	*http://www.noharm.org*
Mercury Free at NIH	*http://www.nih.gov/od/ors/ds/nomercury*
Mercury Thermometers and Your Family's Health	*http://www.noharm.org*
Planning and Holding a Mercury Thermometer Exchange	*http://www.noharm.org*
Sustainable Hospitals	*http://www.sustainablehospitals.org*
Taking a Tympanic Temperature	*http://www.alarismed.com*
Techniques of Vital Signs	*http://hsc.virginia.edu*
Wong on Web Sites of Temperature Measurement in Children	*http://www.us.elsevierhealth.com*

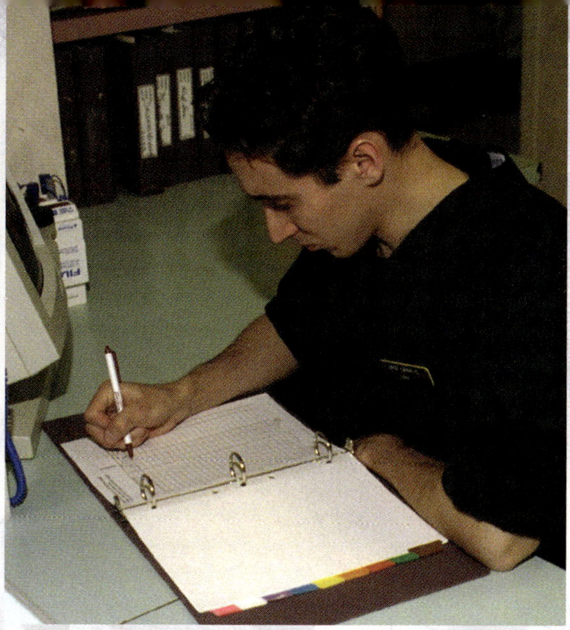

unit 19

Pulse and Respiration

objectives

After completing this unit, you will be able to:

- Spell and define terms.
- Define pulse.
- Explain the importance of monitoring a pulse rate.
- Locate the pulse sites.
- Identify the range of normal pulse and respiratory rates.
- Measure the pulse at different locations.
- List the characteristics of the pulse and respiration.
- Demonstrate the following procedures:
  - Procedure 42 Counting the Radial Pulse
  - Procedure 43 Counting the Apical-Radial Pulse
  - Procedure 44 Counting Respirations

vocabulary

Learn the meaning and the correct spelling of the following words and phrases:

accelerated
apical pulse
apnea
bradycardia
Cheyne-Stokes respirations
cyanosis
dyspnea
expiration
inspiration
pulse
pulse deficit
radial pulse
rales
rate
respiration
rhythm
stertorous
symmetry
tachycardia
tachypnea
volume

INTRODUCTION

The pulse and respiration of the patient are usually counted during the same procedure. Because breathing is partly under voluntary control, a person is able to stop or alter breathing temporarily for a short period. For example, when a patient realizes that her breathing is being watched and counted, she alters her breathing pattern without meaning to do so. To avoid this, the respirations are counted immediately following the pulse count without telling the patient. The patient's hand is kept in the same position, and your fingers remain on the pulse point so that you seem to still be taking the pulse.

THE PULSE

The **pulse** is:

- The pressure of the blood felt against the wall of an artery as the heart alternately contracts (beats) and relaxes (rests).
- More easily felt in arteries that come fairly close to the skin and can be gently pressed against a bone.
- The same in all arteries throughout the body.
- An indication of how the cardiovascular system is meeting the body's needs.

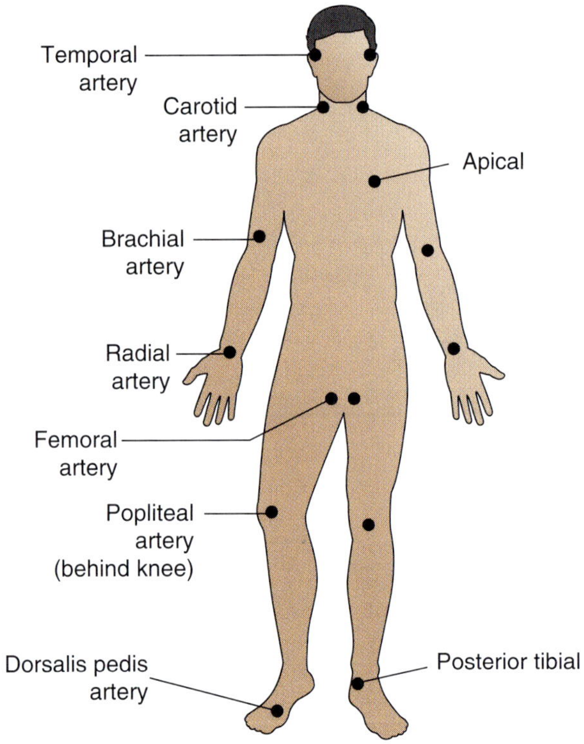

FIGURE 19-1 Common pulse sites of the body.

Radial Pulse

The **radial pulse** is the most commonly measured pulse. It is measured at the radial artery in the wrist. Figure 19-1 shows areas of the body where other large blood vessels come close enough to the surface to be used as sites for counting the pulse. Conscious patients can be checked at the radial artery. (See Procedure 42.) Unconscious patients should be checked at the carotid artery or apically (over the heart).

Pulse measurement includes determining the:

1. Rate or speed
   a. **Bradycardia**—an unusually slow pulse (below 60 beats per minute)
   b. **Tachycardia**—an unusually fast pulse (more than 100 beats per minute)
2. Character
   a. **Rhythm**—regularity
   b. Volume or fullness

Report:

- Pulse rates over 100 beats per minute (bpm) (tachycardia)
- Pulse rates under 60 bpm (bradycardia)
- Irregularities in character (rhythm and volume)

Pulse rates can be affected by:

- Illness
- Emotions
- Age
- Exercise
- Elevated temperature
- Sex
- Position
- Physical training
- Lowered temperature
- Drugs

Table 19-1 shows average pulse rates.

TABLE 19-1 AVERAGE PULSE RATES

Patient	Beats per Minute
Adult men	60–70
Adult women	65–80
Children over 7 years	75–100
Preschoolers	80–110
Infants	120–160

PROCEDURE 42

COUNTING THE RADIAL PULSE

1. Carry out beginning procedure actions.
2. Place the patient in a comfortable position. The palm of the hand should be down and the arm should rest on a flat surface.
3. Locate the pulse on the thumb side of the wrist with the tips of your first three fingers (Figure 19-2). Do not use your thumb—it contains a pulse that may be confused with the patient's pulse.
4. When the pulse is felt, exert slight pressure. Using the second hand of your watch, count for one minute. It is the practice in some hospitals to count for one-half minute and multiply by two and to record the rate for one minute. A one-minute count is preferred and must be done if the pulse is irregular.
5. Remember the reading when counting respirations. Record the reading on your pad as soon as possible.
6. Carry out procedure completion actions.

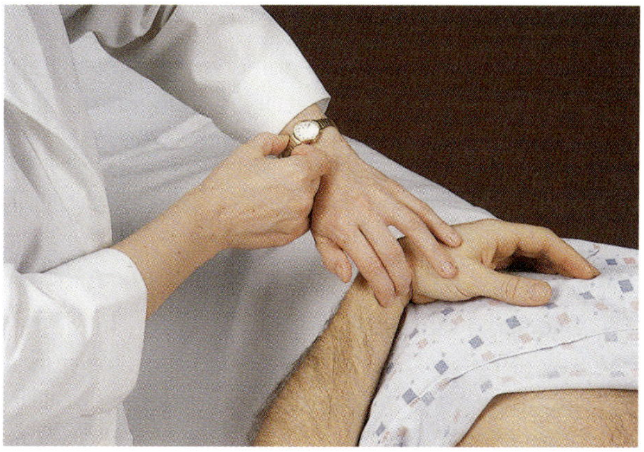

FIGURE 19-2 Locate the pulse on the thumb side of the wrist with the tips of your first three fingers.

The Apical Pulse

An **apical pulse** is measured by counting the heart contractions. The stethoscope is placed over the apex (tip) of the heart. Listen for the heart sounds that indicate closing of the valves. These sounds occur as the heart pumps blood into the arteries. The sounds should occur at the same rate as the pulse that is felt as an expansion of the radial artery. The apex of the heart is found:

- On the left side of the front of the chest
- Between the fifth and sixth ribs
- Just below the left nipple
- In women, under the left breast

Listen carefully for two sounds: lub dub. The louder sound (lub) corresponds to the contraction of the ventricles pushing the blood forward through the arteries, and the closing of the valves to prevent the backflow of blood. This is the sound to be counted. The softer sound (dub) corresponds to the relaxation of the ventricles as they fill with blood before the next contraction and the closing of the semilunar valves to prevent backflow from the arteries.

When documenting an apical pulse reading, write "AP" after the value.

Apical-Radial Pulse Rate

The apical and radial pulse rate is a comparison of the apical rate and the radial rate. Usually they are the same.

Sometimes the contraction of the heart is so weak that it fails to send enough blood to the arteries to expand them. When this happens, no pulse is felt. In this case, the number of loud sounds do not correspond with the number of pulses felt in the radial artery.

The difference between the apical pulse (the loud sounds heard over the heart) and the radial pulse (the expansion felt over the radial pulse) is called a **pulse deficit**. Two people measure the heart rate and the radial pulse at the same time. (See Procedure 43.) The nurse measures the apical pulse while the second person counts the radial pulse for 1 minute. The rates are then compared.

Apical pulse rates are checked:

- Whenever a pulse deficit exists or is suspected.
- Before the registered nurse administers drugs that alter the heart rate or rhythm.
- In children whose rapid rates might be difficult to count at the radial artery.

PROCEDURE 43

COUNTING THE APICAL-RADIAL PULSE

1. Carry out beginning procedure actions.
2. Clean the stethoscope earpieces and bell with disinfectant.
3. Place the stethoscope earpieces in your ears with tips facing slightly forward for better fit.
4. Place the stethoscope diaphragm or bell over the apex of the patient's heart. If it is cold, warm the diaphragm with your hands before placing it on the patient's chest.
5. Listen carefully for the heartbeat.
6. Count the louder sounding beats for one minute.
7. Check the radial pulse for one minute. The best way to obtain these numbers is to have the nurse count the apical pulse while you take the radial pulse (Figure 19-3).
8. Note results on a pad for comparison.
9. Clean earpieces and bell of stethoscope with disinfectant.
10. Carry out procedure completion actions.

    Example: Apical pulse = 108

    Radial pulse = 82

    Pulse deficit = 26 (108 − 82 = 26)

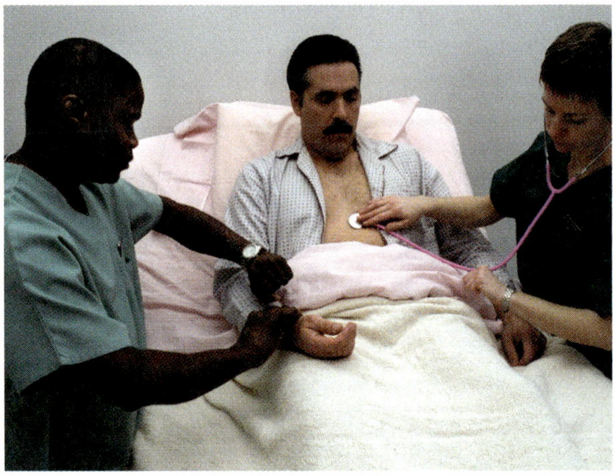

FIGURE 19-3 The nurse takes the apical pulse while the nursing assistant takes the radial pulse.

- For one full minute.
- On any child 12 months of age or younger.
- Whenever you are uncertain of the accuracy of the radial pulse or it is irregular.

Pulse deficits are found in some forms of heart disease.

RESPIRATION

The main function of **respiration** is to supply the cells in the body with oxygen and to rid the body of excess carbon dioxide. When respirations are inefficient, there is less oxygen in the blood available for body needs. In addition, carbon dioxide is released less efficiently. The skin takes on a bluish or dusky color and the patient develops a condition known as **cyanosis**.

There are two parts to each respiration: one **inspiration** (inhalation) followed by one **expiration** (exhalation). Special terms describe different breathing patterns:

- Normal—regular, 16 to 20 breaths per minute
- **Tachypnea**—rapid, shallow breathing
- **Dyspnea**—difficult or labored breathing
- Shallow—breaths that only partially fill the lungs
- **Apnea**—a period of no respirations
- **Cheyne-Stokes respirations**—a period of dyspnea followed by periods of apnea
- **Stertorous**—Snoring-like respirations
- **Rales** (crackles)—moist respirations. At times, fluid (mucus) will collect in the air passages. This causes a bubbling type of respiration. Rales are common in the dying patient.
- Wheezing—difficult breathing accompanied by a whistling or sighing sound due to narrowing of bronchioles (as in asthma) or an increase of mucus in the bronchi.

Respirations should be checked for:

- **Rate**—number of respirations per minute
- Rhythm—regularity
- **Symmetry**—ability of the chest to expand equally as air enters each lung
- **Volume**—depth of respiration
- Character—terms used to describe the character of respirations include:
  - Regular
  - Irregular
  - Shallow
  - Deep
  - Labored (difficult)

PROCEDURE 44

COUNTING RESPIRATIONS

1. When the pulse rate has been counted, you may leave your fingers on the radial pulse and start counting the number of times the chest rises and falls during one minute (Figure 19-4). Count one inhalation and one exhalation as one respiration.
2. Note the depth and regularity of respirations.
3. Record the time, rate, depth, and regularity of respirations.

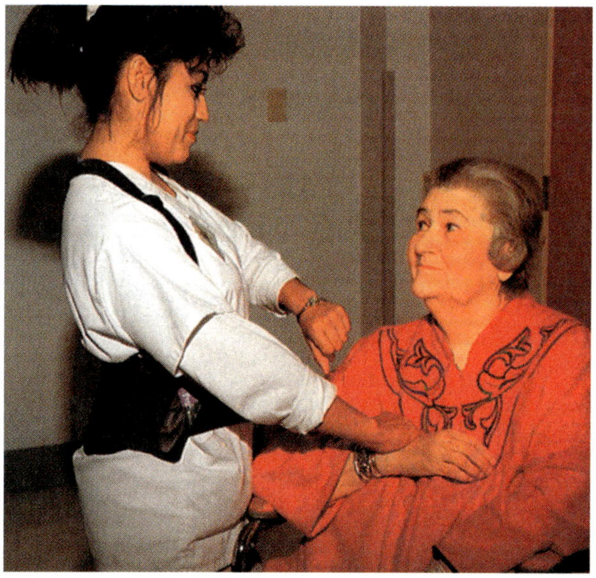

FIGURE 19-4 Continue to rest the back of the hand against the chest wall while counting respirations.

The rate of respiration is determined by counting the rise or fall of the chest for one minute, using a watch equipped with a second hand. (See Procedure 44.)

- The average rate for adults is 16 to 20 respirations per minute.
- If the rate is more than 25 per minute, it is said to be **accelerated**. Accelerated respiration should be reported.
- If the rate is less than 12 per minute, it is too slow. It should be reported.

Remember that, if possible, respirations should be counted without the patient's knowing that you are doing so; the rate and volume may change if the patient knows they are being counted. You might count respirations before or after counting the radial pulse. Continue pressing on the pulse area while counting.

The factors affecting respiratory rates include:

- Illness
- Emotions
- Elevated temperature
- Sex
- Age
- Exercise
- Position
- Drugs

Temperature, pulse, and respiration (TPR) rates and character are recorded in a notebook and then transferred to the patient's chart (Figure 19-5).

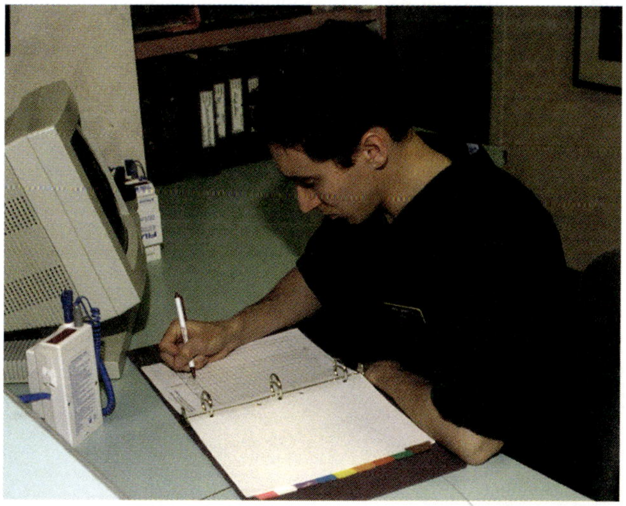

FIGURE 19-5 TPR readings are recorded in the patient's medical record.

REVIEW

A. True/False.

Mark the following true or false by circling T or F.

1. T F A pulse deficit results when there is a difference between the apical and radial pulses.
2. T F The pulse is the pressure of blood against the arterial wall.
3. T F Cheyne-Stokes respirations are deep and regular.
4. T F Pulses differ when counted at different pulse sites.
5. T F The pulse rate of an infant is 110 to 130 bpm.
6. T F An apical pulse should be counted in children.
7. T F The most often used pulse site is the carotid artery.
8. T F The respiratory system rids the body of excess carbon dioxide.
9. T F Mucus in the air passages causes rales.
10. T F A pulse is best counted using the thumb placed over the artery.

B. Matching.

Choose the correct word from Column II to match the words and phrases in Column I.

Column I	Column II
11. ____ Snoring types of respiration	a. accelerated
12. ____ Bluish discoloration to the skin	b. apnea
13. ____ Regularity	c. bradycardia
14. ____ Periods of no respiration	d. cyanosis
15. ____ Difficult breathing	e. dyspnea
16. ____ Rapid respirations	f. rate
17. ____ Increased or speeded up	g. rhythm
18. ____ Expiration	h. stertorous
19. ____ Speed	i. tachypnea
20. ____ Slow pulse	j. inspiration
	k. exhalation

C. Nursing Assistant Challenge.

21. Mrs. Morgan has a heart condition that makes her heart rate irregular and faster than normal. Her respirations are difficult or rapid, labored, and moist. She receives a medication that profoundly alters her heart action. Your orders are to assist in determining the pulse deficit. Answer the statements using the terms in the following list.

apical	rales
dyspnea	tachycardia
radial	tachypnea

   a. The faster heart rate is described as ______.
   b. The difficult respirations can be charted as ______.
   c. Moist respirations are best described as ______.
   d. Rapid respirations are also called ______.
   e. Which pulse rate will you count? ______.
   f. Which pulse rate will a second person count? ______.

22. List two reasons why a radial-apical pulse rate would be ordered.
   a. ______________________________
   b. ______________________________

EXPLORING THE WEB

Description	Location
Assessment	*http://www.delmarhealthcare.com/olcs/white/pnotes.asp* (see Chapter 25)
Measuring vital signs	*http://www.delmarhealthcare.com/olcs/delaune/ppt/DeLaunechapter%2027.ppt*
Techniques of Vital Signs	*http://hsc.virginia.edu*

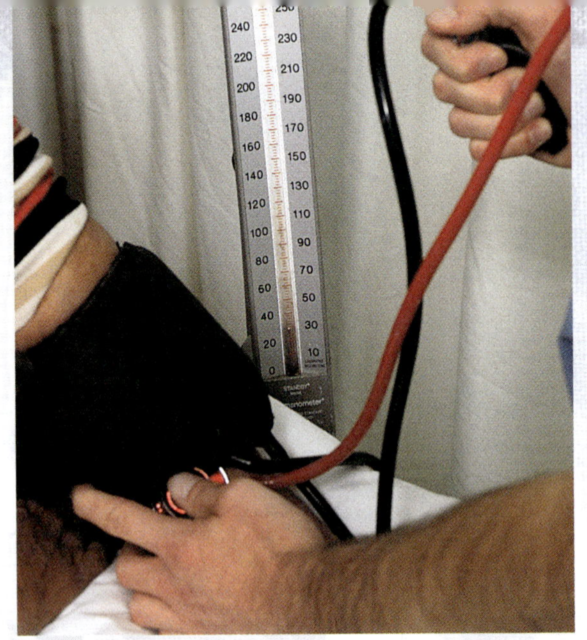

unit 20

Blood Pressure

objectives

After completing this unit, you will be able to:

- Spell and define terms.
- Describe the factors that influence blood pressure.
- Identify the range of normal blood pressure values.
- Identify the causes of inaccurate blood pressure readings.
- Select the proper size blood pressure cuff.
- List precautions associated with use of the sphygmomanometer.
- Demonstrate the following procedure:
  - Procedure 45 Taking Blood Pressure
  - Procedure 46 Taking Blood Pressure with an Electronic Blood Pressure Apparatus

vocabulary

Learn the meaning and the correct spelling of the following words and phrases:

aneroid gauge
auscultatory gap
blood pressure
brachial artery
depressant
diastole
diastolic pressure
elasticity
fasting
hypertension
hypotension
pulse pressure
sphygmomanometer
stethoscope
stimulant
systole
systolic pressure

INTRODUCTION

Blood pressure is the fourth vital sign. It is the measure of the force of the blood against the walls of the arteries. Blood pressure depends on the:

- Volume (amount of blood in the circulatory system).
- Force of the heartbeat.
- Condition of the arteries. Arteries that have lost their **elasticity** (stretch) give more resistance. The pressure is greater in these arteries.
- Distance from the heart. Blood pressure in the legs is lower than in the arms.

Pressure varies with contraction (**systole**) and relaxation (**diastole**) of the ventricles of the heart.

- Systolic blood pressure reading indicates the period when the pressure within the arteries is the greatest, during contraction of the ventricles. The systolic blood pressure is the working pressure.
- Diastolic reading indicates the lowest point of pressure between ventricular contractions. The diastolic blood pressure is the resting pressure.

Blood pressure is elevated by:

- Sex of the patient (males slightly higher than females before menopause)
- Exercise
- Eating
- **Stimulants** (substances that speed up body functions)
- Emotional stress, such as anger, fear, or sexual activity
- Disease conditions, such as arteriosclerosis (hardening of the arteries), elevated cholesterol, or diabetes mellitus
- Hereditary factors
- Pain
- Obesity
- Age
- Condition of blood vessels
- Some drugs

Blood pressure is lowered by:

- **Fasting** (not eating)
- Rest
- **Depressants** (drugs that slow down body functions)
- Weight loss
- Emotions (such as grief)
- Abnormal conditions such as hemorrhage (loss of blood) or shock
- Dehydration and fluid loss
- Some drugs, such as antihypertensives (drugs that lower blood pressure in persons who have hypertension)
- Diuretics (drugs that lower the volume of body fluids)

The factors affecting blood pressure are:

- Age
- Sleep
- Weight
- Emotion
- Heredity
- Gender
- Viscosity of blood
- Condition of blood vessels

EQUIPMENT

The **sphygmomanometer** (blood pressure measuring apparatus) consists of:

- A cuff (different sizes are available) that fits around the patient's arm. There is a rubber bladder inside the cuff. A pressure control button is attached to the cuff. It is important to use the proper size cuff when measuring blood pressure. Cuffs that are too wide or too narrow will give inaccurate readings (Figure 20-1). To check the size of the cuff, compare the length of the rubber bladder inside the cuff (Figure 20-2) with the patient's arm circumference. The bladder should be at least 80% of the circumference of the arm. If it is larger or smaller, obtain a different size cuff.
- Two tubes. One tube is connected to the pressure control bulb and to the bladder inside the cuff. The other tube is connected to the pressure gauge.
- A pressure gauge, which may be a column of mercury (Figure 20-3A) or a round **aneroid gauge** (Figure 20-3B) dial. Both are marked with numbers.

The **stethoscope** (Figure 20-4) magnifies sounds. It consists of:

- A bell or diaphragm.
- Tubing that carries sounds to the listener.
- Earpieces that direct the sounds into the listener's ears. The earpieces and diaphragm must be cleaned with antiseptic before and after each use to prevent transmission of disease.

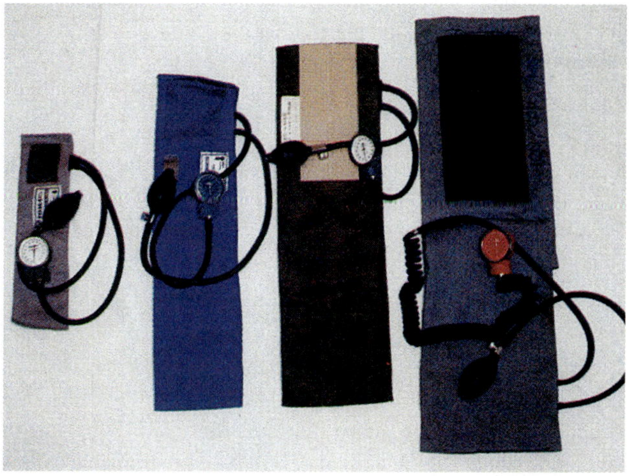

FIGURE 20-1 A variety of cuff sizes are available. The cuff must fit properly for accurate readings.

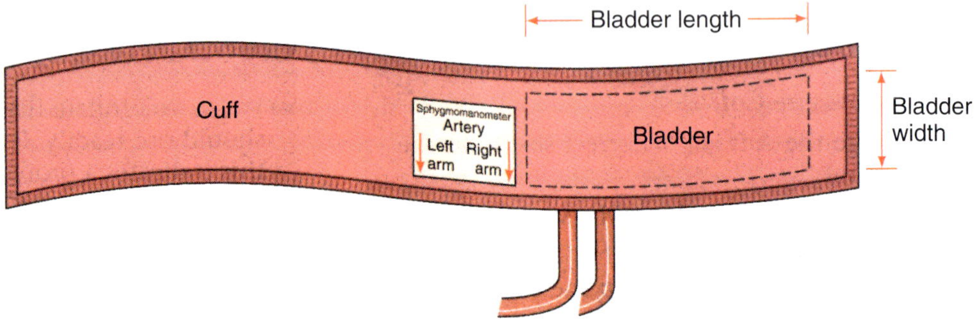

FIGURE 20-2 The bladder inside the cuff should be 80% the circumference of the patient's arm.

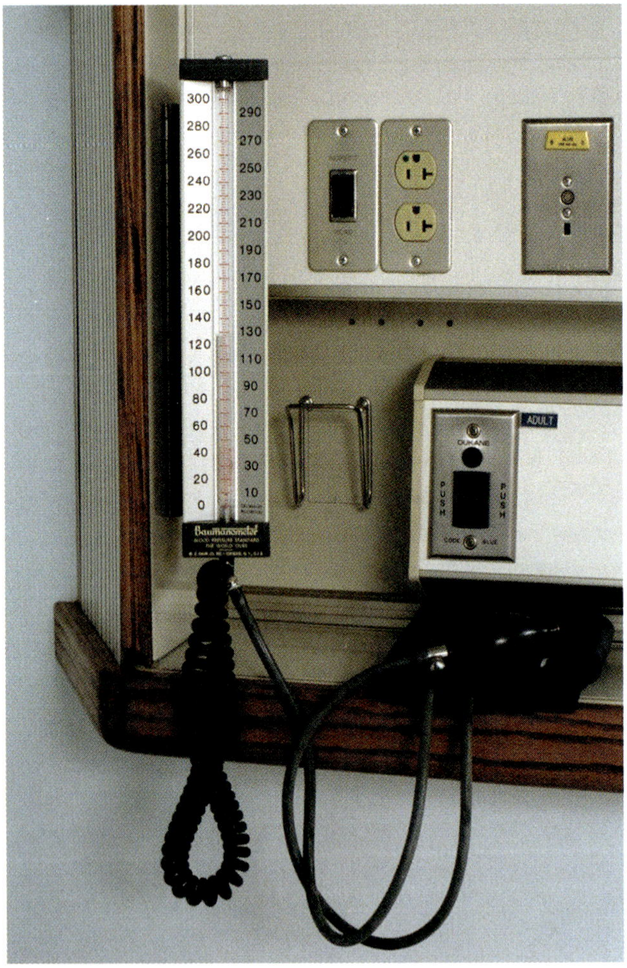

FIGURE 20-3A A mercury gravity sphygmomanometer.

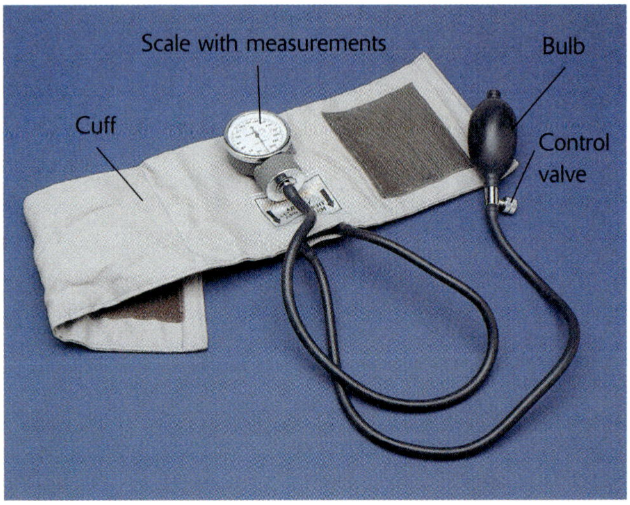

FIGURE 20-3B A dial (aneroid) sphygmomanometer.

Electronic sphygmomanometers with attached cuffs are used in some facilities. You do not have to use a stethoscope with these units, because they automatically register the readings on a digital display. Follow the manufacturer's directions for the type of unit you are using.

Some facilities use an instrument that measures pulse rate, temperature, and blood pressure (Figure 20-5).

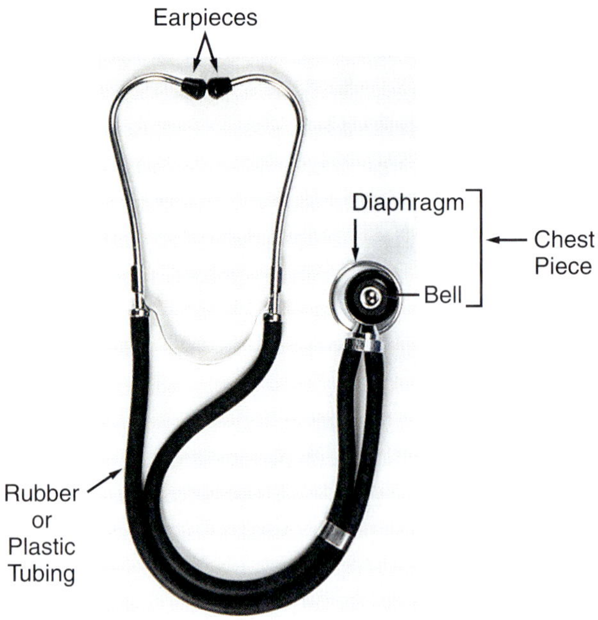

FIGURE 20-4 Stethoscope.

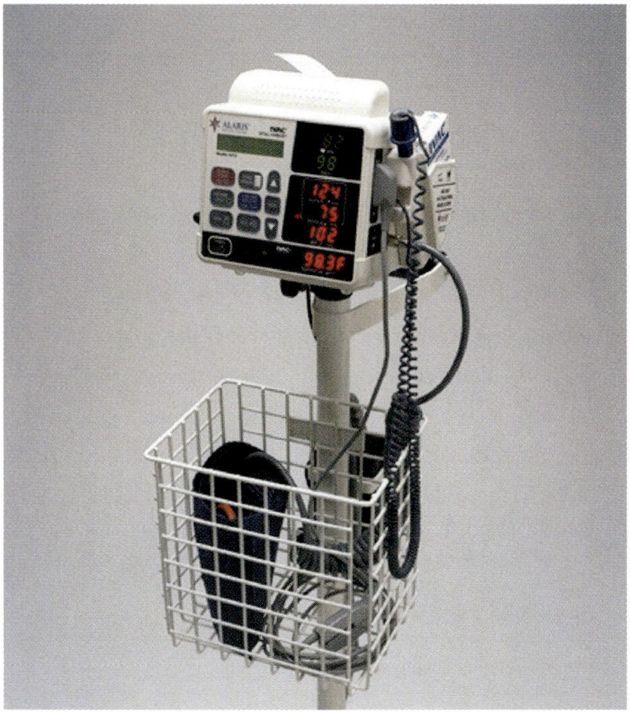

FIGURE 20-5 All vital signs may be checked with a single instrument. *(Vital•Check® patient monitor; photo courtesy of Alaris Medical Systems Inc., San Diego, CA)*

MEASURING THE BLOOD PRESSURE

Blood pressure is usually measured in the upper arm over the brachial artery. Blood pressure readings taken anywhere else must be ordered by a doctor. The values are recorded in millimeters of mercury (mm Hg).

1. The cuff is smoothly applied directly over the **brachial artery** (1 inch above the antecubital area).
2. The stethoscope bell is placed over the brachial artery.
3. Pressure is then increased by inflating the rubber bladder in the cuff to stop the flow of blood through the artery.
4. The pressure is slowly released and the sounds of heart valves closing can be heard. The sounds correspond to pressure changes in the blood.
5. The blood pressure is measured:
   a. At its highest point as the **systolic pressure**. This will be the first regular sound you will hear. This is the sound of the bicuspid and tricuspid valves shutting.
   b. At its lowest point as the **diastolic pressure**. This will be the change or last sound you will hear. This is the sound of the semilunar valves shutting.

guidelines *for*

Preparing to Measure Blood Pressure

Before using the stethoscope:

1. Clean the earpieces with an alcohol wipe (Figure 20-6) and clean the bell with a different alcohol wipe.

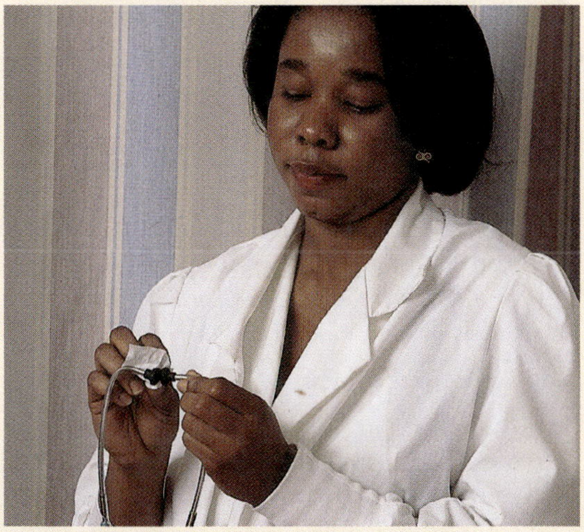

FIGURE 20-6 Clean the earpieces with an alcohol sponge before and after use.

2. Point the earpieces forward when inserting them in your ears.
3. Use the bell portion of the stethoscope (Figure 20-7).
4. Be sure the bell portion is open so you will hear the beats.

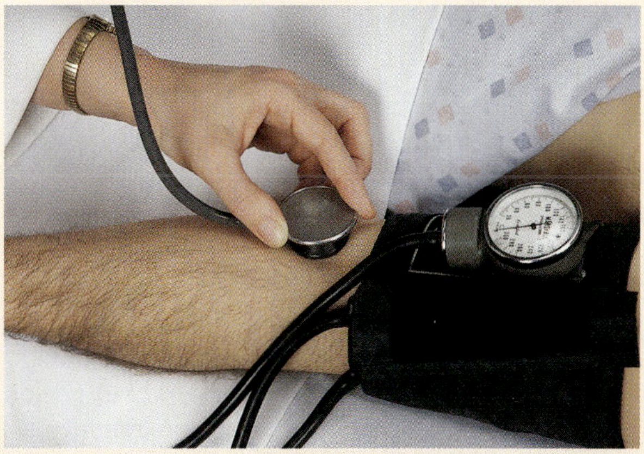

FIGURE 20-7 When taking a blood pressure, use the bell portion of the stethoscope.

continues

guidelines *continued*

Before using a sphygmomanometer:

1. If using a mercury manometer—if the mercury moves up the column very slowly (Figure 20-8), it may have oxidized. Report this to the nurse and use another sphygmomanometer.
2. If using an aneroid manometer—make sure the needle is on zero before you inflate the cuff (Figure 20-9). If it is not, report this to the nurse and use another sphygmomanometer.

Generally:

Turn off radio and television when taking blood pressure. Ask the patient not to talk. Do not take blood pressure on an arm that:

- Has an intravenous feeding or other device inserted
- Is being treated for burns, fractures, or other injuries
- Has a dialysis access device
- Is on the same side as the patient's recent mastectomy (breast removal) or other surgical procedure

SAFETY *Alert*

For accurate blood pressure values, check the stethoscope tubing. Do not use if it has cracks or holes in it. The bell or diaphragm of the stethoscope should not come in contact with the patient's clothing, blood pressure cuff, or other device. Place the bell or diaphragm of the stethoscope flat against the patient's skin and hold it in place. If it is at an angle, you will not be able to hear the sounds. Apply firm but gentle pressure when holding the diaphragm in place. If you press too hard, you will be unable to hear the sound.

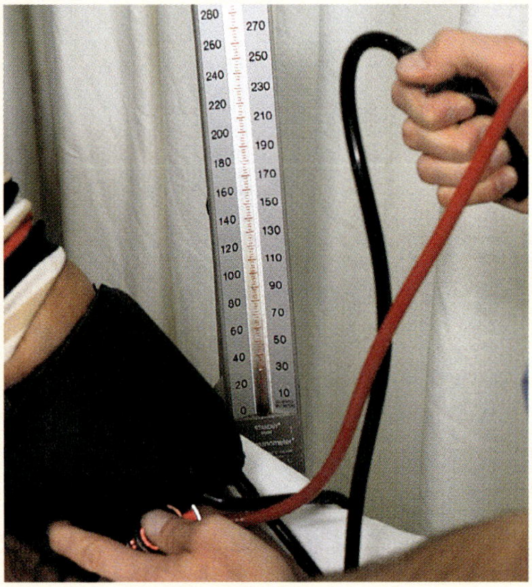

FIGURE 20-8 Do not use the sphygmomanometer if the mercury moves up the column slowly.

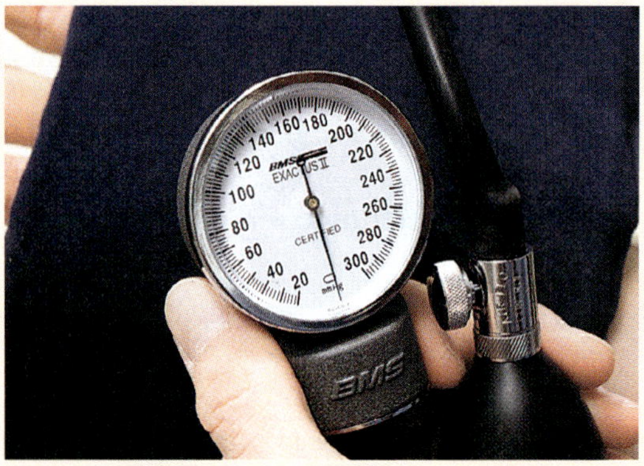

FIGURE 20-9 Make sure the needle is on zero before inflating the cuff on an aneroid sphygmomanometer.

c. The difference between systolic and diastolic pressure is called **pulse pressure**. The pulse pressure gives important information about the health of the arteries. The average pulse pressure in a healthy adult is about 40 millimeters (mm) of mercury (Hg) (range 30–50 mm Hg). However, factors in both health and disease can alter the pulse pressure. An increase in blood volume or heart rate or a decrease in the ability of the arteries to expand may result in an increased pulse pressure.

6. Blood pressure readings are recorded as an improper fraction; for example, systolic/diastolic or 130/92. This means the systolic pressure is 130 and the diastolic pressure is 92. Both numbers in the blood pressure are important, but for people who are 50 or older, systolic pressure gives the most accurate diagnosis of high blood pressure.
7. Blood pressure values:
   a. Average resting adult brachial artery pressure is less than 120 millimeters of mercury (mm Hg) systolic and less than 80 millimeters of mercury (mm Hg) diastolic.
   b. *Prehypertension* is a condition that means you are likely to develop high blood pressure in the future. In this condition, blood pressure is

between 120/80 mm NG and 139/89 mm Hg. People with prehypertension can take steps to decrease their risk.

c. **Hypertension** (high blood pressure) is when values are greater than 140 mm Hg systolic and 90 mm Hg diastolic.
d. **Hypotension** (low blood pressure) is when values are less than 100 mm Hg systolic and 60 mm Hg diastolic. Excessive hypotension can lead to shock.
e. For either hypertension or hypotension, unusual or changed readings must be recorded and reported. (See Procedure 45.)
f. High blood pressure is a dangerous condition. There are no signs and symptoms. It increases the risk of several serious diseases (Unit 39). It can also cause complications of conditions such as diabetes. People with prehypertension and hypertension require regular blood pressure monitoring.
g. Blood pressure classifications are listed in Table 20-1. When systolic and diastolic blood pressures fall into different categories, the higher category is used to classify blood pressure level. For example, 172/78 mm Hg would be stage 2 hypertension (high blood pressure).

Inaccurate Blood Pressure Readings

Causes of inaccurate blood pressure readings include:

- Use of a wrong-size cuff
- An improperly wrapped cuff
- Incorrect positioning of arm
- Not using the same arm for all readings
- Not having the gauge at eye level
- Deflating the cuff too slowly
- Mistaking an **auscultatory gap** (sound fadeout for 10 to 15 mm Hg which then begins again) as the diastolic pressure

TABLE 20-1 BLOOD PRESSURE CLASSIFICATIONS

	Blood Pressure Level (mm Hg)		
Category	**Systolic**		**Diastolic**
Normal	<120	and	<80
Prehypertension	120–139	or	80–89
High Blood Pressure			
Stage I Hypertension	140–159	or	90–99
Stage II Hypertension	≥160	or	≥100

Legend: < means less than; ≥ means greater than or equal to

SAFETY Alert

Do not attempt to measure blood pressure using an arm that is the site of an intravenous infusion, the site of a dialysis access device, paralyzed, injured, or has edema present.

HOW TO READ THE GAUGE

The gauges on sphygmomanometers are marked with a series of lines. The large lines are at increments of 10 millimeters of mercury pressure. The shorter lines are at 2-mm intervals. For example, the first small line above 80 mm is 82 mm. The first small line below 80 mm is 78 mm (Figure 20-10).

To properly read the mercury gauge:

- It should be at eye level.
- It should not be tilted.
- The reading should be taken at the top of the column of mercury. It should not be taken at the "hump" in the middle of the mercury when you hear the first sound.

To properly read the aneroid gauge, observe the gauge at eye level. Do not read it at an angle.

Following completion of the blood pressure measurement, you will record and report the following:

- If you were unable to hear the reading.
- If blood pressure is higher than in a previous reading.
- If blood pressure is lower than in a previous reading.
- If the site where you took the reading was other than brachial artery.

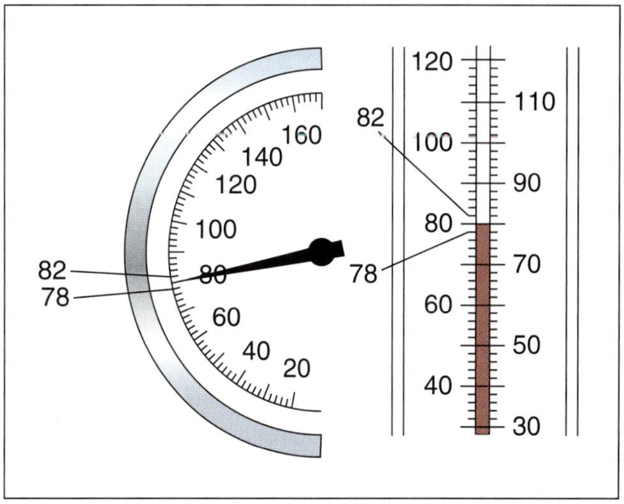

FIGURE 20-10 The aneroid gauge (left) and the mercury gauge (right). Take the reading at the closest line.

PROCEDURE 45

TAKING BLOOD PRESSURE

1. Carry out beginning procedure actions.
2. Assemble equipment:
   - sphygmomanometer with appropriate size cuff
   - stethoscope
   - alcohol wipes
3. Remove the patient's arm from sleeve or roll sleeve 5 inches above the elbow; it should not be tight or binding.
4. Locate the brachial artery with your fingertips (Figure 20-11).
5. Place the patient's arm palm upward, supported on bed or table, at heart level.
6. Wrap the cuff smoothly and snugly around the arm. Center the bladder over the brachial artery. The bottom of the cuff should be 1 inch above the antecubital space (inner elbow) (Figure 20-12).
7. Place the bulb in your dominant hand and feel for the radial pulse with the fingers of your other hand (Figure 20-13). To find out how high to pump the cuff:
   - Rapidly inflate the cuff until you no longer feel the radial pulse.
   - Add 30 mm to that reading. (If you no longer feel the pulse when the mercury or needle reaches 130, add 30 mm for a reading of 160.) Note that point.
8. Quickly and steadily deflate the cuff. Wait 15 to 30 seconds.
9. Place the stethoscope over the brachial artery (Figure 20-14).
10. Reinflate the cuff quickly and steadily to the level you calculated (in the example in step 7, to 160).
11. Release the air at an even pace, about 2 to 3 mm per second. Keep your eyes on the needle or the mercury.
12. Listen for the onset of at least two consecutive beats. Note where the needle is on the sphygmomanometer when you first hear the sound. (Do not stop deflating the cuff.) This is your systolic reading.

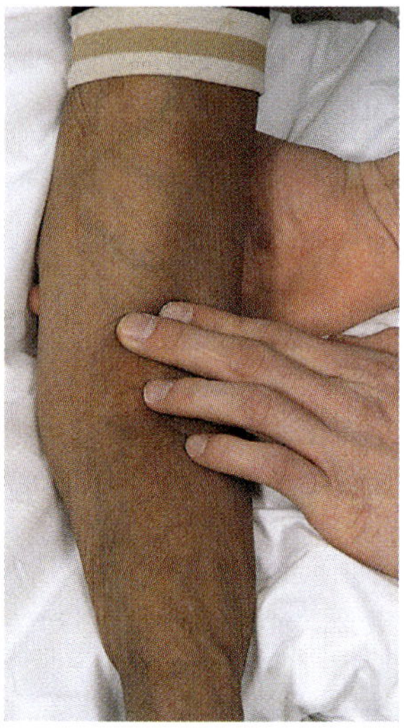

FIGURE 20-11 Locate the brachial artery with your fingertips.

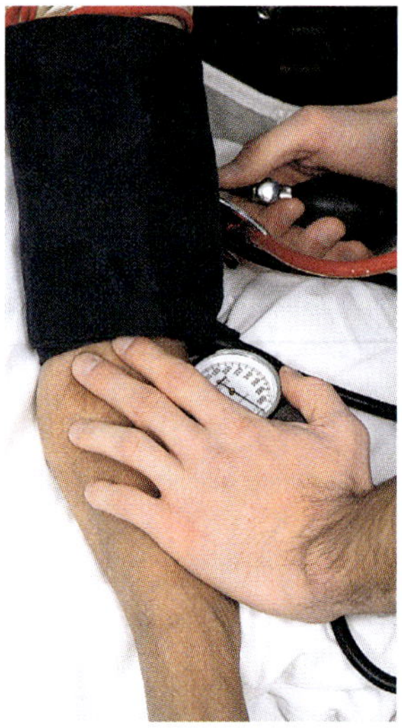

FIGURE 20-12 The bottom of the cuff should be at least 1 inch above the antecubital space (inner elbow).

13. Continue deflating the cuff. The last sound you hear is the diastolic reading. Continue to deflate and to listen for 10 to 20 mm more to make sure you have the correct diastolic reading.
14. Record the reading (blood pressure is always recorded in even numbers, with the systolic on top and the diastolic on the bottom, e.g., 128/82). Indicate the arm used and the position of the patient (sitting, lying down, or standing).
15. If you are not sure of the reading and need to retake the blood pressure, wait 1 to 2 minutes before repeating the procedure.
16. Clean the earpieces of the stethoscope with alcohol wipes. If the tubing has contacted the patient or linen, wipe it as well.
17. Return equipment to the appropriate area.
18. Carry out procedure completion actions.

continues

PROCEDURE 45

continued

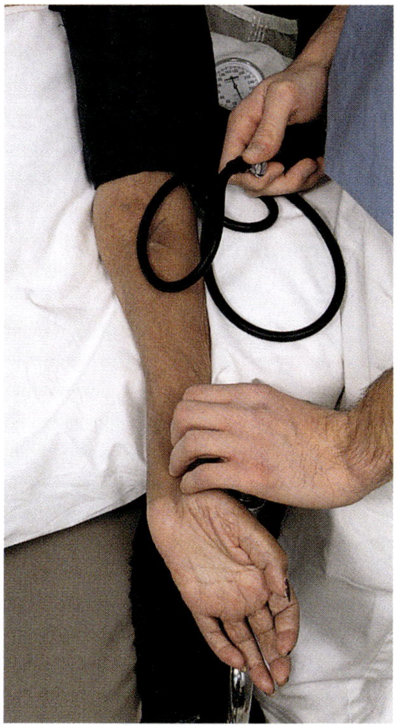

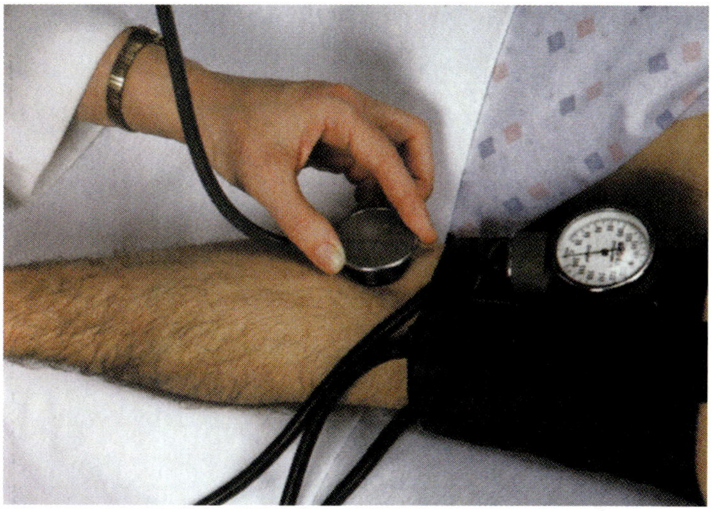

FIGURE 20-14 Position the bell of the stethoscope over the brachial artery.

FIGURE 20-13 Hold the bulb in your dominant hand and feel for the radial pulse with the fingers of the other hand.

guidelines *for*

Electronic Blood Pressure Monitoring

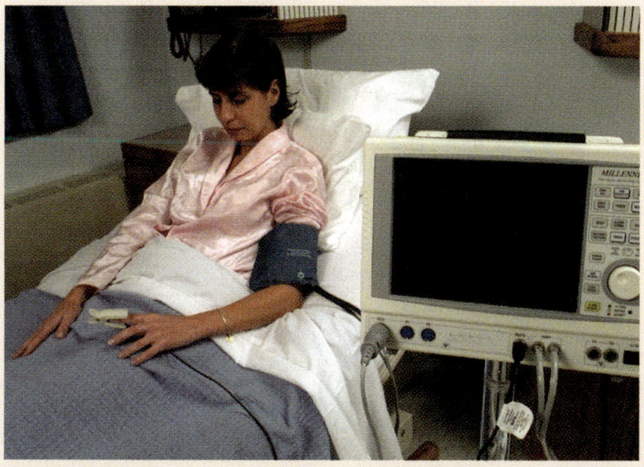

FIGURE 20-15 An electronic blood pressure monitoring unit takes the blood pressure automatically.

Patient Selection (Refer to Figure 20-15)

- This procedure can be done on patients of all ages and sizes, but appropriately sized cuffs must be used.
- At least one blood pressure reading should be taken using the auscultation method before an electronic blood pressure device is used. The auscultation reading is needed as a baseline with which to compare the values from the electronic device.

The procedure is contraindicated in patients with:

- Extreme hypertension or hypotension
- Very rapid heart rates
- Excessive body movement or tremors
- Irregular heart rhythms or atrial dysrhythmias

continues

guidelines *continued*

Patients for whom electronic blood pressure monitoring is not acceptable should be known to all caregivers and identified on the care plan or Kardex. If in doubt, check with the nurse for instructions for patients with very high blood pressure or rapid or irregular heart (pulse) rates.

Do not place the cuff on an arm that:

- Is paralyzed
- Is the site of an intravenous infusion (IV)
- Has a pulse oximeter on it
- Has impaired circulation
- Is the site of a dialysis access device
- Is fractured
- Is burned
- Is on the same side as a recent mastectomy or other surgical procedure site

Application of the Cuff

- Select the proper cuff size. The width should be equal to 40% of the arm circumference.
- The upper arm is the preferred location for the monitoring cuff, but the forearm and ankle may also be used.

PROCEDURE 46

TAKING BLOOD PRESSURE WITH AN ELECTRONIC BLOOD PRESSURE APPARATUS

1. Carry out beginning procedure actions.
2. Assemble equipment:
   - electronic blood pressure device
   - assortment of cuffs and tubes
3. Bring the electronic blood pressure unit to the bedside. Place it near the patient and plug it into a source of electricity.
4. Locate the on/off switch and turn the machine on.
5. Select the appropriate cuff for the machine and size for the patient's extremity.
6. Remove restrictive clothing.
7. Squeeze excess air out of the cuff.
8. Connect the cuff to the connector hose.
9. Wrap the cuff snugly around the patient's extremity, verifying that only one finger can fit between the cuff and the patient's skin. Make sure the "artery" arrow marked on the outside of the cuff is correctly placed over the brachial artery.
10. Verify that the connector hose between the cuff and the machine is not kinked.
11. Set the frequency control for automatic or manual.
12. Press the start button.
13. If the cuff will take periodic, automatic measurements, set the designated frequency of blood pressure measurements.
14. Set upper and lower alarm limits for systolic, diastolic, and mean blood pressure readings.
15. Remove the cuff at least every 2 hours and alternate sites, if possible. Evaluate the skin for redness and irritation. Report abnormalities to the nurse.
16. Carry out procedure completion actions.

REVIEW

A. True/False.

Mark the following true or false by circling T or F.

1. T F The volume of blood in the circulatory system is a factor in the blood pressure.
2. T F Exercise decreases blood pressure.
3. T F To accurately measure blood pressure, you will need both a sphygmomanometer and a stethoscope.
4. T F Blood pressures taken over arteries closer to the heart will be lower than those taken over arteries farther from the heart.
5. T F A blood pressure below 100/70 would signal hypotension.
6. T F The large lines on the blood pressure gauge are in increments of 20 mm of Hg pressure.
7. T F Depressant drugs elevate the blood pressure.
8. T F Using a blood pressure cuff of the wrong size will give an inaccurate reading.
9. T F When measuring a blood pressure, always keep the gauge at eye level.
10. T F Stethoscope earpieces should be cleaned both before and after use.

B. Matching.

Choose the correct word from Column II to match each phrase in Column I.

Column I	Column II
11. G high blood pressure	**a.** brachial
12. F lowest blood pressure reading	**b.** diastolic
	c. stethoscope
13. ____ stretch	**d.** femoral
14. ____ most common artery used to determine blood pressure	**e.** sphygmomanometer
	f. hypotension
	g. hypertension
15. ____ blood pressure apparatus	**h.** elasticity
	i. systolic

C. Completion.

Complete the statements by choosing the correct word.

16. The closing of the heart valves is heard as the ______ sounds.
    (diastolic) (systolic)
17. High blood pressure is known as ______.
    (hypotension) (hypertension)
18. Blood pressure is lowered when weight is ______.
    (gained) (lost)
19. Blood pressure is raised by ______.
    (rest) (exercise)
20. The earpieces of the stethoscope should be pointed ______ as they are placed in the ears.
    (forward) (backward)

D. Nursing Assistant Challenge.

You are assigned to take Mr. King's blood pressure at 12 noon. He is a very heavy man and has an IV inserted in his left arm. His blood pressure was 180/140 at 8 A.M. Answer the following questions:

21. What effect will his size have on your selection of cuff? ____________________
22. On which arm will you apply the cuff? __________
23. Will you report your findings? ______
24. Why? ____________________

EXPLORING THE WEB

Description	Location
Assessment	*http://www.delmarhealthcare.com/olcs/white/pnotes.asp* (see Chapter 25)
Measuring vital signs	*http://www.delmarhealthcare.com/olcs/delaune/ppt/DeLaunechapter%2027.ppt*
National Institutes of Health Guide to Lowering High Blood Pressure	*http://www.nhlbi.nih.gov/hbp*
Systolic blood pressure treatment	*http://www.advancefornurses.com* (see past articles October 27, 2000)
Does Accurate Blood Pressure Depend on Mercury?	*http://www.noharm.org*
The Elimination of Mercury Sphygmomanometers	*http://www.noharm.org*
Mercury Free at NIH	*http://www.nih.gov/od/ors/ds/nomercury*
Sustainable Hospitals	*http://www.sustainablehospitals.org*
Techniques of Vital Signs	*http://hsc.virginia.edu/med-ed*

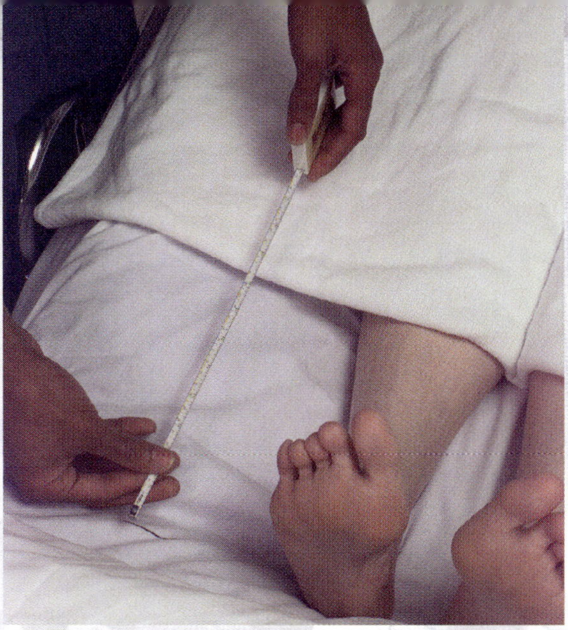

unit 21

Measuring Height and Weight

objectives

After completing this unit, you will be able to:

- Spell and define terms.
- Describe the proper use of an overbed scale.
- Demonstrate the following procedures:
  - Procedure 47 Weighing and Measuring the Patient Using an Upright Scale
  - Procedure 48 Weighing the Patient on a Chair Scale
  - Procedure 49 Measuring Weight with an Electronic Wheelchair Scale
  - Procedure 50 Measuring and Weighing the Patient in Bed

vocabulary

Learn the meaning and the correct spelling of the following words and phrases:

balance bar	**centimeter (cm)**	**kilogram (kg)**
baseline	**increment**	**pound (lb)**

WEIGHT AND HEIGHT MEASUREMENTS

Changes in weight are frequently used as an indicator of the patient's condition.

- A **baseline** (original) measurement of height and weight is usually obtained on admission. These are usually noted on the Kardex.
- Weights are frequently measured when patients are given drugs (diuretics) to increase their urine output.
- Weight is an indicator of the patient's nutritional status.
- Measurements of weight and height must be accurately made and recorded according to facility policy because medications may be ordered according to the patient's size.
- Height measurements may be recorded in feet (') and inches (") or in **centimeters (cm)**.
- Weight measurements may be recorded in **pounds (lb)** or **kilograms (kg)**.

Note: Some facilities use the metric system, so you may be recording weight in kilograms. If your facility uses this measurement system, the scales will be calibrated for the metric system. You will not be required to convert measurements from the inch and pound system to the metric system.

- The upright scale is used for ambulatory patients who can stand unattended on the platform (Figure 21-1).
- A mechanical lift with scale can be used to weigh patients who cannot stand or sit in a wheelchair (Figure 21-2).

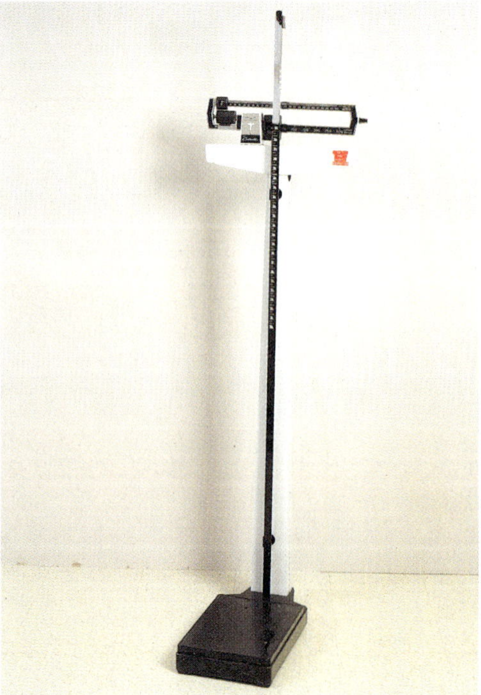

FIGURE 21-1 An upright scale is used only for patients who can stand unaided on the platform.

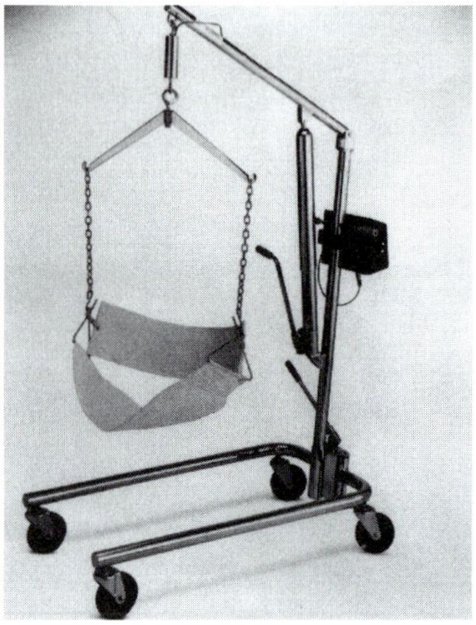

FIGURE 21-2 The scale on the mechanical lift is used when patients are not ambulatory or are too heavy or difficult to move. *(Photo courtesy Health O Meter®)*

- Sling scales can be used to weigh patients whose conditions do not permit the use of a mechanical lift/scale (Figure 21-3).
- Chair scales are used to weigh patients in wheelchairs (Figure 21-4).

(See Procedures 47 to 50.)

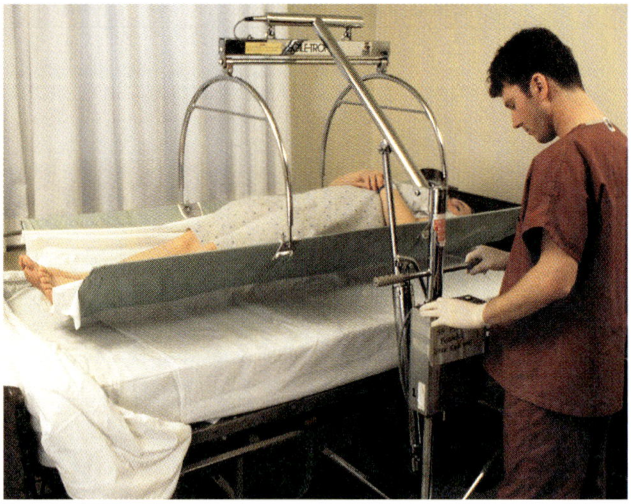

FIGURE 21-3 The sling scale is used for bedfast patients who cannot sit or stand.

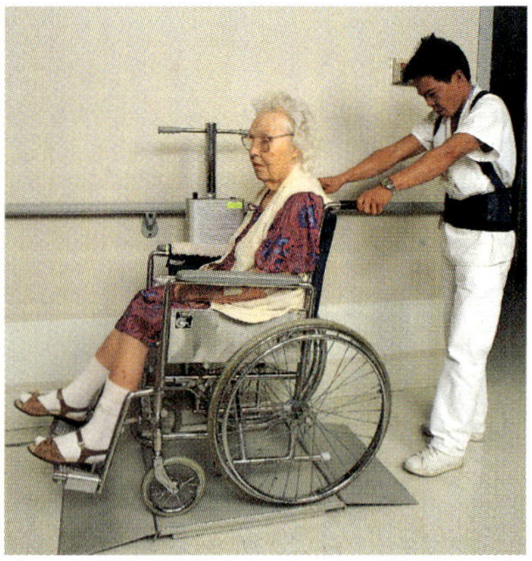

FIGURE 21-4 Electronic chair scales are used for patients who cannot stand on an upright scale.

guidelines *for*

Obtaining Accurate Weight and Height Measurements

To obtain an accurate weight measurement, you must:

- Always balance the scale before using.
- Have the patient empty his or her bladder.
- Weigh the patient at the same time of day each time.
- Have the patient wear the same type of garments each time.
- Use the same method and the same scale each time, if possible.

You must learn to read the scale correctly. There are two bars on the upright scale (see Figure 21-1). The **balance bar** should hang free to start.

- The lower bar indicates weights in 50-pound **increments** (amounts).
- The upper bar indicates one-quarter-pound increments (Figure 21-5).
- The even-numbered pounds are marked with numbers.
- The long line between each number indicates the odd-numbered pounds.
- Each small line indicates one-quarter pound, or 4 ounces.

The two figures are added and recorded as the person's total weight. The sum is recorded according to facility policy in either pounds or kilograms. For example:

Large bar = 100 pounds
Small bar = +22 pounds
Total = 122 pounds

- Height is measured with the ruler attached to an upright scale or with a tape measure when the patient is in bed.

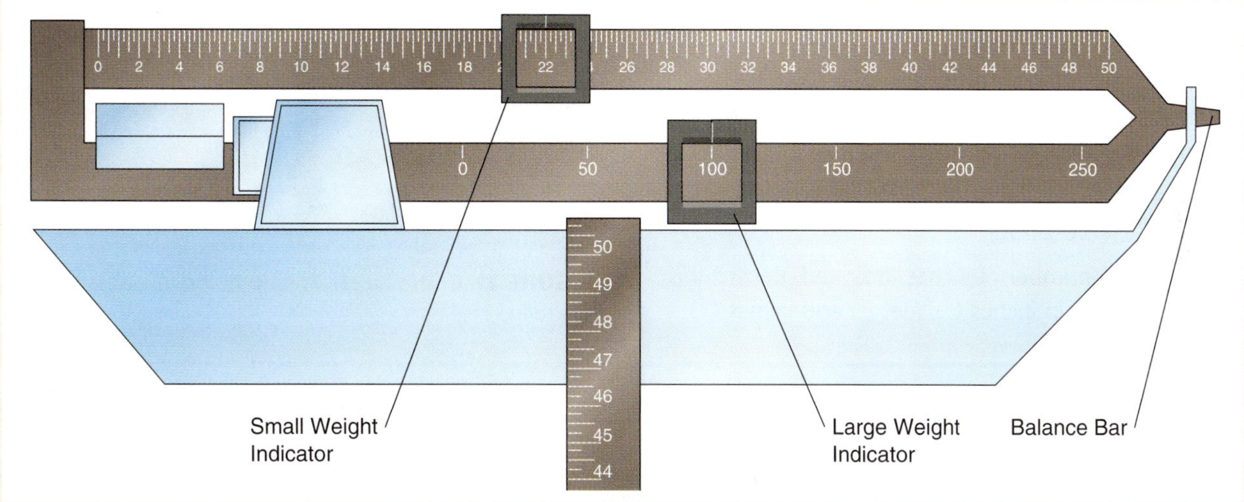

FIGURE 21-5 The upper bar indicates smaller pound weights. The weight shown on the lower bar is measured in 50-pound increments. This figure is added to the amount shown on the upper bar.

PROCEDURE 47

WEIGHING AND MEASURING THE PATIENT USING AN UPRIGHT SCALE

1. Carry out beginning procedure actions.

   ***Note:** Use disposable gloves if there may be contact with open lesions, wet linens, or body fluids.*

2. Check notes or chart for previous weight as documented. Then escort the patient to the scales.

continues

PROCEDURE 47

continued

3. Place a paper towel on the platform of the scale.
4. Be sure the weights are to the extreme left and the balance bar (bar with weight markings) is hanging free.
5. Assist the patient to remove shoes and step up onto the scale platform, facing the balance bar. The balance bar will rise to the top of the bar guide. The patient should not hold the bar or other parts of the scale.
6. Move the large weight to the right to the closest estimated patient weight.
7. Move the small weight to the right until the balance bar hangs freely halfway between the upper and lower bar guides.
8. Add the two figures and record the total as the patient's weight in pounds or kilograms, according to the type of scale used.
9. Assist the patient to turn on the platform until facing away from the balance bar. Raise the height bar until it is level with the top of the patient's head.
10. The reading is made at the movable point of the ruler (Figure 21-6).
11. Note the number of inches indicated. Record this information in inches ("), feet (') and inches ("), or centimeters (cm), according to the type of scale. The height shown in Figure 21-6 is 62 inches. This may be recorded as 62 inches or 5 feet 2 inches (62 ÷ 12 = 5 feet 2 inches). Record the value on your notepad.
12. Assist the patient off the platform. Help the patient to put on shoes, if necessary, and return to the room.
13. Carry out procedure completion actions.

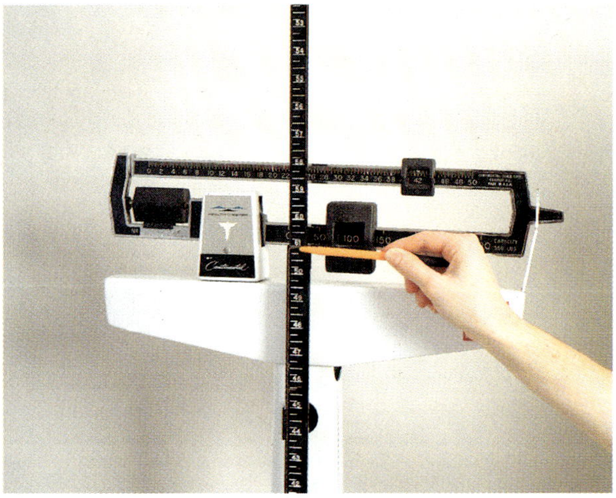

FIGURE 21-6 The height is read at the movable point of the ruler.

PROCEDURE 48

WEIGHING THE PATIENT ON A CHAIR SCALE

1. Carry out beginning procedure actions.
2. Assemble equipment:
   - chair scale
3. Take the patient in a wheelchair to the chair scale. Lock the brakes to the wheelchair. Check the brakes of the chair scale to make sure they are locked in place.
4. Apply a transfer belt to the patient and assist in a pivot transfer to the chair on the scale. Instruct the patient to sit down when the chair is felt against the back of the legs. Be sure the patient's feet are on the footrest of the scale.
5. Walk behind the scale to obtain the reading.
6. Transfer the patient back to the wheelchair.
7. Carry out procedure completion actions.

PROCEDURE 49

MEASURING WEIGHT WITH AN ELECTRONIC WHEELCHAIR SCALE

1. Carry out beginning procedure actions.
2. Assemble equipment:
   - wheelchair scale
3. Determine empty weight of a wheelchair by weighing it on the scale.
4. Take the wheelchair to the patient's room. Help the patient into the wheelchair and take the patient to the electronic wheelchair scale.
5. Open the metal ramp sides the on scale so that they rest on the floor. This allows wheelchair access to the scale.
6. Press the "on" button; the scale zeroes automatically (Figure 21-7).
7. Roll the wheelchair with the patient in it, onto the platform of the scale. Lock wheelchair wheels.
8. The digital readout will show weight.
9. Record weight of the patient and wheelchair. Subtract the wheelchair weight to obtain the patient's weight.
10. Unlock wheelchair wheels. Roll the wheelchair with patient off the scale.
11. Fold the scale ramps back into place.
12. Carry out procedure completion actions.

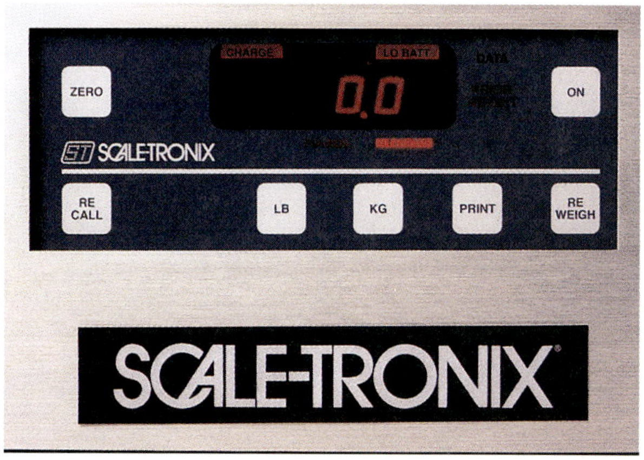

FIGURE 21-7 Press the "on" button to calibrate the scale. This will cause the reading to return to zero. *(Courtesy of Scale-Tronix, White Plains, NY)*

PROCEDURE 50

MEASURING AND WEIGHING THE PATIENT IN BED

1. Carry out beginning procedure actions.
2. Obtain assistance from a coworker.
3. Assemble equipment:
   - overbed scale
   - sheet
   - tape measure
   - pencil
4. Check scale sling and straps for frayed areas or straps that do not close properly.
5. Lower the side rail on your side. Make sure the side rail is up on the other side.
6. Fanfold top linen to foot of bed.
7. Position the patient flat on back with arms and legs straight and body in good alignment. Make sure the sheet is straight and wrinkle-free.
8. Make a small pencil mark at the top of the patient's head on the sheet.

continues

PROCEDURE 50

continued

9. Make a second pencil mark even with the heels (Figure 21-8).
10. Roll the patient on the side. Using the tape measure, measure the distance between the two pencil marks.
11. Note the patient's height in feet and inches on a pad.
12. Cover the canvas sling with a sheet. Balance the scale according to the manufacturer's directions. The scale should be balanced with the sheet, canvas sling, chains, or straps attached.

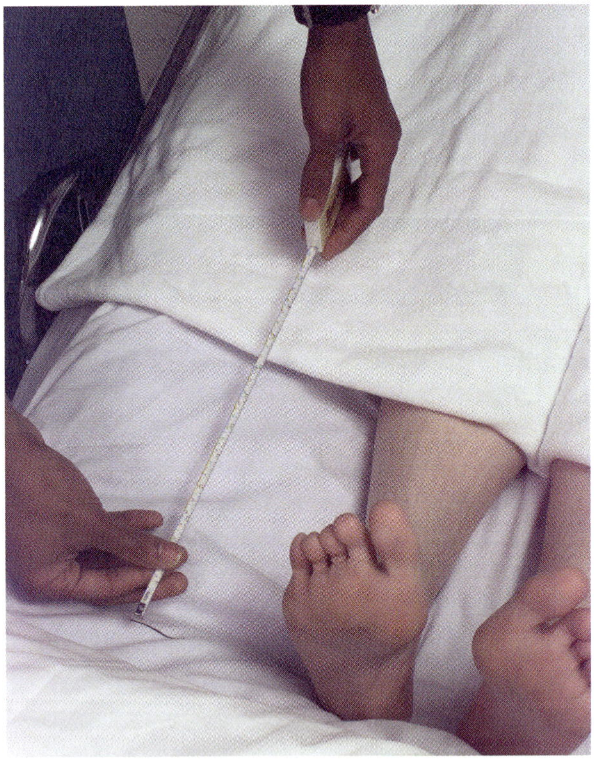

FIGURE 21-8 Measuring the height of the patient in bed. Measure from the pencil line at the heels to the pencil line at the top of the head.

13. Remove the scale sling from the suspension straps and position half of the sheet-covered sling under the patient.
    - Turn the patient away from you.
    - Place the sling, folded lengthwise, under the patient.
    - Return the patient to recumbent position and place the sling so that the patient rests securely within it.
    - Attach the sling to the suspension straps. Check to be sure attachments are secure.
14. Position the lift frame over the bed with base legs in maximum open position, and lock the frame.
15. Elevate the head of the bed and bring the patient to a sitting position.
16. Attach the suspension straps to the frame. Position the patient's arms inside the straps.
17. Slowly raise the sling so the patient's body is off the bed. Be reassuring.
18. Guide the lift away from the bed so that no part of the patient touches the bed.
19. Take and note the reading.
20. Reposition the sling over the center of the bed.
21. Release the knob slowly, lowering the patient to the bed.
22. Remove the sling by reversing the process in step 13.
23. Assist the patient to a comfortable position.
24. Move the overbed scale out of the way.
25. Replace the top bed linen over the patient. Raise the side rail and lower the bed to the lowest horizontal height.
26. Carry out procedure completion actions.

REVIEW

A. True/False.

Mark the following true or false by circling T or F.

1. T F The lower bar on the scale indicates pounds in increments of 25.
2. T F Always check the overbed scale for needed repairs before use.
3. T F To obtain a proper reading, the scale balance bar must hang freely.

4. T F The scale used most often to weigh ambulatory patients in care facilities is the upright scale.

5. T F A patient who cannot get out of bed cannot be measured.

6. T F When using an overbed scale, the patient's body must be free of the bed.

7. T F To measure a patient confined to bed, first help her assume the left Sims' position.

B. Short Answer.

Choose the correct word from the following list to complete each statement in questions 8–12.

ambulatory	inches
centimeters	kilograms
forward	pounds

8. Weights may be measured in ______ or ______.

9. Height measurements may be recorded in feet and ______ or in ______.

10. The upright scale is used to weigh ______ patients.

11. A scale that is calibrated for the metric system will express weights in ______.

12. When a patient is measured on an upright scale, he should face ______.

C. Nursing Assistant Challenge.

Mrs. Haughn is in bed recovering from a stroke. She is unable to walk or stand. She is receiving diuretics. Her doctor wants to order some new medication that is given according to the patient's size. You are assigned to weigh and measure the height of this patient. Answer each of the following by selecting the correct answer.

13. The best way to weigh this patient is with
- **a.** an upright scale.
- **b.** an overbed scale.
- **c.** a wheelchair scale.
- **d.** a chair scale

14. The best way to measure this patient is
- **a.** with a height bar.
- **b.** with a tape measure.
- **c.** to ask the patient.
- **d.** to estimate the height.

15. One reason the physician might have asked for the patient's weight is because the patient
- **a.** is receiving diuretics.
- **b.** has had a stroke.
- **c.** cannot stand.
- **d.** cannot walk.

16. The patient measures 63 inches. This may be expressed as
- **a.** 5 feet 6 inches.
- **b.** 5 feet 8 inches.
- **c.** 5 feet 3 inches.
- **d.** 6 feet 3 inches.

EXPLORING THE WEB

Description	Location
Assessment	*http://www.delmarhealthcare.com/olcs/white/pnotes.asp* (see Chapter 25)
Average height and weight charts (adult)	*http://www.halls.md*
Average height and weight charts (child)	*http://www.halls.md*
Children's growth charts	*http://www.sickkid.net*
Determining body mass index	*http://www.state.ma.us*
Height and weight converter (to metric)	*http://www.mdt.state.mt.us*
Height and weight tables	*http://insurancepage.com*
Notes on the Use of Height and Weight Charts	*http://www.bradfordvts.co.uk*

section 7

Patient Care and Comfort Measures

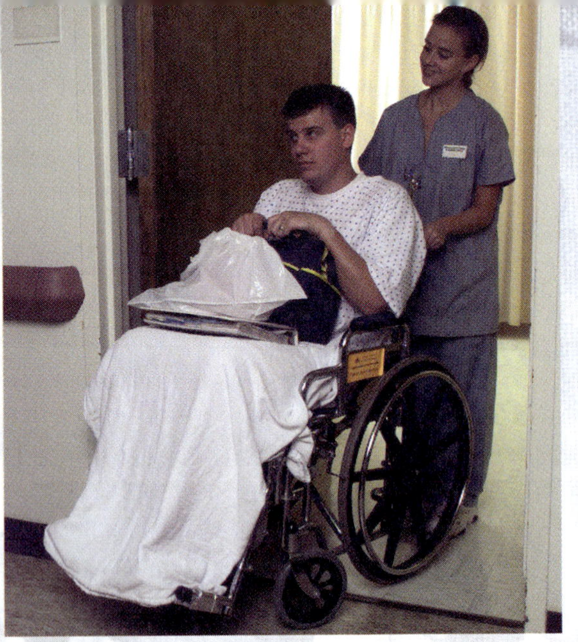

unit 22

Admission, Transfer, and Discharge

objectives

After completing this unit, you will be able to:

- Spell and define terms.
- List the ways the nursing assistant can help in the processes of admission, transfer, and discharge.
- Demonstrate the following procedures:
  - Procedure 51 Admitting the Patient
  - Procedure 52 Transferring the Patient
  - Procedure 53 Discharging the Patient

vocabulary

Learn the meaning and the correct spelling of the following words and phrases:

admission
baseline assessment
discharge
transfer

INTRODUCTION

The nurse is responsible for overseeing and carrying out hospital procedures and physician's orders regarding all admissions, transfers, and discharges. You will usually help the nurse by carrying out the routine procedures associated with these activities.

A nursing assistant, a volunteer, or someone from the admissions office accompanies the new patient to the unit. Someone must always escort the patient to the unit for admission. Also, someone must always escort the patient from the unit during transfer or discharge.

You can do much to make these activities easier for the patient, family, and the other staff members by:

- Having equipment and materials prepared for the activity.
- Being very observant during each activity.
- Documenting observations carefully and accurately. These make a valuable contribution to the nurse's initial **baseline assessment** of the patient's condition.
- Reporting observations directly to the nurse.
- Giving attention to the details of each procedure.
- Being aware of the emotional stress these activities cause patients and their families.
- Being courteous to everyone (Figure 22-1).

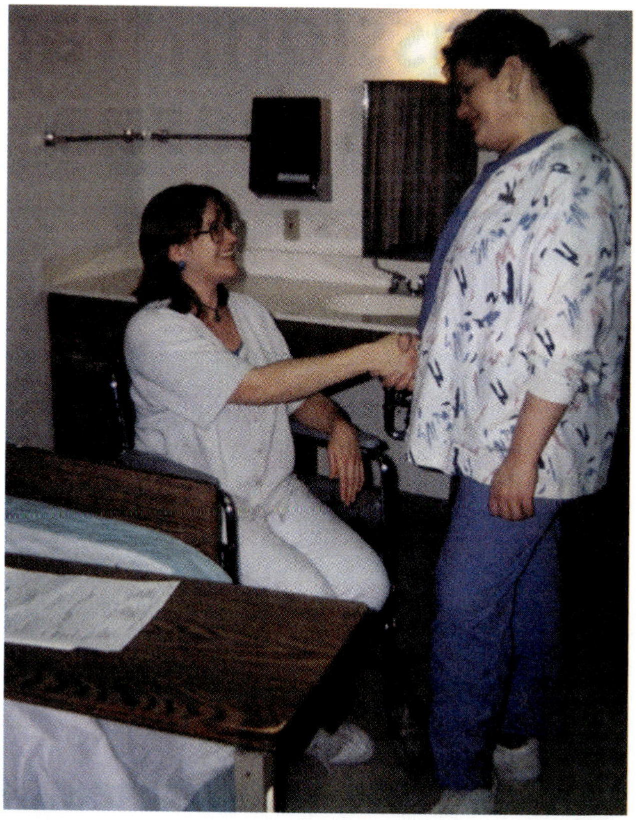

FIGURE 22-1 Treat patients and families with courtesy and respect. First impressions are lasting ones, and you represent your facility to the patient.

ADMISSION

When a person enters a health care facility for treatment of an illness or injury, the **admission** process often causes concern or stress to the patient, family, and friends. The first impression created is very important. You will be one of the first staff members the patient sees, so it is important that you be courteous, confident, and efficient. (See Procedure 51.)

When a patient is ready for admission, ask the nurse if:

- The patient requires a stretcher or wheelchair to reach the unit.
- Any special equipment such as oxygen or a fracture bed is needed.
- There are any special instructions, such as withholding fluids or foods.

Introduce yourself and observe the patient carefully. Listen for complaints as you escort and assist the patient to the room and to bed. Initial observations are very important. They become the basis of comparison for future observations.

Pay particular attention to the patient's skin condition. If you observe rashes, bruises, pressure ulcers, or other abnormalities, inform the nurse and document your findings on the admission record, or according to facility policy.

If it is necessary to ask visitors to leave, do so in a kindly and polite manner. They will be most anxious to remain and see the patient settled and comfortable, so

- Show them where they may wait.
- Let them know about how long they will have to wait.
- Tell them where they can get refreshments.
- Answer questions they may have about where to find a chapel and telephones, and visiting hours.
- After you have completed your part of the admission procedure, locate visitors and let them know they may return to the patient's room.

AGE-APPROPRIATE CARE *Alert*

Pediatric patients may fear separation from the parents. Explain the unit policies for visiting or rooming in. Orient the child and family to the playroom, bathroom, and other areas as appropriate. Speak directly to the child. Show the child how to use the signal or call for help. Ask him or her questions about normal routines. Allow the child to respond before questioning the parents. A primary goal on admission is to make the child and parents as comfortable as possible, relieving anxiety about separation.

COMMUNICATION *Highlight*

Knowing when and how to ask a visitor to leave the room takes tact and diplomacy. Consult the nurse if you are unsure of how to handle a visitor situation. Try to schedule your care for when the patient is alone, if this is possible. If not, ask visitors to leave any time the patient's body will be exposed or a procedure will be performed. If the patient requests that the visitor be allowed to stay, honor the request. However, do not ask the patient if he would like to stay in the presence of others. For an infant or young child patient, parents are generally permitted to remain in the room during procedures. Some adolescent and teenage children will be uncomfortable if parents remain in the room during personal care. Ask the parents to leave the room unless the child asks that they be allowed to stay.

SAFETY *Alert*

Never leave the room until the patient is safe, has the call signal in reach, and knows how to use it.

TRANSFER

It may be necessary for the patient to be moved to another unit (Figure 22-5, see page 333). Preparations for the **transfer** will be handled by the nurse, but you may be asked to assist. (See Procedure 52.)

The transfer may be the patient's own preference, or may be done because a change in the patient's condition requires a different type of care. The transfer may be temporary or permanent. If it is permanent, the patient is discharged from one unit, then admitted to another. The patient may or may not fully understand the reasons for the transfer. Be positive and supportive in your attitude. Recognize that the patient may be feeling very anxious. It would be helpful to know what the patient has been told about the reasons for the transfer. You may learn this from the nurse and by carefully listening to what your patient says.

PROCEDURE 51

ADMITTING THE PATIENT

1. Wash hands.
2. Assemble equipment:
   - equipment for urine specimen collection
   - equipment for taking temperature
   - pad and pencil
   - patient's chart or worksheet
   - stethoscope
   - admission kit
     - water pitcher
     - glass
     - liquid soap
     - washcloth
     - towel
     - basin
     - lotion
     - mouthwash
   - scale
   - blood pressure cuff and manometer
   - watch with second hand
   - disposable gloves (if urine specimen is required)
3. Prepare the unit for the patient by:
   a. Making sure that all necessary equipment and furniture are in their proper places and in good working order.
   b. Checking the unit for adequate lighting.
   c. Loosening the top linen at the foot of the bed. This is called a *toe pleat*.
   d. Opening the bed (Figure 22-2).
4. Identify the patient both by asking the name and checking the identification bracelet.
   a. Introduce yourself.
   b. Take the patient and the patient's family to the unit.
   c. Do not appear to rush the patient.
   d. Be courteous and helpful to the patient and the family.

continues

PROCEDURE 51

continued

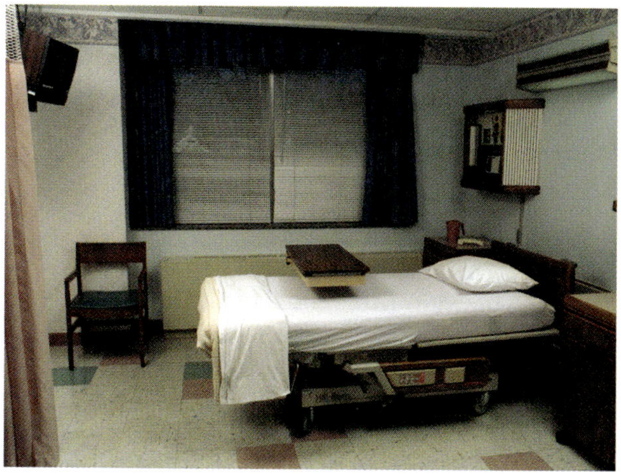

FIGURE 22-2 An open bed notifies everyone that a patient is expected.

5. Ask the patient to be seated, if ambulatory.
   a. Ask the family to go to the lounge or lobby while the patient is being admitted.
   b. Introduce the patient to the other patients in the room, unless it is a private room.
   c. As permitted, explain what will happen in the next hour.
6. Screen the unit to provide privacy (Figure 22-3).
7. Help the patient to undress and put on a hospital gown or night clothes from home. Care for clothing according to facility policy.
8. Check the patient's vital signs, weight, and height.

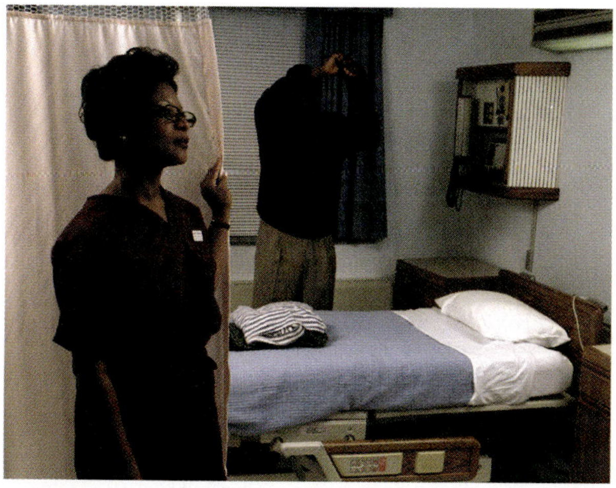

FIGURE 22-3 Provide privacy so the patient can undress.

9. Help the patient get into bed. Adjust the side rails as needed.
10. If the patient is wearing any jewelry or has valuables:
    a. Make a list of them and ask the patient to sign it. This protects the facility and the patient.
    b. Ask the relatives also to sign the list and take the valuables home, or
    c. After checking and signing, give them to the nurse to put in the hospital safe.
11. Tell the patient if a urine specimen is necessary.
    a. Put on gloves and assist the patient as necessary.
    b. Allow the patient to use the bathroom, if ambulatory, or offer the bedpan or urinal.
12. Pour the patient's specimen from the bedpan into the specimen bottle. Put on the cap. Remove gloves and dispose of them according to facility policy. Be sure to label the specimen correctly (see Unit 44).
13. An admission form is usually completed at this time (Figure 22-4). Vital information includes:
    - observations
    - vital signs (TPR, BP, height, weight)
    - known allergies
    - medications being taken
    - food preferences and dislikes
14. If admission is to a long-term care facility, label clothing and complete the personal belongings inventory form according to facility policy.
15. Orient the patient to the unit by explaining:
    - visiting hours
    - how to use the telephone and/or television
    - how to use the call light system for assistance
    - how to operate the bed and light switches, as appropriate
    - standard hospital regulations
    - television rental procedures, if available
    - any questions about facility routines
    - when meals and refreshments are provided
16. Carry out procedure completion actions.

continues

PROCEDURE 51

continued

PATIENT PREFERS TO BE ADDRESSED AS: ____________

FROM: ☐ E.R. ☐ E.C.F. ☐ HOME ☐ M.D.'S OFFICE

COMMUNICATES IN ENGLISH: ☐ WELL ☐ MINIMAL ☐ NOT AT ALL ☐ OTHER LANGUAGE (SPECIFY) ____________

☐ INTERPRETER (NAME PERSON) ☐ NONE

____

MODE OF TRANSPORTATION:

☐ AMBULATORY ☐ OTHER **SMOKER:** ☐ Y ☐ N

☐ WHEELCHAIR ____________

☐ STRETCHER ____________

HOME TELEPHONE NO. ( ) ____________

WORK TELEPHONE NO. ( ) ____________

ORIENTATION TO ENVIRONMENT:

☐ ARMBAND CHECKED ☐ CALL LIGHT

☐ BED CONTROL ☐ PHONE

☐ TV CONTROL ☐ SIDE RAIL POLICY

☐ BATH ROOM ☐ VISITATION POLICY

☐ PERSONAL PROPERTY POLICY ☐ SMOKING POLICY

PERSONAL BELONGINGS: (CHECK AND DESCRIBE)

☐ CLOTHING ____________

☐ JEWELRY ____________

☐ MONEY ____________

☐ WALKER ____________

☐ WHEELCHAIR ____________

☐ CANE ____________

☐ OTHER ____________

DENTURES:

☐ UPPER ☐ PARTIAL

☐ LOWER ☐ NONE

CONTACT LENSES:

☐ HARD ☐ LT ☐ RT

☐ SOFT

GLASSES: ☐ Y ☐ N **HEARING AID:** ☐ Y ☐ N

PROSTHESIS: ☐ Y ☐ N

(DESCRIBE) ____________

DISPOSITION OF VALUABLES:

☐ PATIENT

☐ HOME GIVEN TO: ____________

RELATIONSHIP: ____________

☐ PLACED IN SAFE ____________ (CLAIM NO.)

IN CASE OF EMERGENCY NOTIFY:

NAME: ____________

RELATIONSHIP: ____________

HOME TELEPHONE NO. ( ) ____________

WORK TELEPHONE NO. ( ) ____________

VITAL SIGNS

TEMP: ______ ☐ ORAL ☐ RECTAL ☐ AXILLARY

PULSE: ______ ☐ RADIAL ☐ APICAL RESPIRATORY RATE ______

☐ RT

B/P: ______ ☐ LT ☐ STANDING ☐ SITTING ☐ LYING

HEIGHT: ______ WEIGHT: ______ ☐ BEDSIDE

☐ STANDING

ALLERGIES:

MEDICATIONS: ☐ NONE KNOWN

☐ PENICILLIN ☐ TAPE

☐ SULFA ☐ OTHER (LIST)

☐ IODINE ____________

☐ ASPIRIN ____________

☐ MORPHINE ____________

☐ DEMEROL ____________

FOOD: ☐ NONE KNOWN

(SHELLFISH, EGGS, MILK, ETC.)

____

(PRESCRIPTIVE & NON PRESCRIPTIVE) MEDICATIONS:	DOSE/FREQUENCY	(DATE/TIME) LAST DOSE
1.		
2.		
3.		
4.		
5.		
6.		

DISPOSITION OF MEDICATIONS:

☐ NONE BROUGHT TO HOSPITAL

☐ SENT HOME

WITH ____________

☐ TO PHARMACY: (LIST)

____

ADMITTING DIAGNOSIS: ____________

NURSE'S SIGNATURE: ____________ RN/LVN DATE ______ TIME ______

CHARTER SUBURBAN HOSPITAL
16453 SOUTH COLORADO AVENUE
PARAMOUNT, CALIFORNIA 90723
NURSING ADMISSION ASSESSMENT PAGE 1 of 6

FIGURE 22-4 Accurate admission information is an important part of the nursing assessment.

PROCEDURE 52

TRANSFERRING THE PATIENT

1. Find out which unit the patient will be transferred to. Check to see that it is ready.
2. Learn from the nurse in charge the method of transfer. Get the necessary vehicle (wheelchair, stretcher, or patient's own bed).
3. Check to see if any equipment is to be transferred with the patient.
4. Carry out beginning procedure actions.
5. Explain to the patient what you are doing.
6. Gather all the patient's belongings together.
   a. Place disposables in a paper bag to transport with you.
   b. Check against clothes list.
7. Assist the patient to put on robe and slippers, if permitted. Assist the patient into wheelchair or stretcher, as directed. The entire bed is often used. Make sure the side rails are up during transport.
8. Obtain from the nurse:
   - patient's chart
   - nursing care plan
   - medications
   - paper bag
9. Transport the patient and his belongings to the new unit (Figure 22-5). Use all precautions related to safe transport.
10. Give any transferred medications, the nursing care plan, and the chart to the nurse in charge.
11. Introduce the patient to staff. Proceed to the patient's room.
12. Assist staff in helping the patient into bed. Assist in putting away the patient's belongings and helping the patient to get settled.
13. Before leaving the unit, carry out procedure completion actions.

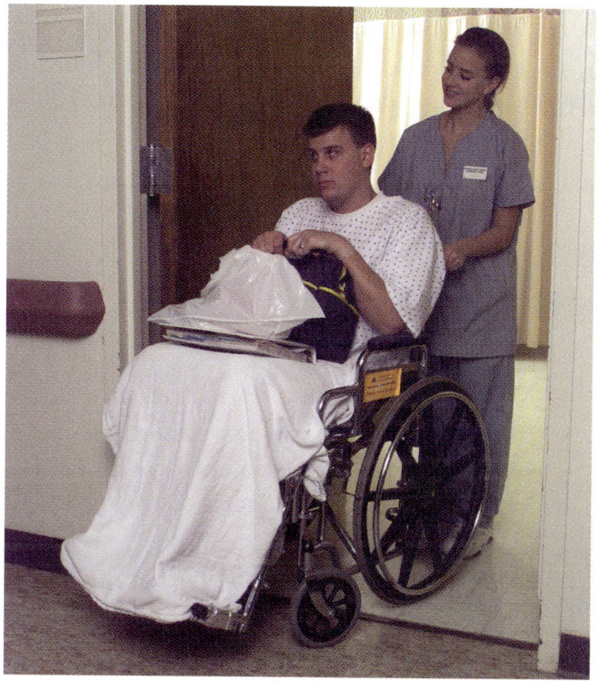

FIGURE 22-5 Transfer the patient calmly and efficiently. Never leave the patient unattended.

All details must be taken care of according to facility policy. Following facility policy ensures that there is no interruption of health care services. Some facilities have transportation services for transferring patients.

After the new unit has been notified and prepared for the move, you will:

- Tell the patient what you are doing.
- Gather all the patient's belongings together. Explain to the patient what you are doing.
- If the patient is expected to return to the unit, you may be asked to gather only a few belongings, such as glasses, dentures, and toiletries.
- Get the patient's medicines, chart, and other personal data from the nurse.
- Assist in the physical transfer.
- Give the records and medication directly to the nurse on the new unit.
- Make sure the patient is safe and comfortable in the new environment before you return to your own unit.

SAFETY Alert

Never leave the patient, the records, or medications unattended.

DISCHARGE

In recent years, the cost of health care has increased steadily. A government program known as *diagnosis-related groups* (*DRGs*) was introduced to control hospital costs. Hospitals are paid a specific amount of money for the care of an individual who has a particular condition or disease that is covered by a DRG.

If the hospital can provide the needed care and discharge the patient early, the hospital saves money and may keep the difference between the actual expenses and the DRG allotted payment. If the patient requires a longer hospital stay than is stated by the DRGs and the costs are higher, the hospital absorbs the additional cost. These standards do not apply to private patients. They apply to patients whose care is being paid for by the federal government, such as Medicare patients. DRGs were developed for Medicare patients, but they are used today by all insurance companies to determine how many hospital days they will pay for. This has resulted in sicker patients being discharged from acute care facilities sooner.

Following hospitalization, many patients are discharged to subacute units or to long-term care facilities for further care, or to home to finish recuperation.

The discharge procedure is usually simple if the patient is going to another facility. The social worker and nurse relay information to the receiving facility. The patient and the patient's belongings are sent to the new facility. Discharge to the patient's home is more complicated and requires a number of actions called *discharge planning* (covered in Unit 34).

The Discharge Process

The **discharge**, or authorized release, of a patient requires a written order from the physician. If a patient indicates an intention to leave without an order, report it to your supervisor immediately. The nurse will make the necessary arrangements. Health care facilities have special policies that must be followed in these cases.

The patient should be spared any fatigue or unnecessary delay when being routinely discharged. (See Procedure 53.) You can help if you:

PROCEDURE 53

DISCHARGING THE PATIENT

1. Check to be sure the physician has ordered the patient to be discharged. If a discharge order has not been written, check with the supervisor before proceeding.
2. Carry out beginning procedure actions.
3. Assemble equipment
   - wheelchair
   - cart to transport items
4. Help the patient to dress, if necessary.
5. Collect the patient's personal belongings. Help the patient check them against the admission list.
   a. Pack, if necessary.
   b. Check valuables against the admission list according to facility policy.
   c. Make sure that all of the patient's belongings have been removed from the closet and bedside stand.
   d. Check to see if medications or other equipment are to be sent home with the patient.
   e. Verify that the patient has received discharge instructions from the nurse, physician, or discharge coordinator.
6. Tell the patient or a member of the family how to collect valuables from the facility safe, if valuables were put there.
7. Help the patient into a wheelchair.
8. Take the patient to the discharge entrance of the facility.
   a. Help the patient to transfer safely into the vehicle.
   b. Be gracious as you say goodbye.
9. Return the wheelchair.
10. Return to the patient unit.
    a. Strip the bed. Dispose of linen according to facility policy.
    b. Clean and replace equipment used in patient care, according to facility policy.
11. Wash your hands.
12. Record the discharge in accordance with facility policy. Include:
    - time
    - method of transport
    - patient's reaction
    - signature
13. Report completion of task to nurse.

- Check with the nurse to make sure that the physician has written an order for discharge before preparing the patient.
- Gather all the patient's belongings and assist in packing, if necessary. Patients who are well enough usually prefer to assemble their own things. You will need to do this activity completely for other patients.
- Carefully check the closet and bedside table. Disposable equipment is often sent home with the patient. If this is the policy in your facility, be sure that the equipment is clean.
- Check with the nurse for any medications or other treatment-related equipment that should be sent home with the patient.
- Verify that the patient has received discharge instructions from the nurse, physician, or discharge coordinator.
- Never allow a patient to leave the health care facility unassisted. The patient is the staff's responsibility until she has left the building.

REVIEW

A. True/False.

Mark the following true or false by circling T or F.

1. T F When transferring a patient, it is all right to leave the patient unattended and return immediately to your own unit.
2. T F Use all precautions related to safe transport when admitting or discharging a patient.
3. T F You do not need to waste time introducing a new patient to others, because facility stays are very short anyway.
4. T F It is all right to allow patients to leave a health care facility at any time.
5. T F After discharge, the patient's unit is stripped, cleaned, and restocked.
6. T F The patient's unit should be prepared as soon as you are notified that there will be an admission.
7. T F During a transfer, the patient's medications remain on the original unit.
8. T F Measuring the patient's height and weight is part of the admission procedure.
9. T F The discharge order is written by the physician.
10. T F You should observe the patient carefully during the admission procedure.

B. Multiple Choice.

Select the one best answer for each of the following.

11. The assistant can do much to help facilitate the admission procedure by
    - **a.** preparing equipment after the patient arrives on the unit.
    - **b.** letting the nurse make all the observations.
    - **c.** giving attention to the details of the procedure.
    - **d.** recognizing that admission to the facility causes more anxiety to the staff than to the patient.
12. When dealing with the newly admitted patient's family, you should
    - **a.** treat them with courtesy and consideration.
    - **b.** send them home.
    - **c.** let the nurse deal with them.
    - **d.** allow them to stay at the patient's bedside at all times.
13. Part of the admission procedure includes
    - **a.** securing a stool specimen.
    - **b.** obtaining a sputum specimen.
    - **c.** working in a hurried manner so the patient knows you are efficient.
    - **d.** measuring vital signs.
14. Valuables that accompany the patient to her unit should be
    - **a.** taken away.
    - **b.** listed and signed for.
    - **c.** left in the bedside stand.
    - **d.** tucked under the pillow for safety.
15. When a patient is transferred, you should always include his
    - **a.** personal belongings.
    - **b.** bed.
    - **c.** pillow.
    - **d.** blood pressure cuffs.

C. Nursing Assistant Challenge.

Mrs. Leon is being admitted because her emphysema is making it very difficult for her to breathe. She is accompanied by her husband and both are obviously nervous. The next morning, her condition worsens. She is moved to the intensive respiratory care unit. Answer the following questions yes or no.

_____ **16.** The anxiety of the patient and family is not natural.

_____ **17.** You should answer questions about facility routines during admission.

____ **18.** When taking vital signs, you should use an oral thermometer.

____ **19.** When Mrs. Leon is transferred, take all of her personal articles with her.

____ **20.** One way to prepare the unit for admission might include checking for the need for oxygen.

____ **21.** You should turn Mrs. Leon's oxygen up to at least 6 liters to assist with her breathing.

EXPLORING THE WEB

Description	Location
Emory University MedWeb	*http://www.medweb.emory.edu*
Health Care Professionals Network Policies, Procedures, Guidelines	*http://www.wlm-web.com*
National Institutes of Health Nursing Policy Manual	*http://www.cc.nih.gov/nursingnew/nursingresources/nursingpolicies.shtml*
Nursing Managers Policies	*http://www.4nursingmanagers.com*
UAMS Clinical Programs Nursing Manual	*http://www.uams.edu*
UTMB Nursing Practice Standards	*http://www.wahoo.utmb.edu*

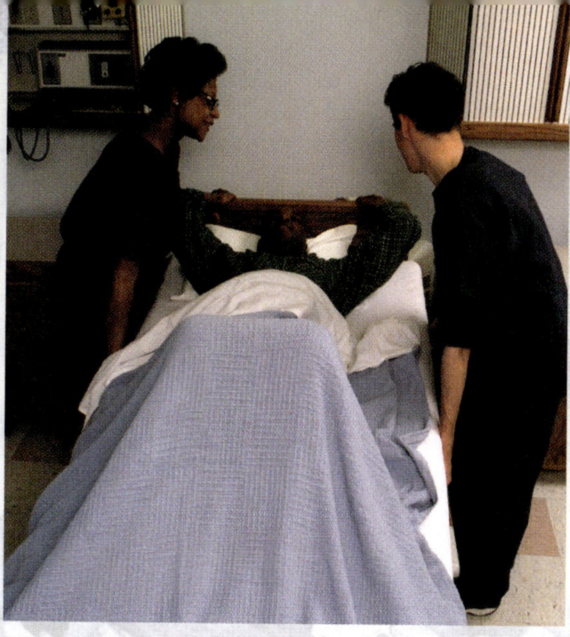

unit 23

Bedmaking

objectives

After completing this unit, you will be able to:

- Spell and define terms.
- List the different types of beds and their uses.
- Operate each type of bed.
- Properly handle clean and soiled linens.
- Demonstrate the following procedures:
  - Procedure 54 Making a Closed Bed
  - Procedure 55 Opening the Closed Bed
  - Procedure 56 Making an Occupied Bed
  - Procedure 57 Making the Surgical Bed

vocabulary

Learn the meaning and the correct spelling of the following words and phrases:

box (square) corner	closed bed	gatch bed	open bed
CircOlectric® bed	electric bed	mitered corner	Stryker frame

INTRODUCTION

The room, especially the bed, is the patient's home while he or she is in the hospital or health care facility. A well-made bed offers both comfort and safety. It is an extremely important contribution to the well-being of the patient.

OPERATION AND USES OF BEDS IN HEALTH CARE FACILITIES

The types of beds and the methods used to operate them may vary in different health care facilities, but the basic principles of bedmaking are the same. The most common beds are the:

- **gatch bed**—a stationary bed about 26 inches high. Modern facilities are equipped with beds that can be raised to the desired height for bedside nursing or lowered to 13 inches to accommodate the out-of-bed patient. The position of the head and knee areas of the bed can be adjusted for comfort. This operation may be done manually by turning the cranks.
- **electric bed**—a bed similar to the gatch bed, in that it can be raised or lowered and the knee and head areas can be adjusted. It is operated electrically (Figure 23-1). You will be using this bed most often in a large facility.
- low bed—low beds are commonly used in health care facilities for patients who are at risk of falls, for whom use of side rails is not desirable. The bed frame is 4 to 6 inches from the floor to the top of the frame deck. These beds reduce the risk of injury if the patient falls from the bed. Some facilities place pads on the floor next to the bed to further reduce the risk of injury. Nursing assistants must use good body mechanics and mechanical lifts when assisting patients into and out of these beds, to prevent back injuries.

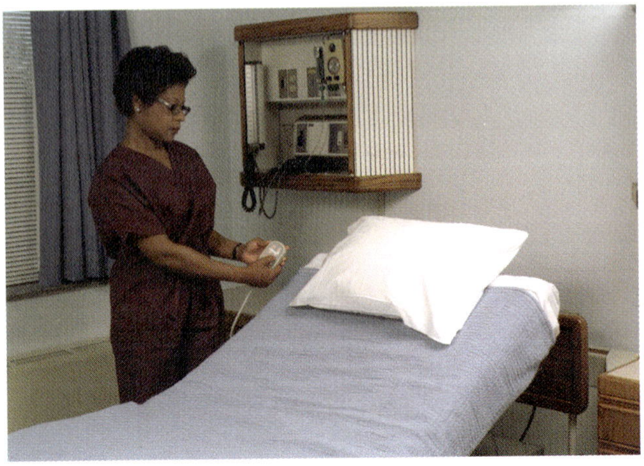

FIGURE 23-1 The typical hospital bed is electronically operated. The head and foot can be adjusted for patient comfort. The height of the bed can be raised, making it easier to give care.

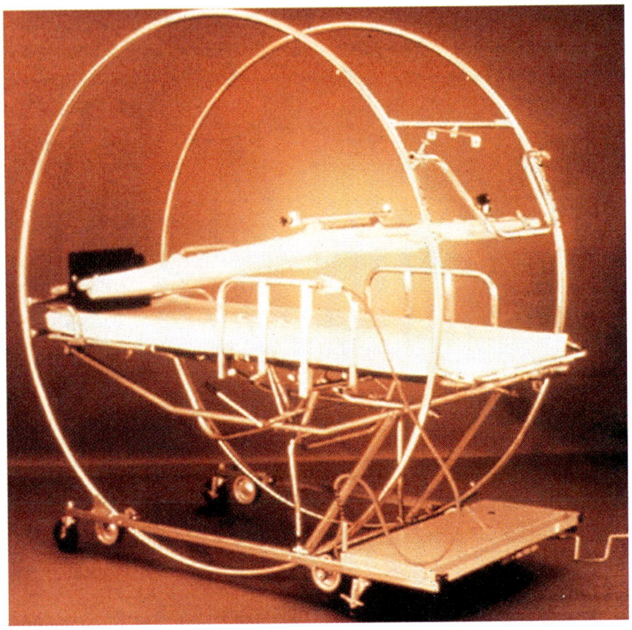

FIGURE 23-2 Turning may be frightening for patients who are in a CircOlectric® bed. Provide calm reassurance. *(Courtesy of Stryker Corporation, Kalamazoo, MI)*

- **CircOlectric® bed**—a special bed frame placed within a circular frame (Figure 23-2). This bed is operated electrically. The circular frame can be rotated. The patient is secured on the inner frame before the bed is moved. The entire inner frame is rotated forward. This allows for position change without any stress on the patient. After rotating, the patient is on the abdomen.
- **Stryker frame**, spinal bed, or wedge bed—a turning frame that serves the same purpose as the CircOlectric® but is operated manually. Once the patient is secured by placement of the upper frame, a crank is used to turn the entire frame and the patient. After turning, the patient is on the abdomen. The patient lies on the frame until turned once more (Figure 23-3).

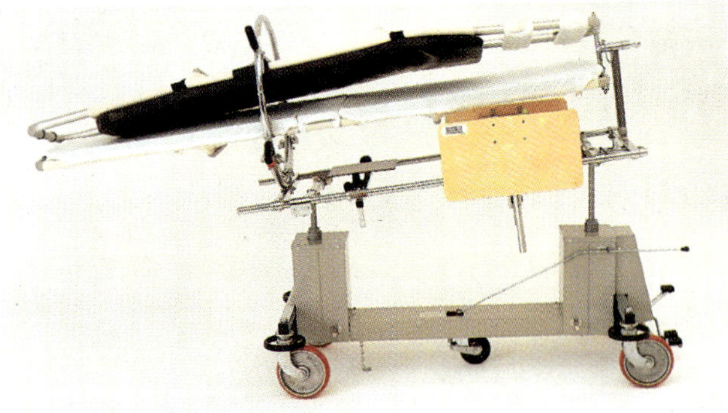

FIGURE 23-3 The Stryker® frame is similar to the CircOlectric® bed, but is manually operated. It is used for patients with pressure ulcers, paralysis, and spinal cord injuries. The patient is sandwiched between two boards when being turned, and may become very frightened. Reassure the patient when turning the frame. *(Courtesy of Stryker Corporation, Kalamazoo, MI)*

SAFETY *Alert*

Use the special turning beds only if you have been trained and are permitted to use them. In most facilities, two or more staff must be present when a patient is turned on a special bed. Make sure to follow the manufacturer's directions for use of the bed, and be certain that all safety straps are fastened properly before you move the patient. When using the Stryker frame, always turn the patient in the direction of the narrow wedge, to reduce the risk of falls. Turn the frame quickly and smoothly. Close the locks and replace the pins after the patient has been turned. If the perineal section of the frame must be removed for patient elimination, remember to replace it promptly.

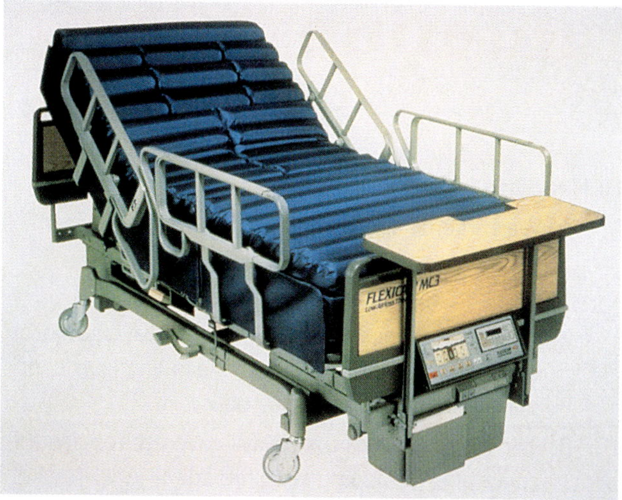

FIGURE 23-4 The low air loss bed is used for pressure ulcer prevention and treatment. Although these beds exert less pressure on the skin than a regular mattress, patients must still be turned and repositioned frequently to prevent skin breakdown. *(Courtesy of Hill-Rom, Charleston, SC)*

Patients with severe burns or spinal injuries are often placed on special beds like the CircOlectric® or Stryker frame, for safety. These beds allow patients to be repositioned with minimal handling of their bodies.

The turning procedure is frightening for many patients. Reassure the patient that he is secure and that turning will proceed without incident. In most facilities, a licensed nurse must be present during turning.

Other types of beds are available for the treatment of patients with multiple or advanced pressure ulcers, flaps, grafts, burns, and intractable pain. For example, one special unit that supports the patient's body evenly is filled with a sand-like material. Warm, dry air circulates through the material to maintain an even temperature and support the body evenly.

A low air loss bed (Figure 23-4) provides pressure relief for patients who have pressure ulcers, those who are at risk of pressure ulcers, and some patients with burns. This mattress is designed to keep the patient cooler and drier than other types of beds. Low air loss beds reduce pressure to the patient's skin, and reduce friction and shearing, which contribute to skin breakdown. These beds use a system of air-filled pillows in which inflation pressure can be adjusted so the characteristics of the support surface are matched to those of the body being supported. The pillows can be inflated and deflated to adjust the level of pressure relief. The design of the bed allows slight air escape upon movement, which reduces pressure.

Patients using a low air loss bed must still be turned and positioned regularly to prevent skin breakdown, which can occur despite the pressure-reducing mattress. Avoid tucking the bottom sheet in tightly, as this increases pressure within the bed. Some facilities use these beds with nylon covers only, without sheets. The nylon cover reduces friction and shearing. Follow the care plan and facility policies. Special underpads are used with the low air loss bed.

Correct operation of any bed or equipment is important for patient safety. Always seek help and instruction from the nurse or another health care professional when using any specialized beds. Never try to operate any bed or equipment with a patient in it without first practicing and gaining security and skill in the procedures. Although different types of hospital beds may be similar in design, the operating instructions vary. For safety, always follow the manufacturers' directions in operating the various therapeutic beds.

SAFETY *Alert*

Become familiar with the features of the low air loss bed used by your facility. Some have bed scales built in, making it possible to weigh the patient without moving her from the bed. CPR is not effective in a low air loss bed, even with a back board. The beds have a switch that rapidly deflates the air pillows in an emergency. Become familiar with the location and operation of the features of the bed.

BEDMAKING

Bed linen is always changed when soiled. It is routinely changed:

- daily in the acute care facility.
- two or three times a week in long-term care facilities.

Residents in long-term care may prefer to use their own pillows, blankets, and spreads.

guidelines *for* Handling Linens and Making the Bed

Handling Linens

1. Wash hands and use gloves if necessary; other personal protective equipment may also be required.
2. Laundry hampers placed in the hallway should be at least one room away from clean linen carts, or placed according to facility policy.
3. The clean linen cart is always covered; replace the cover after removing required linen.
4. Take only the linens you need into the patient's room.
5. Linens that touch the floor are considered dirty and are placed in the laundry hamper; they are not used.
6. Avoid contact between the linens and your uniform (for both clean and soiled linens).
7. Unused linen is never returned to the clean linen cart; it is placed in the laundry hamper.
8. As soiled linen is removed from the bed, keep the soiled areas on the inside and fold or roll the linen toward the center.
9. Never shake bed linens, because microbes will be released into the air.
10. Soiled linen is never placed on environmental surfaces in the room, such as the overbed table, chair, or floor; soiled linens are placed in the appropriate laundry hamper (follow facility policy).
11. Fill laundry hampers no more than two-thirds full. Keep the lid of the hamper on tightly at all times.
12. Many facilities do not permit laundry hampers or barrels to be taken into the patient's room. Soiled linen may be placed in a plastic bag or a pillowcase in the room. Make a cuff at the top of the bag or open end of the pillowcase and place the cuff over the back of the chair. When the bag or case is two-thirds full, secure the top and place it in the hamper in the hallway.
13. Laundry hampers or barrels are returned to the utility room after use, or as directed by facility policy.

Making the Bed

1. Use proper body mechanics at all times to prevent back injury.
2. Work on one side of the bed at a time to complete removal of soiled linen and placement of clean linen.
3. Make sure the bottom sheet and draw sheet (if used) are smooth and unwrinkled (wrinkles in bed linens can lead to skin breakdown, especially for patients who must remain in bed).
4. Follow the care plan for positioning the head and foot of the bed, the number of pillows to be used, and the use of pillows for positioning.

OSHA *Alert*

Elevating the bed to a working height that is comfortable for you takes a minute, but it is one of the most important things you will do to protect your back. Stay on one side of the bed until it is completely made before moving to the other side. This helps organize your time and conserves energy.

SAFETY *Alert*

Be alert when removing bed linen. Look carefully for items that are a potential source of injury to yourself or the patient, such as lancets and needles. Make sure the patient's personal items are not accidentally sent to the laundry with the bed linen.

Closed Bed

The **closed bed** is made following discharge of a patient and after the unit is cleaned (terminal cleaning). It remains closed until a new patient is to be admitted. Details are important. The same procedure is followed when making an unoccupied bed, but the bed is opened as a final step when a patient is to occupy it shortly. (Refer to Procedure 54.)

PROCEDURE 54

MAKING A CLOSED BED

1. Wash your hands and assemble equipment:
   - 2 pillowcases
   - pillow
   - spread
   - blankets, as needed
   - 2 large sheets (90" × 108") (substitute one fitted sheet, if used)
   - cotton draw sheet or half sheet (if used)
   - plastic or rubber draw sheet (if used in your facility)
   - Mattress pad and cover, if mattress is not plastic-treated

Note: *Mattresses that are treated with plastic do not require a moisture-proof sheet or cotton half sheet (draw sheet). In selected cases, the half sheet is used as a lifter to assist in moving the patient. It is sometimes used simply to keep the bottom sheet clean. Some facilities use fitted bottom sheets. If this is so, use a fitted sheet in place of one of the large sheets.*

2. Elevate the bed to a comfortable working height in the horizontal position. Lock bed wheels so the bed will not roll. Place a chair at the side of the bed.
3. Arrange the linen on the chair in the order in which it is to be used.
4. Position the mattress to the head of the bed by grasping the mattress handles (or the edge of the mattress, if no handles are present).
5. If used, place a mattress cover on the mattress. Adjust it smoothly for corners. You will work entirely from one side of the bed until that side is completed. Then go to the other side of the bed. This conserves time and energy.
6. Place the mattress pad even with the top of the mattress and unfold it.
7. Place the bottom sheet on the bed and unfold it, seam side down and wide hem at the top. The small hem should be brought to the foot of the mattress (Figure 23-5). The center fold should be at the center of the bed. If a fitted bottom sheet is used, fit it smoothly around one corner (Figures 23-6A and B).

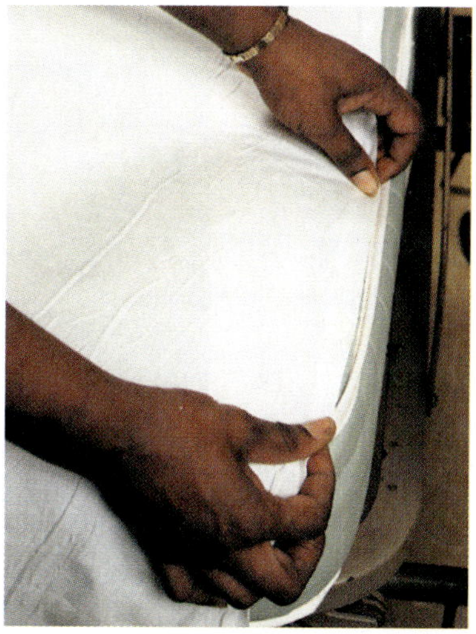

FIGURE 23-5 Place the flat bottom sheet even with the end of the mattress at the foot of the bed.

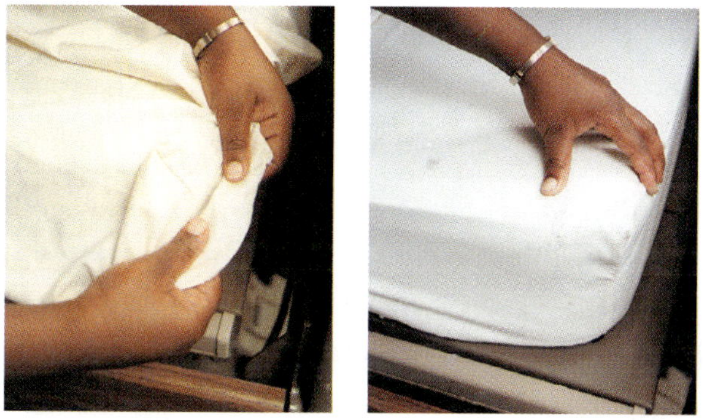

A B

FIGURE 23-6A and **B** If a fitted bottom sheet is used, pull and smooth it around the corner.

8. Tuck 12 to 18 inches of sheet smoothly over the top of the mattress (Figures 23-7A to C).
9. Make a **mitered corner** (Figure 23-8). The square corner, preferred by some facilities, is made in a way similar to the mitered corner.
10. Tuck in the sheet on one side, keeping the sheet straight. Work from the head to the foot of the bed. If using a fitted sheet, adjust it over the head and bottom ends of the mattress.
11. If used, place the plastic draw sheet and half sheet with upper edge about 14 inches from the head of the mattress and tuck under one side. Be sure that the half sheet covers the plastic sheet.

continues

PROCEDURE 54

continued

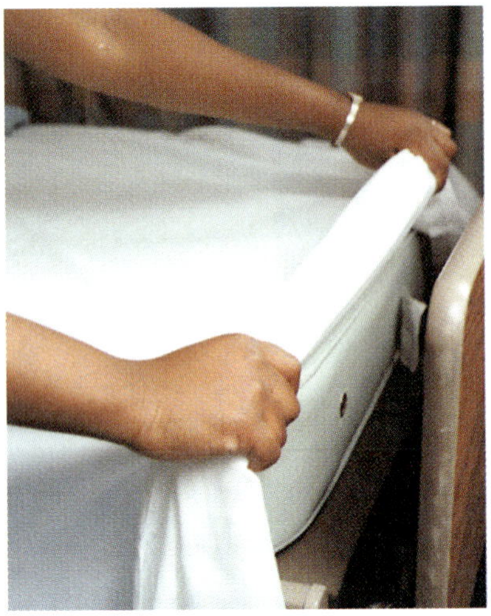

FIGURE 23-7A Gather about 12 to 18 inches of the top sheet at the bottom of the bed.

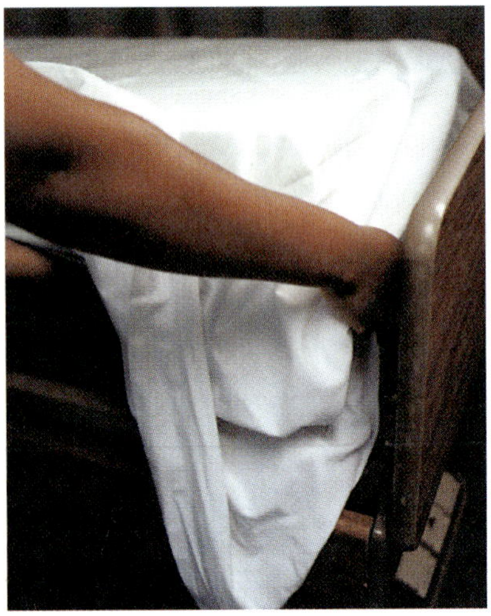

FIGURE 23-7B Face the foot of the bed and lift the mattress with your near hand.

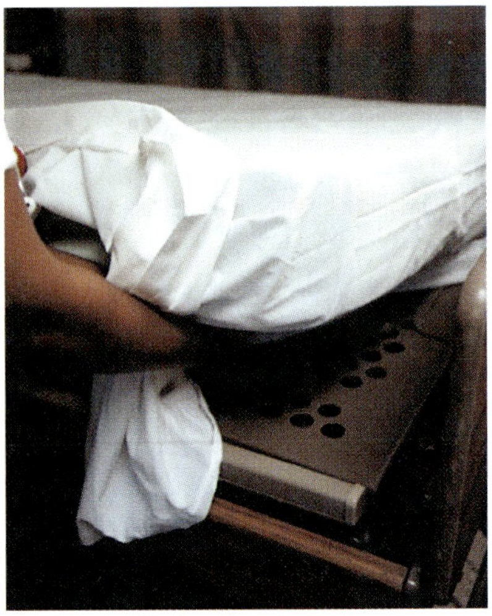

FIGURE 23-7C Bring the sheet smoothly over the end of the mattress with your opposite hand.

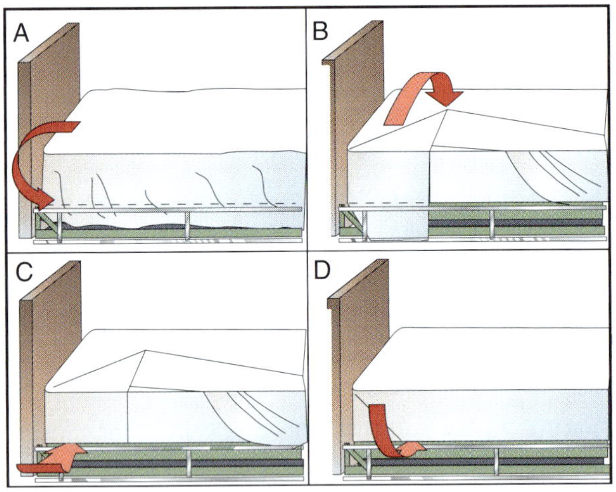

FIGURE 23-8 Making a mitered corner. A. The sheet is hanging loose at the side of the bed. B. Pick up the sheet about 12 inches from the head of the bed to form a triangle. C. Tuck in the sheet at the head of the bed. Pick up the triangle and place your other hand at the edge of the bed near the head to hold the edge of the sheet in place. Bring the triangle over the edge of the mattress and tuck it smoothly under the mattress. Tuck in the rest of the sheet along the side of the mattress. Make sure the sheet is wrinkle-free.

It should cover the area from above the patient's shoulders to below the hips.

12. Unfold and place the top sheet on the bed, seam up, top hem even with the upper edge of the mattress and the center fold in the center of the bed.
13. Spread the blanket over the top sheet and foot of mattress. Keep the blanket centered.
14. Tuck the top sheet and blanket under the mattress at the foot of the bed as far as the center only. Make a **box (square) corner** (Figures 23-9A to C).
15. Place the spread with its top hem even with the head of the mattress. Unfold the spread to the foot of the bed.
16. Tuck the spread under the mattress at the foot of the bed and miter the corner. Sometimes the spread may be placed directly on top of the sheet. Rather than tucking the sheet, blanket, and/or spread under the end of the mattress separately and forming separate corners, all of the covers may be tucked under at the same time and one corner formed (Figures 23-10A to E).
17. Go to the other side of the bed. Fanfold the top covers to the center of the bed so you can work with the lower sheets and pad.
18. Tuck the bottom sheet under the head of the mattress and miter the corner. Working from top to bottom, smooth out all wrinkles and tighten these sheets as much as possible to provide comfort. (Adjust a fitted bottom sheet smoothly and securely around the mattress corners.)

continues

PROCEDURE 54

continued

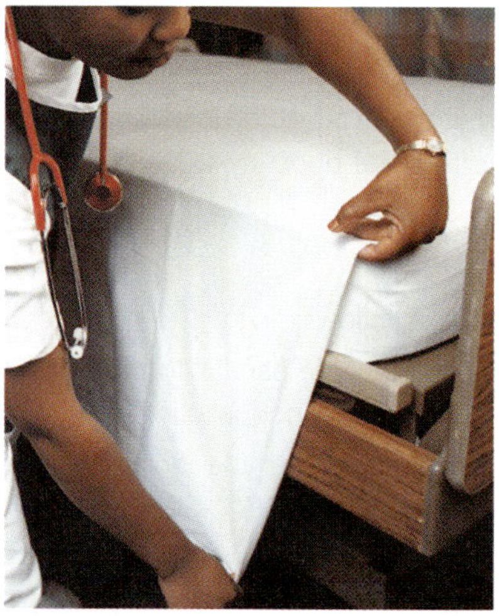

FIGURE 23-9A Make the square (box) corner following the steps shown in Figures 23-8A–C. Then, holding the corner with your left hand, grasp the bottom of the sheet and pull it straight down until the fold is even with the edge of the mattress.

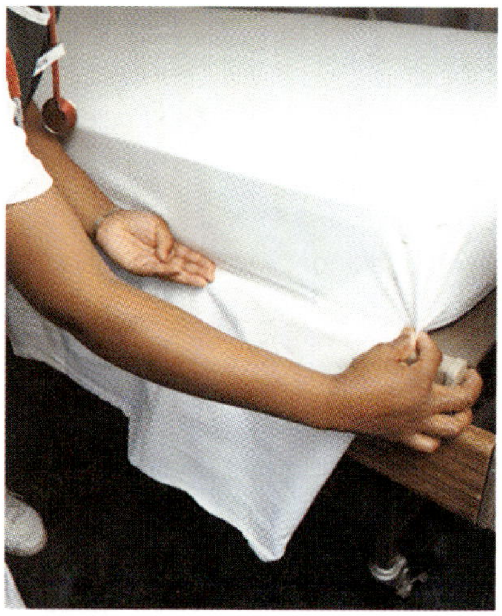

FIGURE 23-9B Holding the square corner in place, tuck the remaining sheet under the mattress.

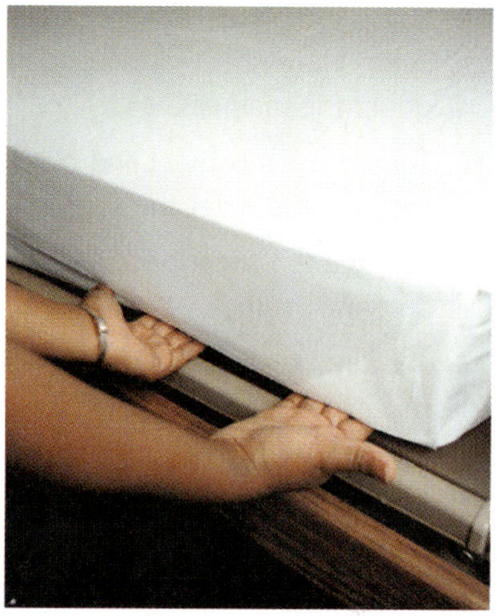

FIGURE 23-9C The finished square corner should look like this.

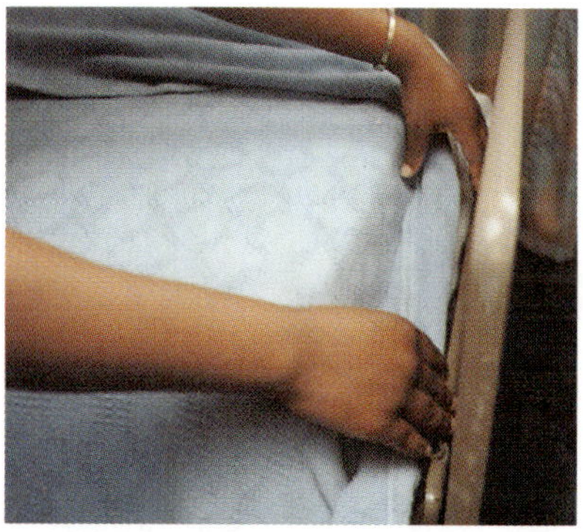

FIGURE 23-10A Gather the top sheet and bedspread together. Smooth evenly over the end of the mattress.

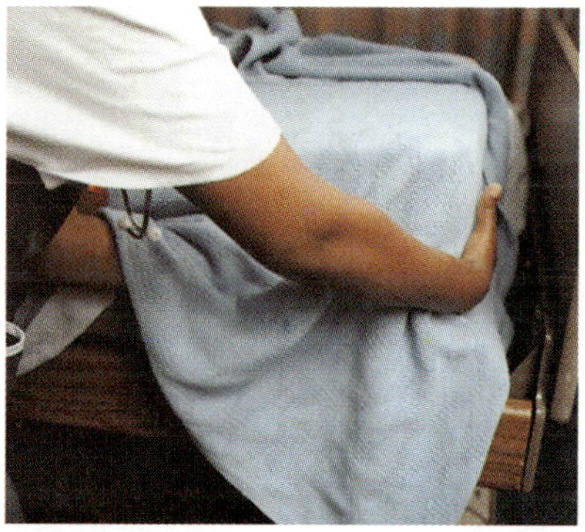

FIGURE 23-10B Tuck the sheet and spread under the mattress together.

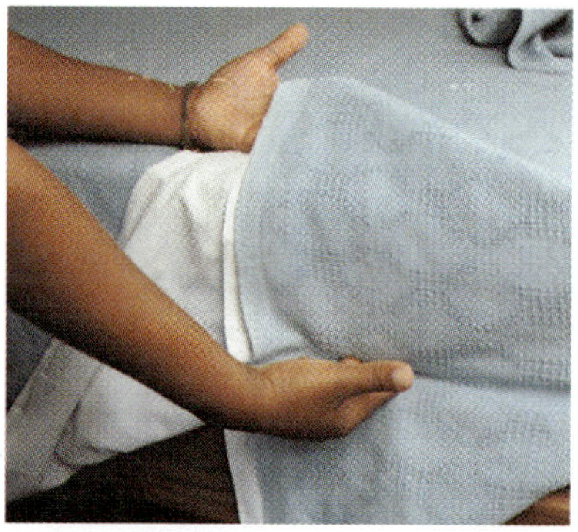

FIGURE 23-10C Continue as with the procedure for a mitered corner.

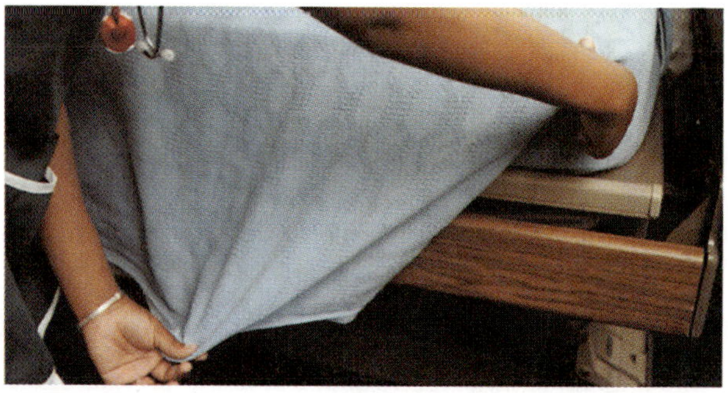

FIGURE 23-10D Slide your finger to the end to make a smooth edge.

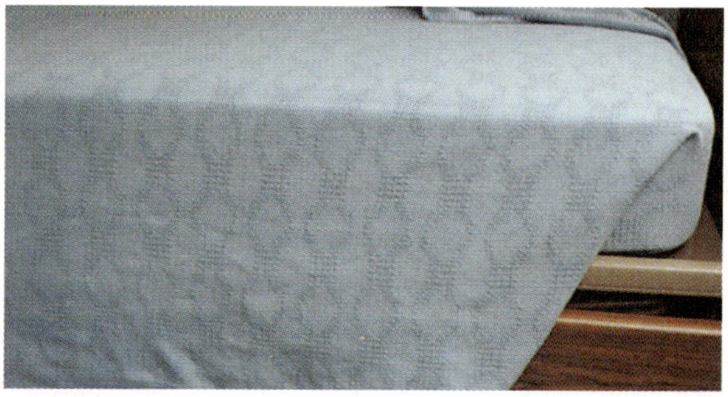

FIGURE 23-10E The completed top bedding. Repeat the procedure on the other side of the bed.

continues

PROCEDURE 54

continued

19. Grasp the protective draw sheet (if used) and cotton draw sheet in the center. Tuck these sheets under the mattress.
20. Tuck in the top sheet and blanket at the foot of the bed and miter the corner.
21. Fold the top sheet back over the blanket, making an 8-inch cuff.
22. Tuck in the spread at the foot of the bed and miter the corner. Bring the top of the spread to the head of the mattress.
23. Insert the pillow into a pillowcase:
    a. Place your hands in the clean case, freeing the corners.
    b. Grasp the center of the end seam with hand outside the case and turn the case back over your hand (Figure 23-11A).
    c. Grasp the pillow through the case at the center of one end. Pull the case over the pillow with your free hand (Figures 23-11B and 23-11C). (Do not allow the pillow to touch your uniform.)
    d. Adjust the corners of the pillow to fit in the corners of the case.
24. Place the pillow at the head of the bed with the open end away from the door.
25. Lower the bed to the lowest horizontal position.
26. Arrange the room as follows:
    a. Replace the bedside table parallel to the bed. Place the chair in its assigned location.
    b. Place the overbed table over the foot of the bed opposite the chair.
    c. Place the signal cord within easy reach of the patient.
    d. Leave the side rails down.
    e. Check for possible hazards, such as gatch handles that are out of place.
27. Leave the unit neat and tidy.
28. Wash your hands.
29. Report completion of the task to your supervisor.

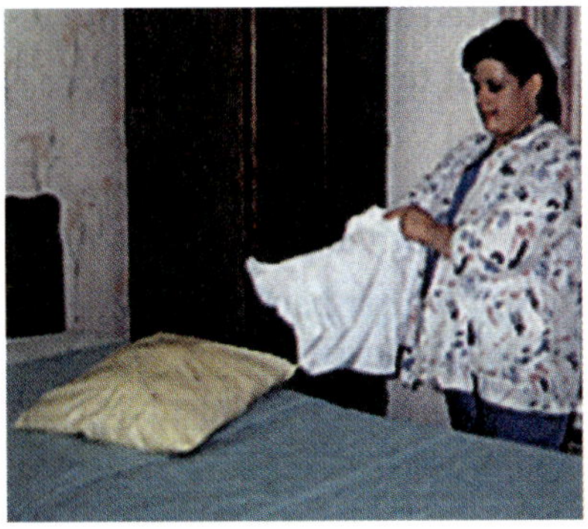

FIGURE 23-11A Grasp the pillowcase at the seam and fold it back and over your wrist, inside out.

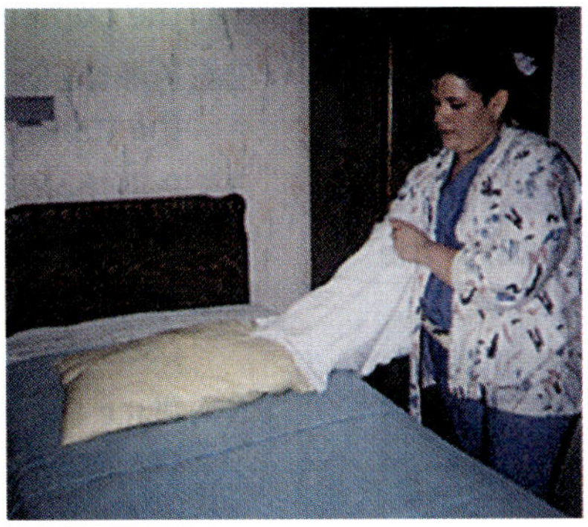

FIGURE 23-11B Grasp the end of the pillow in the center with your pillowcase-covered hand.

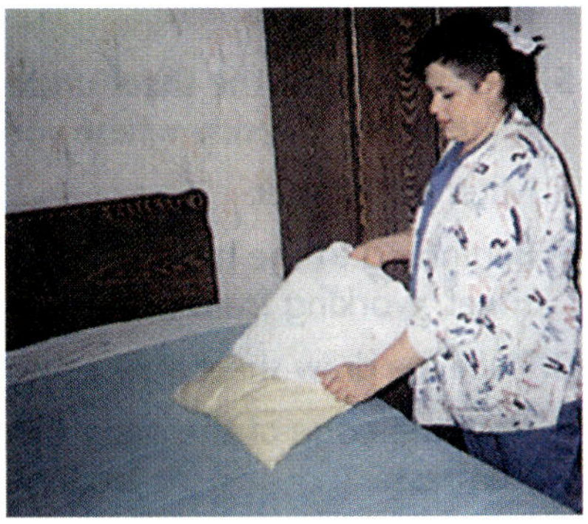

FIGURE 23-11C Unfold and smooth the pillowcase over the pillow.

INFECTION CONTROL *Alert*

Wear gloves when removing bed linen that is wet or soiled. Place the soiled linen in a plastic bag or linen hamper. Avoid contaminating environmental surfaces with gloves that have handled soiled linen. Remove one glove, if necessary. Follow facility policy for disinfecting the mattress. Allow it to dry. Discard your gloves and wash your hands. It is not necessary to wear gloves when you are handling clean linen. Cracks in the mattress are a potential source of odors and contamination. Report cracks in the mattress to the proper person in your facility.

The Unoccupied Bed

Beds are often made while patients are up in a shower or chair. Follow the procedure for making a closed bed but then fanfold the top bedding halfway down. This "opens" the bed and makes it easier for the person to get into it.

The Open Bed

The **open bed** is like a sign saying "welcome" to the new patient (Figure 23-12). It indicates that the patient's arrival has been made known to the assistant. It also shows that the unit has been prepared. In long-term care facilities, the bed is not opened unless the resident is going to bed soon. (See Procedure 55.)

The Occupied Bed

Unless the patient is permitted out of bed by physician's order, the bed is made with the patient in it. (See Procedure 56.) Bedmaking usually follows the bed bath, while the patient is covered with a bath blanket. It may, however, be done any time it would add to the comfort of the patient.

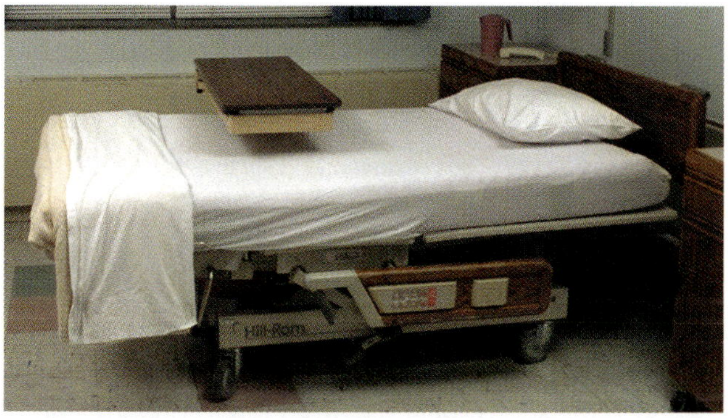

FIGURE 23-12 Open the closed bed by drawing the bedding to the foot of the bed and fanfolding it.

SAFETY *Alert*

Never turn your back on the patient or leave the bedside when the bed is in the high position and the side rail is down.

Surgical Bed

The surgical bed provides a safe, warm environment to receive the postsurgical patient. It must be made in such a way that movement from stretcher to bed is made with maximum safety and minimum effort. For this reason, the bed should be left open and at stretcher height. (See Procedure 57.)

All equipment needed to monitor vital signs and to supervise recovery should be in place and ready for use. You should also keep alert for the patient's return so you can help make a safe transfer from stretcher to bed.

Modern surgical techniques have shortened the time many patients stay in an acute care facility after surgery. Patients are often admitted on the morning of surgery to special units, have the surgery performed, return to these same units immediately after surgery, and are discharged the same day to recuperate at home. These units are called ambulatory, short-term, or day-care units. To prepare a postsurgical bed in one of these units:

- Tighten the bottom linen.
- Fanfold the top linen to the side or foot of bed.
- Raise the bed to stretcher height and lock the wheels.
- Place the equipment to check vital signs, emesis basin, and tissues by the recovery bed.

PROCEDURE 55

OPENING THE CLOSED BED

1. Wash your hands.
2. Check assignment for bed location.
3. Raise the bed to a comfortable working height in the horizontal position. Move the overbed table to one side.
4. Lock the bed wheels.
5. Loosen the top bedding.
6. Facing the head of the bed, grasp the top sheet and spread and fanfold it to the foot of the bed.
7. Return the bed to the lowest horizontal position. Place the overbed table over the foot of the bed.
8. Place the call bell near the pillow or within easy reach. It should be visible and within reach of the patient at all times.
9. Leave the unit neat and tidy.
10. Wash your hands.
11. Report completion of the task to the nurse.

PROCEDURE 56

MAKING AN OCCUPIED BED

1. Carry out beginning procedure actions.
2. Assemble the equipment needed:
   - disposable gloves (if linens are soiled with blood, body fluids, secretions, or excretions)
   - cotton draw sheet or turning sheet for selected patients
   - 2 large flat sheets (or one large flat sheet and one fitted bottom sheet)
   - 2 pillowcases
   - laundry hamper
3. Place the bedside chair at the foot of the bed.
4. Arrange the clean linen on the chair in the order in which it is to be used.
5. The bed should be flat, with wheels locked, unless otherwise indicated. Raise the bed to working horizontal height. Lower the side rail on your side of the bed.
6. If the bed linens are soiled with blood or other body fluids, wash your hands and put on disposable gloves.
7. Loosen the bedclothes on your side by lifting the edge of the mattress with one hand and drawing the bedclothes out with the other. Never shake the linen. This spreads germs.
8. Put the side rail up and go to the opposite side of the bed.
9. Adjust the mattress to the head of the bed (Figure 23-13). Get help, if necessary.
10. Remove the top covers except for the top sheet, one at a time. Fold to bottom. Pick up in the center. Place them over the back of chair if they are to be reused.

Note: *Carefully check each piece of linen for foreign articles (such as patient care equipment, eyeglasses, dentures, items of food, or eating utensils). Remove any such items.*

11. Place the clean sheet or bath blanket over the top sheet. Have the patient hold the top edge of the clean sheet if able. If the patient is unable to help, tuck the sheet beneath the patient's shoulder.

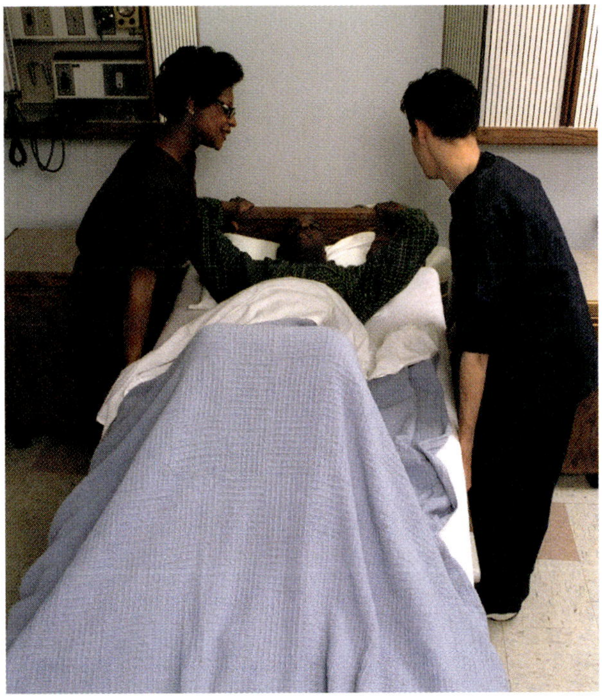

FIGURE 23-13 The patient grasps the head of the bed and pushes in with the heels while two nursing assistants pull the mattress to the head of the bed.

12. Slide the soiled sheet out, from top to bottom. Put it in a hamper or plastic bag.
13. Ask the patient to move to the side of the bed toward you. Assist if necessary. Move one pillow with the patient and remove the other pillow. Pull up the side rail. (Alternatively, you may ask the patient to turn toward the opposite side of the bed, holding onto the raised side rail. You would then fanfold the sheet, as in step 15, but there would be no need to go to the other side of the bed.)
14. Go to the other side of the bed. Fanfold the soiled cotton draw sheet, if used, and bottom sheet close to the patient (Figure 23-14).
15. Straighten the mattress pad. If the bottom sheet is to be changed, place a clean sheet on the bed so that the narrow hem comes to the edge of the mattress at the foot. The seamed side of the hem is toward the bed. The lengthwise center fold of

continues

PROCEDURE 56

continued

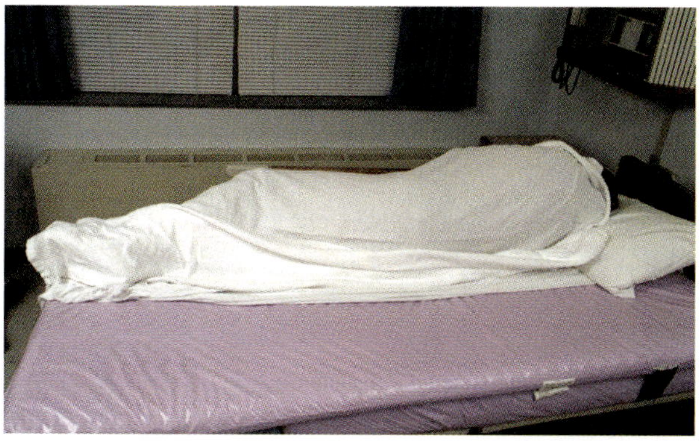

FIGURE 23-14 Fanfold the soiled bottom sheet to the center of the bed as close to the patient as possible. Note that the bottom linen is flat and the patient is positioned to the far side of the bed.

the sheet is at the center of the bed. Fanfold the opposite side of sheet close to patient.

16. Tuck the top of the sheet under the head of the mattress.
17. Make a mitered corner.
18. Tuck the side of the sheet under the mattress, working toward the foot of the bed.
19. Position a fresh draw sheet, if used. Tuck it under the mattress.
20. Ask or assist the patient to roll toward you, over the fanfolded linen. Move the pillow with the patient.
21. Raise the side rails. Test for security.
22. Go to the other side of the bed. Lower the side rail. Remove the soiled linen by rolling the edges inward. *Keep soiled linen away from your uniform.* Placed soiled linen in the hamper or plastic bag. (Raise the side rail if leaving the bedside.)
23. Remove gloves, if worn, and discard according to facility policy.
24. Wash your hands.
25. Pull the clean bottom sheet into place. Tuck it under the mattress at the head of the bed. Make a mitered corner.
26. Pull gently to eliminate wrinkles. Then tuck the side of the sheet under the mattress, working from top to bottom.
27. Pull the draw sheet smoothly into place. Tuck it firmly under the mattress.
28. Place the top sheet over the patient. Remove the bath blanket.
29. Complete the bed as an unoccupied bed. To reduce pressure on toes, grasp the top bedding over the toes and pull straight up. Some patients prefer not to have the blanket and top sheet or spread tucked in.
30. Assist the patient to turn on his or her back. Place a clean pillowcase on the pillow that is not being used. Replace that pillow. Change the other pillowcase.
31. Carry out procedure completion actions.

PROCEDURE 57

MAKING THE SURGICAL BED

1. Wash your hands.
2. Check assignment for unit location.
3. Assemble the following equipment:
   - disposable gloves (if linens are soiled with blood or body fluids)
   - articles for basic bed
   - one extra draw sheet
   - bath blanket for warmth
   - one protective (rubber or plastic) draw sheet (if used in facility)
   - roll of one-inch gauze bandage
4. Lock the bed.
5. Apply gloves if linen is wet or soiled with blood or body fluids.

continues

PROCEDURE 57

continued

6. Strip and discard used linen.
7. Remove gloves and discard according to facility policy.
8. Wash your hands.
9. Make the bottom foundation bed (steps 1–11 in Procedure 54). Repeat on the opposite side of the bed.
10. Place a protective draw sheet over the head of the mattress sheet. Cover with a cotton draw sheet. Miter the corners and tuck them in on the sides.
11. Place the top sheet, blanket, and spread in the usual manner. Do not tuck them in.
12. Fold the linen back at the foot of the bed even with the edge of the mattress.
13. Fanfold the upper covers and top sheet to the far side of the bed (Figure 23-15).
14. Tie a waterproof pillow to the head of the bed with gauze bandaging or place according to facility policy.
15. Arrange the bed so there is adequate room to position a stretcher next to it. Leave the bed locked and at the same height as a stretcher.
16. Check the unit for obvious hazards.
17. Leave the room neat and tidy.
18. Wash your hands.
19. Report completion of the task to nurse.

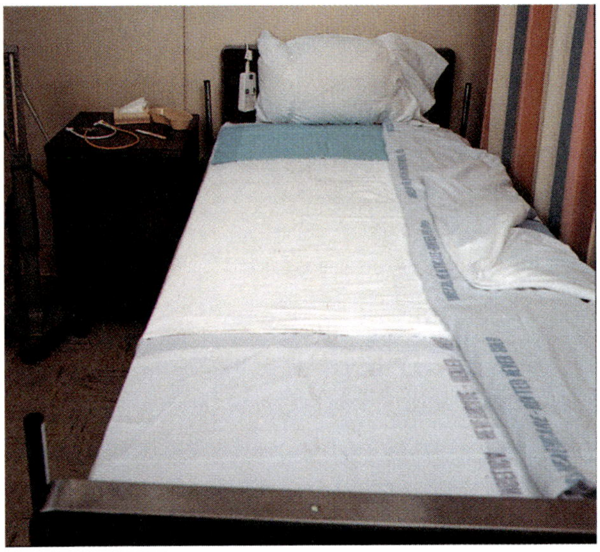

FIGURE 23-15 Prepare the surgical bed by fanfolding the covers to the far side of the bed. Raise the bed to stretcher height.

REVIEW

A. True/False.

Mark the following true or false by circling T or F.

1. T F The patient is most comfortable in a closed bed.
2. T F The Stryker frame is used to turn patients easily.
3. T F You should not attempt to operate a bed until you have been thoroughly supervised.
4. T F The closed bed is made after terminal cleaning is finished.
5. T F Bottom bed linen can be loosely tucked as long as there are no wrinkles when you have finished.
6. T F A mitered corner is tucked in, forming a triangle.
7. T F Shaking linen as you change the bed spreads germs.
8. T F The open bed is like a sign saying "welcome."
9. T F Before making an occupied bed, adjust the mattress to the head of the bed.
10. T F The side rail opposite you must be up as you make an occupied bed.

B. Multiple Choice.

Select the one best answer for each of the following.

11. Loosening the top bedding at the foot of the bed is done
    - **a.** to improve the appearance of the bed.
    - **b.** in unoccupied beds.
    - **c.** as folds in the bottom sheet.
    - **d.** to reduce pressure on the toes.

12. When making an unoccupied bed, make the
  a. entire bottom first.
  b. far side of the bottom and top first.
  c. near side of the entire bed first.
  d. far side of the bottom first.

13. Before making an unoccupied bed,
  a. elevate it to a comfortable working height.
  b. keep the bed at the lowest horizontal height.
  c. raise the head portion.
  d. raise the side rails on the opposite side.

14. Before making any bed, always
  a. raise the side rails.
  b. lower the bed to the lowest horizontal height.
  c. lock the bed wheels.
  d. raise the head of the bed.

15. Sheets should be smoothly tucked in over the head of the mattress
  a. 5 to 7 inches.
  b. 12 to 18 inches.
  c. 20 to 24 inches.
  d. 26 to 30 inches.

16. If a draw sheet or lift sheet is used, it should be placed so that it covers the area under the patient's
  a. head and shoulders.
  b. heels and lower legs.
  c. buttocks only.
  d. shoulders to buttocks.

17. When placing the case on the pillow,
  a. tuck it under your chin.
  b. lay the pillow on the chair.
  c. pull the case over while grasping the pillow with the opposite hand.
  d. lay the pillow on the bedside stand.

18. When opening a closed bed,
  a. fanfold top bedding to the foot.
  b. loosen all top bedding.
  c. leave the bed at its highest horizontal height.
  d. raise the head of the bed.

19. The top bedding in a surgical bed is
  a. untucked and draped.
  b. tucked in on two sides.
  c. untucked and fanfolded.
  d. made with toe pleats.

20. A common element to all bedmaking is
  a. fanfolding the linen.
  b. leaving the unit neat and tidy.
  c. leaving the bed in the high position.
  d. using the same linen and equipment.

C. Nursing Assistant Challenge.

21. You are assigned to make a closed bed. You have washed your hands and assembled the following equipment: pillow, blanket, spread, mattress pad, and mattress cover. What else will you need?

EXPLORING THE WEB

Description	Location
Hospital bed and bedrail safety advice	*http://www.ecri.org*
Hospital bed safety	*http://www.fda.gov/cdrh/beds*
Safe linen handling information	*http://www.nailm.com*
A Guide to Bed Safety	*http://www.patientsafety.com*
Hill-Rom Beds	*http://www.hill-rom.com*
Stryker Corporation	*http://www.strykercorp.com*
Stryker Medical	*http://www.med.strykercorp.com*

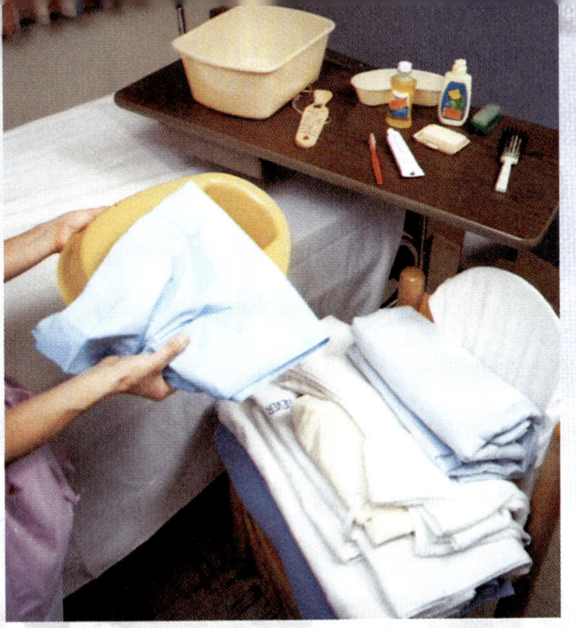

unit 24

Patient Bathing

objectives

After completing this unit, you will be able to:

- Spell and define terms.
- Describe the safety precautions for patient bathing.
- List the purposes of bathing patients.
- State the value of whirlpool baths.
- Demonstrate the following procedures:
  - Procedure 58 Assisting with the Tub Bath or Shower
  - Procedure 59 Bed Bath
  - Procedure 60 Changing the Patient's Gown
  - Procedure 61 Waterless Bed Bath
  - Procedure 62 Partial Bath
  - Procedure 63 Female Perineal Care
  - Procedure 64 Male Perineal Care
  - Procedure 65 Hand and Fingernail Care
  - Procedure 66 Bed Shampoo
  - Procedure 67 Dressing and Undressing the Patient

vocabulary

Learn the meaning and the correct spelling of the following words and phrases:

axilla	**genitalia**	**perineum**
cuticle	**perineal care**	**pubic**

INTRODUCTION

A daily bath is as important for the patient as it is for you. Following the bath, the patient feels relaxed, clean, and refreshed. A bath with warm water and mild soap:

- Removes dirt and perspiration
- Increases circulation
- Provides the patient with mild exercise
- Provides an opportunity for close observation

You as the caregiver are able to see firsthand how the patient's condition is improving, declining, or changing in any way. Your observations are valuable aids to accurate nursing assessments.

With the physician's permission, the patient may be allowed to take regular tub baths or showers. Other patients will be bathed in bed.

Bathing may be performed as:

- Tub bath
- Shower bath
- Complete bed bath
- Partial bed bath
- Self-sponge bath or waterless bath
- Whirlpool bath
- Perineal care

During bathing, special attention should be given to skin areas that touch, including:

- Between the legs
- Under the arms
- Under the breasts
- Under the scrotum
- Between the buttocks
- Around the anus
- For obese people, under folds of skin or fat

Gently sponge and pat these areas dry. Follow facility policy for the use of talcum or corn starch.

A partial bath cleans the hands, face, back, axillae, buttocks, and genitals. It is very refreshing. Many patients will be able to help with bathing. Whenever possible, encourage patients to do so.

Waterless Bath

Some facilities are taking a new approach to bathing called *waterless bathing*. It may also be called *basinless bathing* or *bag bath*. The only equipment needed is a package of premoistened disposable washcloths (Figure 24-1). Each package contains washcloths moistened with a special cleansing solution that evaporates quickly after being applied so that drying is not necessary. Eight washcloths are supplied so that separate parts of the body (face, arms, legs, torso, and genitalia) can be washed. The washcloths can be warmed in the microwave for comfort. This equipment can be used by the nursing assistant to administer a bath or by the patient to self-bathe.

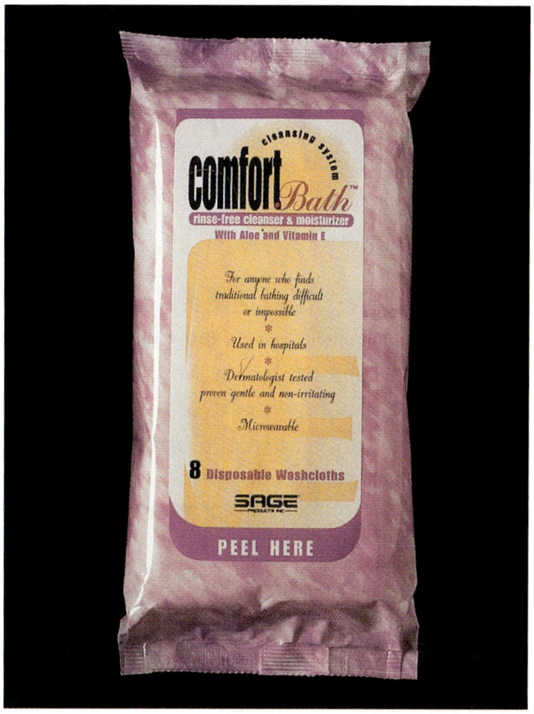

FIGURE 24-1 The waterless bathing system may be used at room temperature, or warmed for comfort. Although the product is more expensive than more conventional methods of bathing, the time savings make it worthwhile. It is gentle on the patient's skin. *(Courtesy of Sage Products, Inc.)*

The procedure is similar to a bed bath, with cleansing done in the same order:

- Face and neck
- Chest and abdomen
- Far arm and hand
- Near arm and hand
- Far leg and foot
- Near leg and foot

INFECTION CONTROL Alert

Waterless bathing products are designed to be used for one bath. Smaller kits containing four cloths are also available for partial baths and perineal care. The package may be resealed if not all of the cloths are used. However, the open package should be dated and discarded in 48 to 72 hours, or according to facility infection control guidelines. Follow facility policy for discarding unused cloths after the bath is completed. Discard used cloths properly, according to facility policy. Avoid flushing them down the toilet. A plastic bag at the bedside works well for cloth disposal.

- Back and buttocks
- Perineum

The waterless bathing system has several advantages:

- It is faster and more economical for the facility; each bath takes approximately 8 to 10 minutes.
- It is less fatiguing for the patient.
- It conserves moisture, reduces drying, and is gentler to skin than soaps.
- It creates less friction, because the cloths are softer than regular washcloths and towels, and drying is eliminated.

The following precautions are used when bathing patients with the waterless bathing system:

- The washcloths may be used at room temperature, but many facilities microwave them for comfort. Monitor the temperature carefully to prevent overheating and intermittent hot spots that could injure the patient.
- Peel the label back or open the package before heating to avoid bursting in the microwave.
- Follow manufacturers' directions for heating the package. One minute is usually sufficient to warm the contents to a comfortable temperature.
- The cloths in the package are for single use only.
- Discard unused cloths within 72 hours of opening the package, or immediately if they are dry.

Whirlpool Bath

The most stimulating form of bathing for patients is a therapeutic bath that is given in a whirlpool tub (Figure 24-2). The whirlpool bath benefits patients because:

- The temperature of the water can be regulated to a constant 97°F.

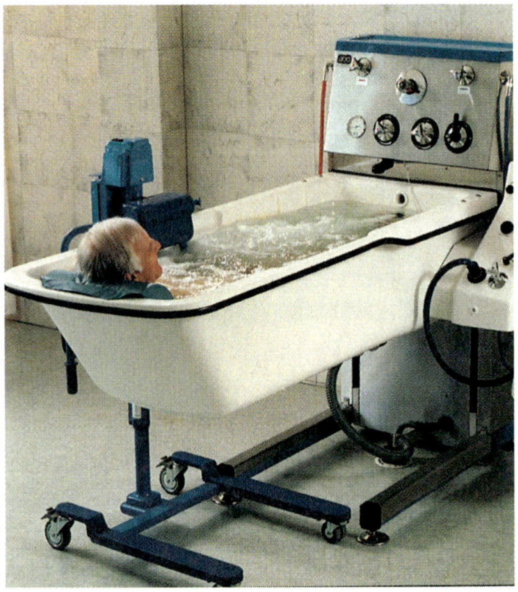

FIGURE 24-2 The water in the whirlpool circulates, maintaining a constant temperature and stimulating circulation. *(Courtesy of Arjo-Century, Inc.)*

INFECTION CONTROL *Alert*

The jets in some whirlpool tubs have the potential to harbor dangerous pathogens. Follow facility policies for carefully cleaning the tub with the proper disinfectant solution. Make sure that you follow directions correctly and run the disinfectant through the tub for the correct length of time.

INFECTION CONTROL *Alert*

Check with the nurse before giving a whirlpool bath to a patient with a surgical incision or pressure ulcer.

- The movement of the water stimulates circulation.
- Warm, circulating water is relaxing and invigorating.
- It provides the value of whirlpool activity with cleansing.

Tips: Never pour liquid soap or shampoo into a whirlpool tub. A tiny bit of liquid soap will result in an abundance of suds. If the patient accidentally creates a suds problem, rub a bar of soap against the walls of the tub to reduce the bubbles.

Care of the hair, teeth, and nails usually follows the bath procedure, but may be carried out as independent procedures. Range-of-motion exercises frequently follow bathing.

PATIENT BATHING

Nursing assistants are frequently assigned to bathe patients. It is important to follow the guidelines and the procedures for bathing carefully to ensure patient comfort and safety. (Refer to Procedures 58, 59, and 61 to 64.)

SAFETY *Alert*

Make sure a chair is available next to the tub or shower in case the patient needs to sit quickly. Turn the hot water on last and off first to prevent injury.

Safety Measures for Special Treatments

Patients receiving special treatments can be bathed. They include, for example, the patient who is receiving an IV, has drainage tubes, or is receiving oxygen. These patients, however, need special care.

Be careful, as you bathe and move the patient, that you:

- Do not put stress on the tubes.
- Never lower the IV container below the level of the infusion site.
- Never raise the drainage tube above the drainage site.

INFECTION CONTROL *Alert*

Think about what precautions are necessary as you perform the procedures in this chapter. Apply the principles of standard precautions. However, avoid overkill. Patients need to be touched. Do not wear gloves for the entire bathing procedure unless there is a reason to do so. When bathing patients, remove the gloves and put on a clean pair immediately prior to contact with mucous membranes and nonintact skin. Do not cross-contaminate body sites by wearing the same pair of gloves for the entire procedure. Avoid contaminating the environment with your used gloves. Discard gloves properly. Wash your hands after removing gloves.

AGE-APPROPRIATE CARE *Alert*

Most patients, young and old, have some independence with activities of daily living when they are in the home. Sometimes they are able to continue to do all or part of these skills. If so, encourage them to continue, unless contraindicated. Provide the supplies needed and arrange them conveniently so the patient can use them. Supervise the patient and assist if needed. This may take longer, but you will reinforce the patient's feelings of self-worth by allowing her to do these things. Organize your work so that you can do something else while the patient is performing self-care skills, as appropriate. This makes good use of your time. If the patient is unable to complete the task, finish it promptly without complaint.

guidelines *for*

Patient Bathing

- Wear disposable gloves if there may be contact with open lesions, blood, body fluids, secretions, or excretions.
- Make sure the shower or tub is cleaned before and after each use (Figure 24-3).
- Check that all safety aids, such as hand rails, shower chairs, tub seats/benches, and hydraulic lifts are in good repair and proper working order.
- Always fasten the safety belt when moving a patient into or out of a whirlpool tub with a hydraulic lift seat.
- Protect patients from fatigue by transporting patients to and from the tub room and carrying out the bathing procedure as efficiently as possible.
- Make sure the patient's body is covered during transport.
- If a patient falls in the tub or shower room or feels faint during bathing, do not leave him alone.

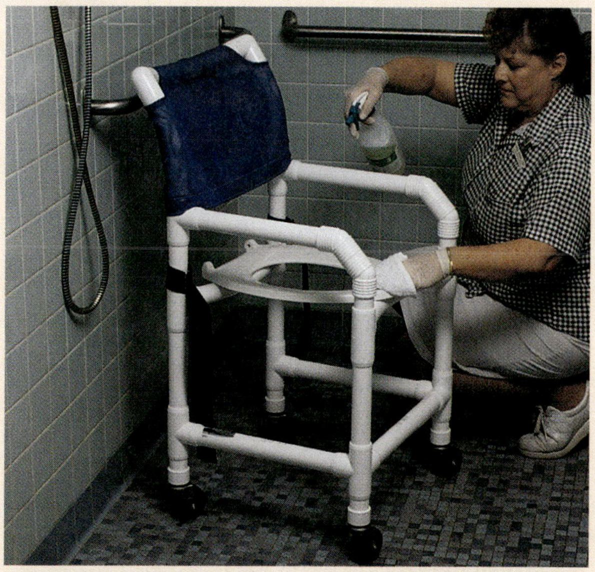

FIGURE 24-3 Clean the tub or shower chair before and after use. Wipe all areas, including the hand rails.

continues

guidelines *continued*

Signal for help, using the emergency call button in the bathroom. Do not lock the bathroom door.

- Use good body mechanics to protect yourself and the patient.
- Nonskid strips placed in the tub and on the floor of the shower prevent slipping.
- Hand rails secured to the walls help prevent falls as the patient transfers into and out of the tub.
- The patient should be assisted in all transfer activity related to the bath. Be sure to have enough help.
- The use of a shower chair will prevent patient stress and fatigue, but it must be secured so that it does not move as the patient transfers into and out of it.

SAFETY *Alert*

Never leave the patient alone in the tub or shower. A call signal in the bathing area is used to call for emergency help.

- Wipe up all water spilled or dripped on the floor immediately, to prevent falls.
- The room should be comfortably warm (about 70°F) and free from drafts, to prevent chilling the patient.
- Cotton bath blankets should be used to cover the patient during a bed bath. They may also be used for added warmth following the tub bath or shower.
- Drape the patient's genital area with a bath towel for modesty during a tub bath or shower.
- Wrap the patient with a bath blanket for warmth and modesty immediately at the end of the tub bath or shower.
- The temperature of the water for a shower, tub bath, or bed bath should be maintained at about 105°F. The temperature of the whirlpool is set at 97°F because the whirlpool maintains a constant temperature. Use a bath thermometer to check the temperature of the water.
- Observe the patient's skin for any changes or irregularities. Note any reddened areas. Do not disturb or injure warts or moles. Report anything unusual.

Tips: It is important to use a bath blanket and towels to drape the patient during all bathing and personal care procedures, even if the room is completely private. Being exposed is uncomfortable for most people. Draping the patient properly provides a sense of dignity, reduces feelings of vulnerability, and protects the patient's modesty and self-esteem. Do not omit this important step for any patients, regardless of their age.

PROCEDURE 58

ASSISTING WITH THE TUB BATH OR SHOWER

1. Carry out beginning procedure actions.
2. Assemble equipment needed:
   - disposable gloves
   - liquid soap
   - washcloth
   - 2–3 bath towels
   - bath blanket
   - bath lotion
   - deodorant
   - chair or stool beside shower or tub
   - bath or shower chair, as needed
   - patient's gown, robe, and slippers
   - bath mat
3. Take the supplies to the bathroom. Prepare the bathroom for the patient. Make sure the tub is clean.
4. Fill the tub half full of water at 105°F or adjust the shower flow. If a bath thermometer is available, check the water temperature. If a bath thermometer is not available, test the water with

continues

PROCEDURE 58

continued

your wrist or elbow. The water should feel comfortably warm.

5. Help the patient put on a robe and slippers. Escort the patient to the bathroom. Cover the nonambulatory patient with a bath blanket when going to or from the bath or shower.
6. Help the patient to undress. Give the patient a towel to wrap around the waist.
7. Position a shower chair in tub or shower, if needed (Figure 24-4).
8. Assist the patient into the tub or shower. For the patient's safety, the bottom of the tub and the shower floor are covered with a nonskid surface.
9. Put on disposable gloves if the patient has open skin lesions.
10. Encourage the patient to wash the rest of his or her body. Assist in washing, as needed.
11. Wash the patient's back.
    - Observe the skin for signs of redness or breaks. See Unit 37 for information on caring for pressure sores or other skin lesions.

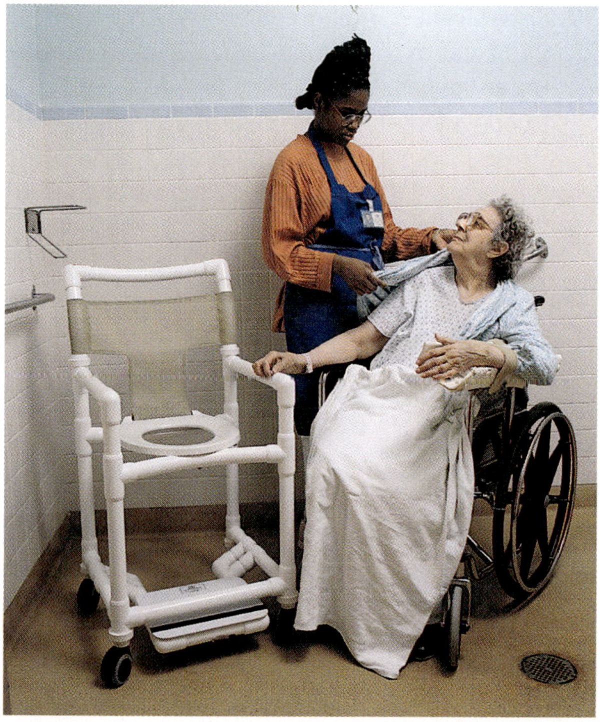

FIGURE 24-4 The shower chair is used to enable the patient to bathe safely.

12. The patient may wash the **genitalia** (external reproductive organs), if able.
    - If the patient is not able to wash the genitalia, then you will also perform this part of the bath. Apply disposable gloves before bathing the genital area.
    - After washing the genitalia, remove gloves, if worn, and discard according to facility policy.
    - Wash your hands.
13. If the patient shows any signs of weakness:
    - Get help. Use the call button.
    - Remove the plug and let the water drain.
    - Turn off the shower.
    - Allow the patient to rest until feeling better before making any attempt to assist the patient out of the tub or shower.
    - Keep the patient covered with a bath blanket to avoid chilling.
14. If the patient wants a shampoo and you have permission to do so:
    - Ask the patient to hold a washcloth over eyes.
    - Pour a small amount of water on hair (enough to wet hair thoroughly).
    - Use a small amount of shampoo to lather hair.
    - Massage scalp gently.
    - Rinse hair with warm water.
    - Repeat lathering, massaging, and rinsing, if necessary.
    - Towel hair dry.
15. Hold the bath blanket around the patient as he or she steps out of the tub. The patient may choose to remove the wet towel from under the bath blanket.
16. Assist the patient to dry, apply deodorant, dress, and return to the unit.
17. Escort the patient back to his or her unit. Return supplies to the patient's unit.
18. Carry out procedure completion actions.
19. Return to the bath or shower room. Put on gloves and clean and disinfect the tub, shower chair, and hand rails.
20. Discard soiled linen.
21. Wash your hands.

PROCEDURE 59

BED BATH

Note: *Disposable gloves should be worn if the patient has draining wounds, nonintact skin, or if contact with blood, body fluids, mucous membranes, secretions, or excretions is likely.*

1. Carry out beginning procedure actions.
2. Assemble equipment needed:
   - disposable gloves
   - bed linen
   - bath blanket
   - laundry bag or hamper
   - bath basin
   - bath thermometer
   - soap and soap dish, or liquid soap
   - washcloths
   - face towel
   - 2 bath towels
   - hospital gown/patient's night clothes
   - lotion
   - equipment for oral hygiene
   - nail brush, emery board, and orangewood stick (if needed)
   - deodorant
   - brush and comb
   - bedpan and cover or urinal
   - paper towel or protector
3. Close the windows and door to prevent chilling the patient.
4. Close the privacy curtain.
5. Put clean towels and linen on a chair in the order of use (Figure 24-5). Place a laundry hamper nearby.
6. Offer the bedpan or urinal. If the patient wants to use the bedpan or urinal, put on gloves. Empty and clean the bedpan or urinal before proceeding with the bath. Remove gloves and discard according to facility policy. Wash your hands.
7. Lower the head of the bed and the side rail on the side where you are working.
8. Loosen the top bedclothes. Remove and fold the blanket and spread and place them over the back of the chair.

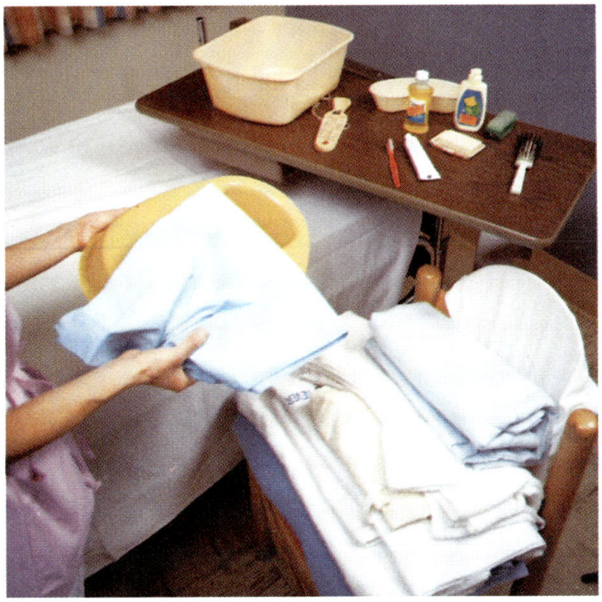

FIGURE 24-5 Assemble equipment. Place bed linens on the chair and remaining items (except bedpan) on the overbed table. If used, the bedpan or urinal should be cleaned immediately, then returned to the bedside stand.

9. Place a bath blanket over the top sheet (Figure 24-6) and remove the sheet by sliding it out from under the bath blanket. Place the sheet in a laundry hamper.

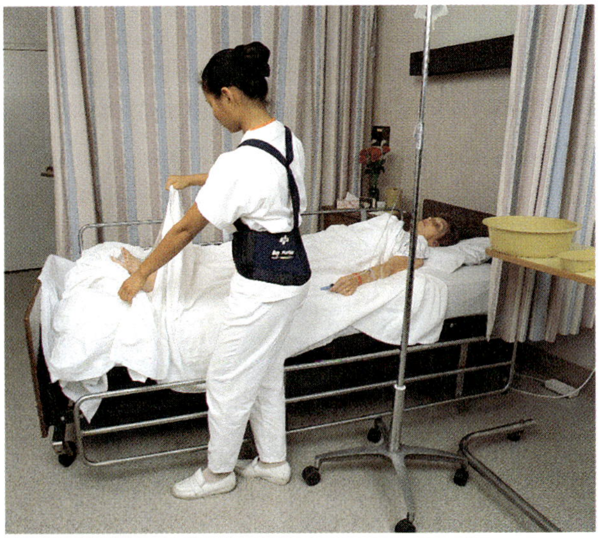

FIGURE 24-6 Replace the top bedding with a bath blanket.

continues

PROCEDURE 59

continued

10. Leave one pillow under the patient's head. Place the other pillow on a chair.

11. Remove the patient's night wear and place it in a laundry hamper (assuming the patient has no IV).

12. Fill a bath basin two-thirds full with water at 105°F. Use a bath thermometer, if available, to be sure of the proper temperature.

13. Assist the patient to move to the side of the bed nearest you.

14. Fold a face towel over the upper edge of the bath blanket to keep the blanket dry. Put on gloves.

15. Form a mitt by folding a washcloth around your hand (Figure 24-7 shows a mitt being made on a gloved hand).

- **a.** Wet the washcloth.
- **b.** Wash eyes, using separate corners of the cloth for each eye.
- **c.** Wipe from inside to outside corner.
- **d.** Do not use soap near eyes.
- **e.** After you have washed the eyes, remove gloves and discard according to facility policy.
- **f.** Do not use soap on the face unless the patient requests it.

16. Rinse the washcloth and apply soap if the patient desires. Squeeze out excess water. Do not leave soap in water.

17. Wash and rinse the patient's face (Figure 24-8), ears, and neck well. Use a towel to dry.

18. Remove gloves and discard according to facility policy.

19. Expose the patient's far arm. Protect the bed with a bath towel placed underneath the arm (Figure 24-9).

- **a.** Wash, rinse, and pat dry arm and hand.
- **b.** Be sure **axilla** (armpit) is clean and dry.
- **c.** Repeat for other arm.
- **d.** Apply deodorant if the patient requests it.

20. Care for hands and nails as necessary. Check with the nurse first to see if there are any special instructions.

- **a.** Place the patient's hands in a basin of water. Wash each hand carefully. Rinse and dry. Push **cuticle** (base of fingernails) down gently with a towel while wiping the fingers. Be sure to dry between fingers.
- **b.** Clean under the nails with orangewood stick. Shape the nails with emery board. Be careful not to file nails too close. Do not cut nails if the patient is diabetic. Inform the nurse if attention is needed.

21. Discard used bath water and refill the basin two-thirds full with water at 105°F.

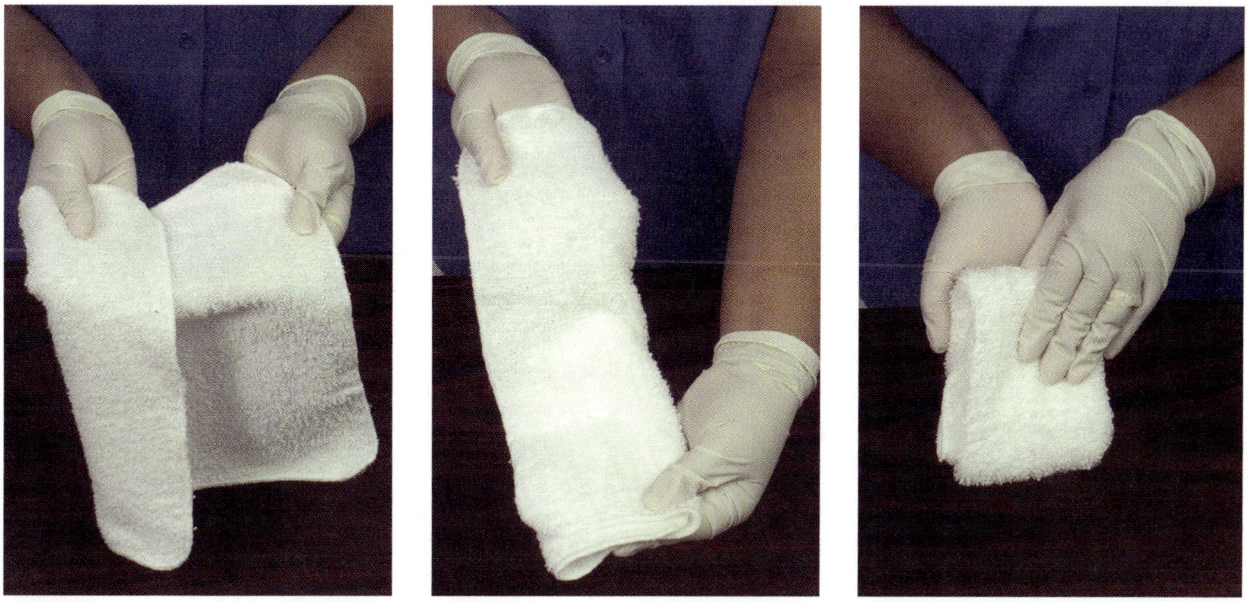

FIGURE 24-7 To make a mitt over a gloved hand, wrap the washcloth in thirds around one hand. Then bring the free end over the palm and tuck in the end. The thumb is free to hold the washcloth in place.

continues

PROCEDURE 59

continued

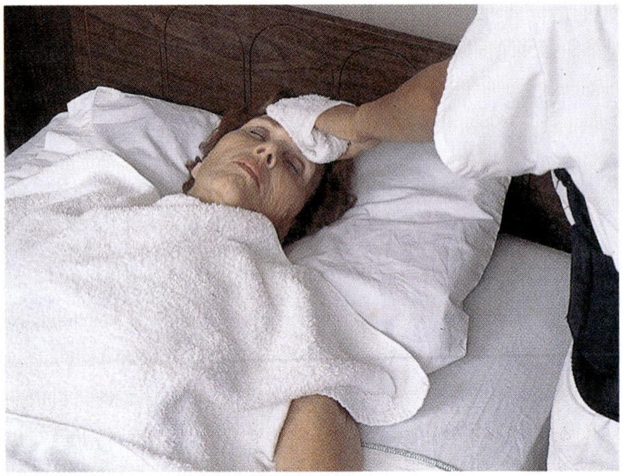

FIGURE 24-8 Wash the face carefully, doing each eye separately. Avoid soap in the eye area. Some patients do not use soap on the face.

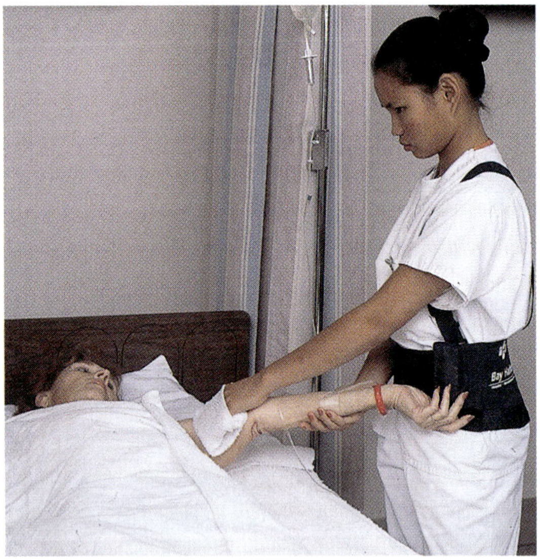

FIGURE 24-9 Place the towel under the patient's arm. Support the arm as you wash it.

22. Put a bath towel over the patient's chest. Then fold the blanket to waist. Under the towel:
    a. Wash, rinse, and pat dry chest (Figure 24-10).
    b. Rinse and dry folds under the breasts of a female patient carefully to avoid irritating the skin.
23. Fold the bath blanket down to the **pubic** area (location of external genitalia). Wash, rinse, and pat dry abdomen. Fold the bath blanket up to cover the abdomen and chest. Slide the towel out from under the bath blanket.

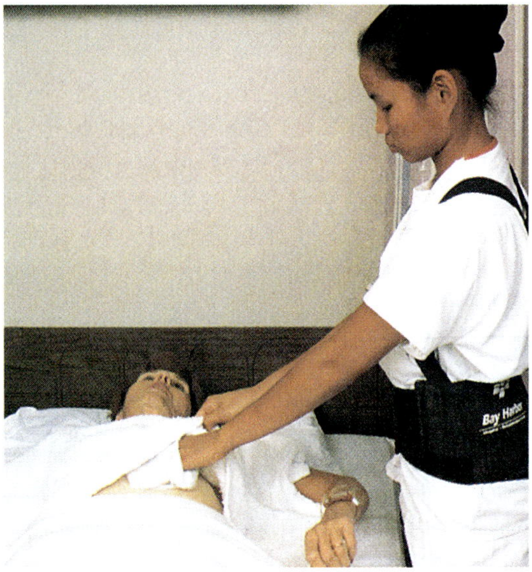

FIGURE 24-10 Lift the towel with one hand. Wash underneath with the other hand.

24. Ask the patient to flex the far knee, if possible. Fold the bath blanket up to expose the thigh, leg, and foot. Protect the bed with a bath towel.
    a. Put the bath basin on the towel.
    b. Place the patient's foot in the basin (Figure 24-11).
    c. Wash and rinse the leg and foot.
    d. When moving the patient's leg, support it properly.
25. Lift the leg and move the basin to the other side of the bed. Dry the leg and foot. Dry well between toes.
26. Repeat for the other leg and foot. Take the basin off the bed before drying the leg and foot.
27. Care for toenails as necessary. Check with the nurse for any special instructions. Apply lotion to the feet of a patient with dry skin. Do not apply lotion between the toes, as this keeps the area moist and promotes fungal growth.
    - Do not attempt to cut thickened nails.
    - File nails straight across.
    - Do not round edges.
    - Do not push back the cuticle, because it is easily injured and infected.
    - If the patient is diabetic, inform the nurse if toenail care is required.

continues

PROCEDURE 59

continued

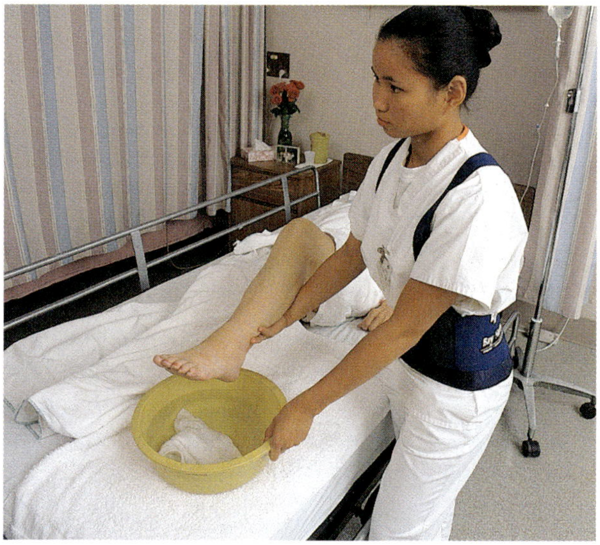

FIGURE 24-11 Support the leg and place the patient's foot in the basin.

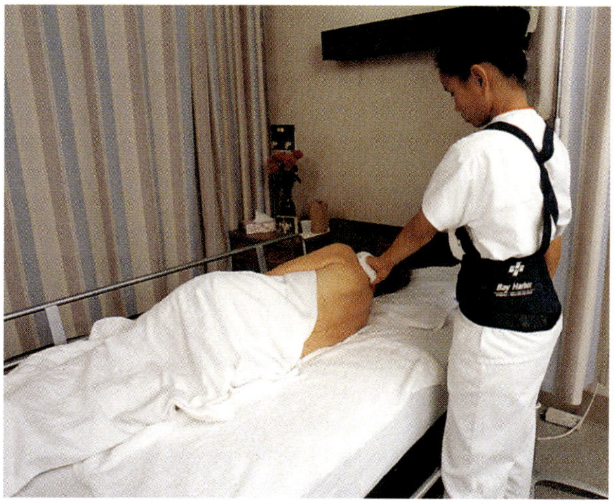

FIGURE 24-12 Change the water and wash the patient's back.

28. Change water and check for the correct temperature with a bath thermometer. It may be necessary to change the water before this point in the patient's bath if it becomes cold or too soapy.
29. Help the patient to turn on the side away from you. Help her to move toward the center of the bed. Place a bath towel lengthwise next to the patient's back.
    - Wash, rinse, and dry neck, back, and buttocks (Figure 24-12).
    - Use long, firm strokes when washing the back.
30. A back rub is usually given at this time (see Unit 25).
31. Help the patient to turn on the back.
32. Place a towel under the buttocks and upper legs. Change the water in the basin and check for the correct temperature. Place a washcloth, soap, basin, and bath towel within convenient reach of the patient. Have the patient complete the bath by washing the genitalia. Assist the patient if necessary. You must take responsibility for the procedure if the patient has difficulty. Many times patients are reluctant to acknowledge the need for help. If assisting a patient with genital washing, always put on disposable gloves.
    - For a female patient, wash from front to back, drying carefully.
    - For a male patient, carefully wash and dry the penis, scrotum, and groin area. If the patient is not circumcised, gently push the foreskin back and carefully wash and dry the penis. Then gently pull the foreskin down to its original position.
33. Remove gloves and discard according to facility policy.
34. Carry out range-of-motion exercises as ordered (see Unit 40 for procedures).
35. Cover the pillow with a towel. Comb or brush the patient's hair. Oral hygiene is usually given at this time (see Unit 25).
36. Discard towels and washcloth in a laundry hamper.
37. Provide a clean gown.
38. Clean and replace equipment according to facility policy.
39. Put clean washcloth and towels in the bedside stand, or hang according to facility policy.
40. Change the bed linen, following the procedure for making an occupied bed. Replace and discard soiled linen in a laundry hamper.
41. Remove and discard disposable gloves according to facility policy. Wash your hands.
42. Raise the side rails, if required.
43. Carry out procedure completion actions.

PROCEDURE 60

CHANGING THE PATIENT'S GOWN

Note: *Wear disposable gloves if the patient has draining wounds, nonintact skin, or if contact with mucous membranes, blood, body fluids, secretions, or excretions is likely.*

1. Carry out beginning procedure actions.
2. Assemble equipment needed:
   - disposable gloves
   - bath blanket
   - clean gown
   - laundry bag or hamper
3. Place a bath blanket over the top sheet. Pull the sheet down by sliding it out from under the bath blanket.
4. Loosen gown from the patient's neck.
5. Slip the gown down the arms.
6. Make sure the patient is covered by a bath blanket (Figure 24-13).

Note: *This procedure is to be used only when the patient has an IV that is NOT run through an electric pump. When a pump is used, the patient may wear a gown that snaps at the shoulder. In this case, the gown can be removed without touching the IV bag or tubing. If the patient is wearing a nonsnap gown, call the nurse if the gown is to be changed. Never disconnect the tubing from the pump.*

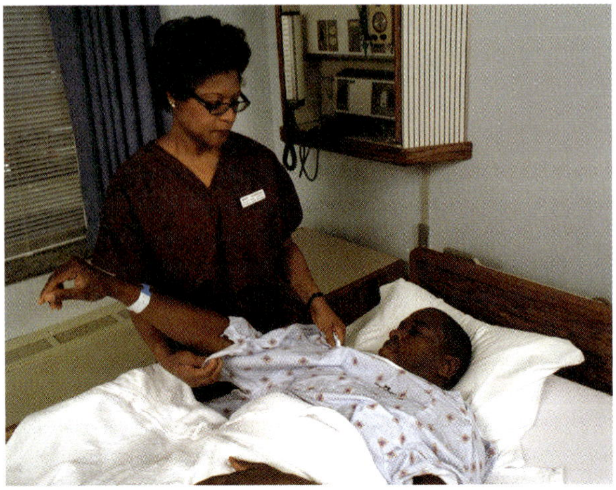

FIGURE 24-13 Keeping the patient covered with the bath blanket, remove the patient's gown.

7. For a patient wearing a regular gown (nonsnap):
   a. Remove the gown from the arm without the IV and bring the gown across the patient's chest to the other arm.
   b. Place a clean gown over the patient's chest to avoid exposure.
   c. On the arm with the IV, gather the gown material in one hand so there is no pull or pressure on the IV line (Figure 24-14A), and slowly draw the gown over the tips of the patient's fingers.
   d. With your free hand, lift the IV free of the standard and slip the gown over the bag of fluid (Figure 24-14B), removing the gown from the patient's body. **Never allow the bag of fluid to be lower than the patient's arm.**
   e. Take the sleeve of a clean gown and slip it over the bag of fluid, over the tubing, and up the patient's arm.
   f. Replace the bag of fluid on the IV standard.
   g. Remove the soiled gown and place it at the end of the bed. Finish putting the clean gown on the patient's other arm. Secure the neck ties.
   h. Place the soiled gown in a laundry hamper.

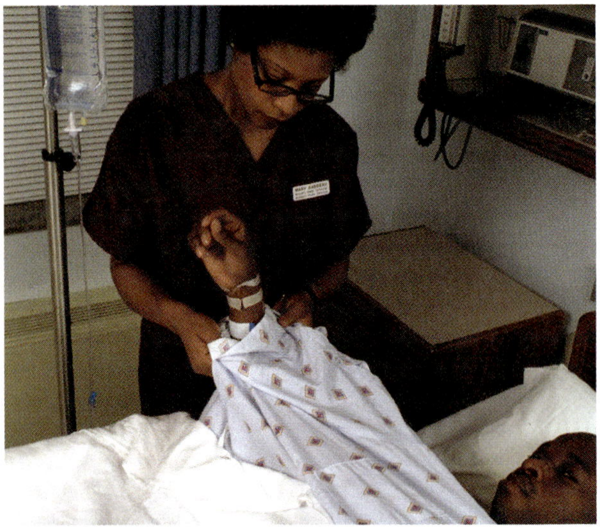

FIGURE 24-14A Gather the material of the gown in one hand so there is no traction on the IV line. Slowly draw the gown over the tips of the patient's fingers.

continues

PROCEDURE 60

continued

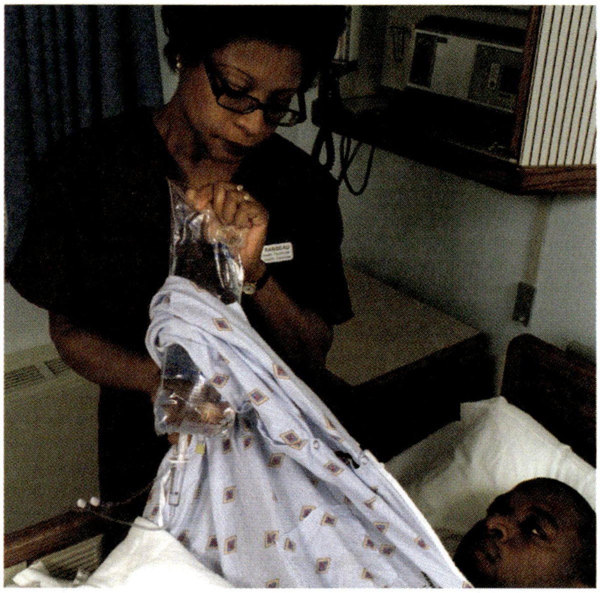

FIGURE 24-14B With your free hand, lift the IV off the standard and slip the gown over the bag of fluid.

   i. Make sure the IV is dripping at the required rate and that the tubing is not kinked or twisted.

8. If the patient has a weak or paralyzed arm, always undress the patient in the following manner:
   a. Untie the gown and remove the back sides of the gown from underneath the patient.
   b. Remove the gown from the stronger arm first.
   c. Bring the gown across the patient's chest and slide the gown down over the weak arm.
   d. Gently lift the patient's weak arm to finish removing the gown over the patient's hand.
   e. Reverse the procedure to put a clean gown on the patient, by putting the gown over the weaker arm first.
9. Pull the sheet up over the bath blanket. Remove the bath blanket.
10. Carry out procedure completion actions.

PROCEDURE 61

WATERLESS BED BATH

1. Carry out beginning procedure actions.
2. Assemble equipment:
   - disposable gloves
   - bed linen
   - bath blanket
   - laundry bag or hamper
   - hospital gown/patient's night clothes
   - bath towel
   - lotion for back rub
   - waterless bathing product, heated according to facility policy or patient wishes
   - basin of warm water for soaking hands (optional)
   - comb, brush
   - bedpan or urinal with cover, as needed
   - supplies for oral hygiene, as needed
   - supplies for nail care, as needed
   - small plastic bag to discard used bathing cloths
   - large plastic bag or hamper for soiled linen
3. Close the windows and door to the room.
4. Pull the privacy curtain. Place clean supplies on the overbed table.
5. Offer the bedpan or urinal. Put on gloves if you will be assisting with this procedure.
6. Lower the head of the bed and the side rail on the side where you will be working.
7. Loosen the top bedclothes. Remove and fold the blanket and spread and place them over the back of the chair.

continues

PROCEDURE 61

continued

8. Place a bath blanket over the top sheet and remove the sheet by sliding it out from under the bath blanket. Place the sheet in the laundry hamper.
9. Leave one pillow under the patient's head. Place the other pillow on the chair.
10. Remove the gown (see Procedure 60) and place it in the laundry hamper.
11. Assist the patient to move to the side of the bed near you.
12. Warm the package according to facility policy and manufacturer's directions. Open the package. (If you used a microwave to heat the package, check the cloths for hot spots.) Remove one cloth and cleanse the patient's face and neck. (The solution on these cloths can safely be used around the eyes.)
13. Place a towel over the patient's chest. Fold the bath blanket down to the waist and cleanse the chest. Be sure the area under a female patient's breasts is carefully cleaned.
14. Fold the bath blanket down to the pubic area and wash the abdomen. Replace the bath blanket over the abdomen and chest. Remove the towel by sliding it out from under the bath blanket. Discard the used cloth in the plastic bag.
15. Uncover the far arm. Remove another cloth from the package and wash the arm and hand. It is nice to soak each of the patient's hands separately in a basin of warm water while you wash the opposite arm. This is refreshing for the patient who cannot be out of bed to bathe. Wash each axilla. Apply deodorant if the patient desires. Discard the used cloth in the plastic bag. Cover the arm with the bath blanket.
16. Uncover the near arm. Remove a new cloth from the package. Wash the arm, hand, and axilla. Apply deodorant. Discard the used cloth in the plastic bag. Cover the patient with the bath blanket.
17. Provide nail care as needed.
18. Ask the patient to flex the far leg, if possible. Fold the bath blanket up to expose the thigh, leg, and foot. Remove a new cloth from the package. Cleanse the thigh, leg, and foot. Be sure the area between the toes is left dry. Discard the used cloth in the plastic bag. Cover the leg and foot with the bath blanket.
19. Repeat step 18 with the near thigh, leg, and foot.
20. Make sure the side rail on the opposite side of the bed is up. Help the patient turn onto the side away from you. Place a bath towel lengthwise next to the patient's back.
21. Remove a new cloth from the package. Draw the bath blanket back to expose the back. Wash the back and buttocks. Discard the used cloth in the plastic bag. A backrub may be given at this time. Cover the patient with the bath blanket.
22. Assist the patient to turn onto the back. Position a towel under the buttocks by asking the patient to lift the hips, if possible. Remove a new cloth from the package. Hand the patient the cloth and instruct the patient to wash the perineum. Assist if necessary. (Wear gloves if you will be assisting.) Discard gloves and the used cloth in the plastic bag. Remove the towel.
23. Wash your hands.
24. Assist the patient to put on a clean gown.
25. Cover the pillow with a towel. Comb or brush the patient's hair. Assist with oral hygiene, if needed.
26. Change the bed linen, following the procedure for making an occupied bed (see Procedure 56). Put soiled linen in a plastic bag or linen hamper.
27. Carry out procedure completion actions.

PROCEDURE 62

PARTIAL BATH

1. Carry out beginning procedure actions.
2. Assemble equipment needed:
   - disposable gloves
   - bed linen
   - bath blanket
   - bath thermometer
   - soap and soap dish or liquid soap
   - washcloth
   - face towel
   - bath towel
   - gown and robe
   - laundry bag or hamper
   - bath basin
   - lotion
   - equipment for oral hygiene
   - nail brush, emery board, and orangewood stick
   - brush, comb, and deodorant
   - bedpan or urinal and cover
   - paper towels or protector

Note: *A package of premoistened washcloths can be substituted for the basin of water, soap, washcloth, and towel if the facility has approved the use of the waterless bath. The nursing assistant or the patient (condition permitting) can use the premoistened washcloths for the partial bath.*

3. Close windows and door and turn off fans to prevent chilling the patient.
4. Put the towels and linen on the chair in the order of use. Make sure a laundry hamper is available.
5. Put on disposable gloves.
6. Offer the bedpan or urinal (see Unit 25). Empty and clean it before proceeding with the bath. Remove gloves and discard according to facility policy. Wash your hands.
7. Elevate the head of the bed, if permitted, to a comfortable position.
8. Loosen the top bedclothes. Remove and fold the blanket and spread and place them over the back of the chair. Place a bath blanket over the top sheet. Remove the top sheet by sliding it out from under the bath blanket.
9. Leave one pillow under the patient's head. Place the other pillow on the chair.
10. Assist the patient to remove the gown. Place the gown in the laundry hamper. Make sure the patient is covered with a bath blanket.
11. Place paper towels or a bed protector on the overbed table.
12. Fill a bath basin two-thirds full with water at 105°F. Place the basin on the overbed table.
13. Push the overbed table comfortably close to the patient.
14. Place towels, washcloth, and soap on the overbed table within easy reach.
15. Instruct the patient to wash as much as she is able and tell her that you will return to complete the bath.
16. Place the call bell within easy reach. Ask the patient to signal when ready.
17. Wash hands and leave unit.
18. Wash hands and return to unit when the patient signals. Put on a new pair of gloves.
19. Change the bath water. Complete bathing those areas the patient could not reach. Make sure the face, hands, axillae, buttocks, back, and genitals are washed and dried.
20. Remove gloves and discard according to facility policy.
21. Wash your hands.
22. Give a backrub with lotion.
23. Assist the patient in applying deodorant and a fresh gown.
24. Cover the pillow with a towel. Comb or brush the patient's hair. Assist with oral hygiene, if needed (see Unit 25).
25. Clean and replace equipment according to facility policy.
26. Put a clean washcloth and towels in the bedside stand, or hang according to facility policy.
27. Change the bed linen, following the procedure for making an occupied bed. Put soiled linen in the laundry hamper.
28. Carry out procedure completion actions.

Perineal Care

The **perineum** is the area between the legs. In females, it is the area between the vagina and the anus. In males, it is the area between the scrotum and the anus.

Perineal care may be performed as part of general bathing or as a separate procedure, as needed. **Perineal care** means to wash the area including the genitals and anus (see Procedures 63 and 64). Always wear gloves and use standard precautions when caring for the perineal area.

Tips: If the patient has been incontinent, remove the wet pad or linen and replace with a dry pad before beginning perineal care. Clean excess stool off with toilet tissue before beginning.

COMMUNICATION *Highlight*

Patients who need assistance with perineal care and those who become incontinent may feel guilty and embarrassed. Avoid showing disgust. Be sensitive to the patient's feelings. Communicate with the patient tactfully. Use proper terms when referring to body parts and excretions.

INFECTION CONTROL *Alert*

Providing perineal care is one of the most important procedures you will perform as a nursing assistant. Always apply the principles of standard precautions. Remember that there are mucous membranes in the genital area. If you are wearing gloves, change them before beginning care. Using proper technique is critical because of the high risk of contamination and infection. Avoid scrubbing back and forth. Always wipe from clean to dirty with a single wipe, then turn or discard the cloth, according to facility policy. Guidelines for female perineal care vary with the institution. In some facilities, you will be instructed to clean the center first, then each side. In others, you will clean the sides of the genitalia first, then the center. Know and follow your facility policies. Discard your gloves properly and avoid contaminating environmental surfaces with your used gloves.

PROCEDURE 63

FEMALE PERINEAL CARE

1. Carry out beginning procedure actions.
2. Assemble equipment:
   - disposable gloves
   - bath blanket or top sheet
   - bedpan and cover
   - liquid soap
   - basin
   - bath thermometer
   - bed protector
   - washcloth and towel
   - plastic bag(s), if needed to discard linen or trash
   - laundry barrel or hamper
3. Lower the side rail on the side where you will be working. Be sure the opposite side rail is up and secure.
4. Remove the bedspread and blanket. Fold and place them on the back of the chair.
5. The patient is to be on her back. Cover the patient with a bath blanket and fanfold the sheet to the foot of the bed.
6. Put on disposable gloves. Fill a basin with water at 105°F.
7. Ask the patient to raise her hips while you place a bed protector underneath the patient.
8. Offer the bedpan to the patient.
   a. If used and the patient is on intake and output, record the amount.
   b. Empty and clean the bedpan before continuing with the procedure.

continues

PROCEDURE 63

continued

   c. Remove gloves and discard according to facility policy.
   d. Wash your hands and put on a new pair of gloves.
9. Position the bath blanket so that only the area between the legs is exposed.
10. Ask the patient to separate her legs and flex her knees.

Note: *If the patient is unable to spread her legs and flex her knees, turn the patient on her side with the legs flexed. This position provides easy access to the perineal area.*

11. Wet the washcloth, make a mitt, and apply a small amount of liquid soap.

Note: *Heavy soap application may be difficult to rinse off completely. Soap residue is irritating.*

12. Use one gloved hand to stabilize and separate the vulva (Figure 24-15). With the other gloved hand, proceed as follows.
   a. Bring the soaped washcloth in one downward stroke along the far side of the outer labia to the perineum.
   b. Rinse the washcloth, remake the mitt, and rinse the area just cleaned.
   c. Repeat steps a and b, washing and rinsing the inner far labia.
   d. Repeat steps a and b, washing and rinsing the inner near labia.
   e. With gloved hands, separate the labia. Clean and rinse the inner part of the vulva to the perineum.
   f. Dry the washed area with a towel.
13. Turn the patient away from you. Flex the upper leg slightly if permitted.
14. Make a mitt, wet it, and apply soap lightly.
15. Expose the anal area. Wash the area, stroking from perineum to coccyx (front to back) (Figure 24-16).
16. Rinse well in the same manner.
17. Dry carefully.
18. Return the patient to her back.
19. Remove and dispose of the bed protector according to facility policy.
20. Cover the patient with a sheet or bath blanket.
21. Remove and dispose of gloves according to facility policy. Wash your hands.
22. Remove, fold, and store the bath blanket according to facility policy.
23. Replace the top covers, tuck them under the mattress, and make mitered corners. (Some patients prefer that the top covers not be tucked in.)
24. Put up the side rail.
25. Put on gloves. Empty the water. Clean equipment and dispose of or store it, according to facility policy.
26. Remove gloves and discard according to facility policy. Wash your hands.
27. Carry out procedure completion actions.

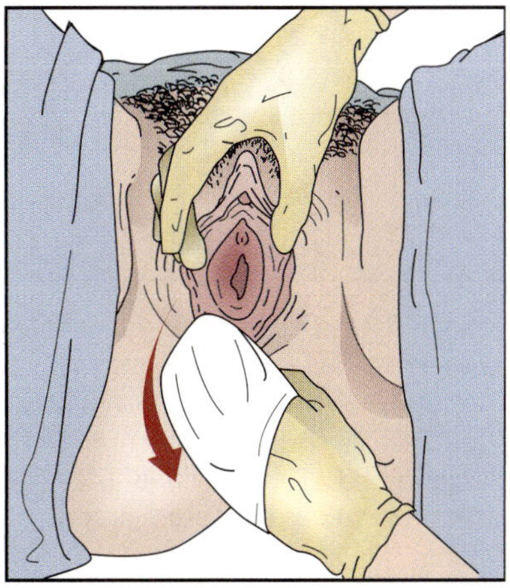

FIGURE 24-15 Spread the vulva with one hand. With the washcloth in the other hand, start in the front and stroke downward along the outer labia.

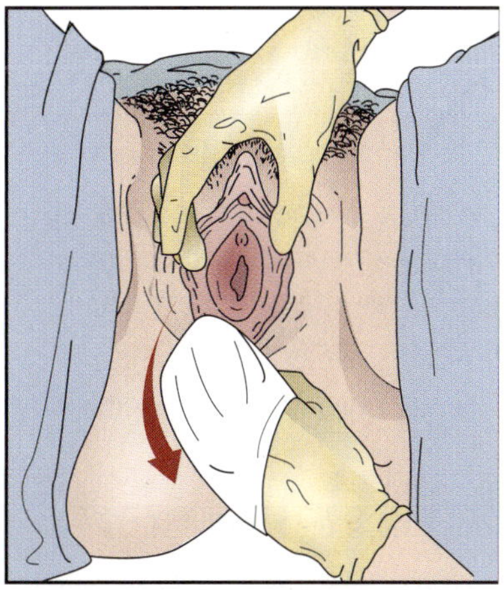

FIGURE 24-16 With one hand, lift up on the buttocks to expose the anal area. Wipe from the perineum back toward the anus.

PROCEDURE 64

MALE PERINEAL CARE

1. Carry out beginning procedure actions.
2. Assemble equipment:
   - disposable gloves
   - bath blanket
   - bath thermometer
   - urinal and cover or bedpan and cover
   - soap, washcloth, and towel
   - plastic bag
   - bed protector or bath towel
   - ordered solution (if other than water)
   - basin
   - laundry hamper
3. Fill a basin with warm water at approximately 105°F.
4. Lower the side rail on the side where you will be working.
5. Fanfold the blanket and spread to the foot of the bed. Remove, fold, and place them on the back of the chair.
6. Cover the patient with a bath blanket and fanfold the sheet to the foot of the bed.
7. Put on disposable gloves.
8. Place a bed protector under the patient's buttocks.
9. Offer the bedpan or urinal.
   a. If used and the patient is on intake and output, record the amount.
   b. Empty and clean the bedpan or urinal before continuing with the procedure.
   c. Remove gloves and discard according to facility policy.
   d. Wash your hands and put on a new pair of gloves.
10. Have the patient flex and separate his knees.

Note: *If the patient is unable to spread his legs and flex the knees, the perineal area can be washed with the patient on his side with the legs flexed. This position provides easy access to the perineal area.*

11. Draw the bath blanket upward to expose the perineal area only.
12. Make a mitt with a washcloth and apply a small amount of soap.

Note: *Heavy soap application may be difficult to rinse off completely. Soap residue is irritating.*

13. Grasp the penis gently with one hand and wash. Begin at the meatus and wash in a circular motion (Figure 24-17).
14. If the patient is not circumcised, draw the foreskin back (Figure 24-18). Be sure the entire penis is washed. Rinse thoroughly.
15. Continue to wash down the penis and the rest of the perineal area, including the scrotum, using downward strokes and working outward to the thighs. Lift the scrotum and wash the perineum.
16. Rinse the washcloth and remake a mitt. Rinse the urethral and perineal areas well, working in the same direction until the entire area is clean and soap-free.
17. Dry the washed area with a towel. Reposition the foreskin if necessary.

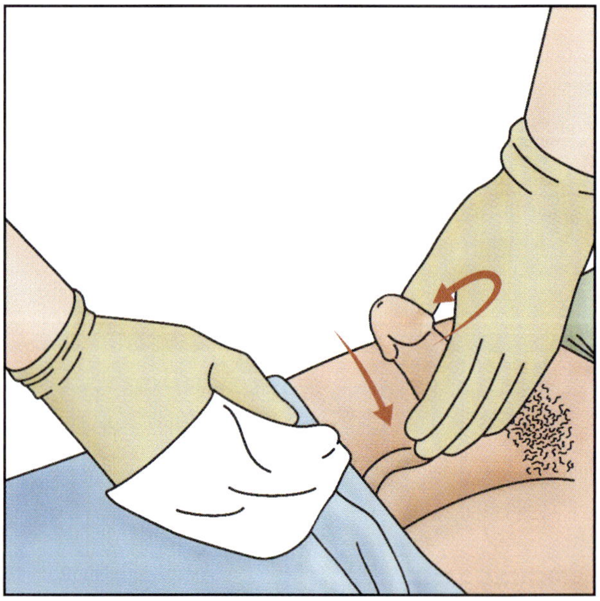

FIGURE 24-17 Grasp the penis gently with one hand. With the other, wipe in a circular motion, beginning with the urinary meatus, working outward over the glans (head of the penis). Continue to wash down the penis and the rest of the perineal area, including the scrotum, using downward strokes and working outward to the thighs.

continues

PROCEDURE 64

continued

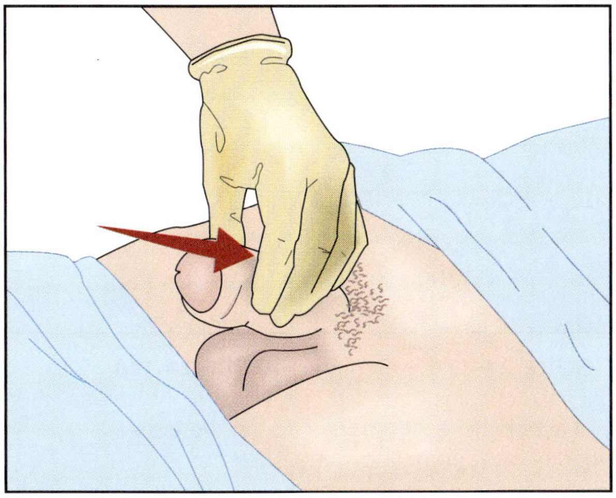

FIGURE 24-18 If the patient is not circumcised, gently push the foreskin back so the glans can be washed. Once the penis is washed and dried, return the foreskin to its normal position.

18. Turn the patient away from you. Flex his upper leg slightly if permitted.
19. Make a mitt, wet it, and apply soap lightly.
20. Expose the anal area. Wash the area, stroking from perineum to coccyx.
21. Rinse well in the same manner.
22. Dry carefully.
23. Return the patient to his back.
24. Remove and dispose of the bed protector according to facility policy.
25. Cover the patient with a sheet.
26. Remove and dispose of gloves according to facility policy. Wash your hands.
27. Remove, fold, and store the bath blanket, according to facility policy.
28. Replace the top covers, tuck them under the mattress, and make mitered corners. (Some patients prefer that the top covers not be tucked in.)
29. Put up the side rail, if required.
30. Put on gloves. Empty the water. Clean equipment and dispose of or store it, according to facility policy.
31. Remove gloves and discard according to facility policy. Wash your hands.
32. Carry out procedure completion actions.

PROCEDURE 65

HAND AND FINGERNAIL CARE

Note: Check with the nurse and nursing care plan to learn if this procedure is permitted for the patient or if it is to be modified because of the patient's condition.

This procedure can be carried out independently or can be modified and added to the bath procedure.

1. Carry out beginning procedure actions.
2. Assemble equipment:
   - basin
   - bath thermometer
   - soap
   - bath towel and washcloth
   - lotion
   - plastic protector
   - nail clippers
   - emery board
   - orangewood stick
   - nail polish (optional)
3. Elevate the head of the bed, if permitted, and adjust the overbed table in front of the patient. If the patient is allowed out of bed, assist the patient to transfer to a chair and position the overbed table waist-high across the patient's lap.
4. Place a plastic protector on the overbed table.

continues

PROCEDURE 65

continued

5. Fill a basin with warm water at approximately 105°F, using the bath thermometer to test temperature. Place the basin on the overbed table.
6. Instruct the patient to put hands in the basin and soak for approximately 5 minutes. Place a towel over the basin to help retain heat. Add warm water if necessary. Remember to remove the patient's hands before adding water.
7. Wash the patient's hands. Push cuticles back gently with a washcloth or an orangewood stick (Figure 24-19A). (A cream may be used to soften the cuticles first.) Use a soft brush or orangewood stick to clean under nails. (Check with the nurse before using an orangewood stick for a patient with diabetes.)
8. Dry the patient's hands with a towel. Remember to dry between the fingers.
9. Use nail clippers to cut fingernails straight across, if permitted by facility policy (Figure 24-19B).
   - Do not cut below the tips of the fingers.
   - Keep nail clippings on the protector to be discarded.

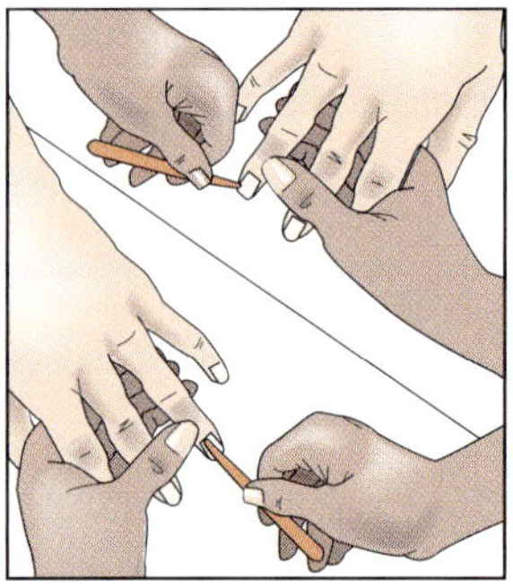

FIGURE 24-19A Gently push the cuticles back with a washcloth, or orangewood stick, if permitted.

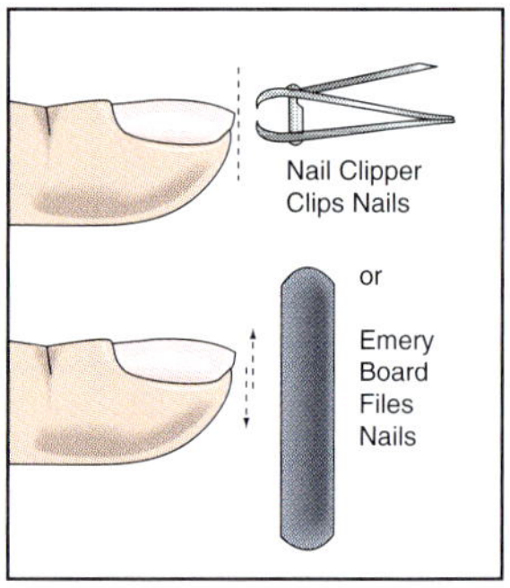

FIGURE 24-19B Clip the nails straight across, then round the edges.

10. Shape and smooth the fingernails with an emery board. Apply polish to nails if the patient desires.
11. Pour a small amount of lotion in your palms and gently smooth it on the patient's hands.
12. Empty the basin of water. Gather equipment. Clean and store it according to the facility policy.
13. Return the overbed table to the foot of the bed. If the patient has been sitting up for the procedure, assist the patient to get into bed.
14. Carry out procedure completion actions.

PROCEDURE 66

BED SHAMPOO

1. Carry out beginning procedure actions.
2. Assemble equipment needed:
   - shampoo tray
   - shampoo
   - washcloths
   - 3 bath towels
   - bath blanket
   - pitcher of water (105°F)
   - safety pin
   - 2 bed protectors
   - waterproof covering for pillow
   - large bucket to collect used water
   - hair dryer, if available (portable)
   - hairbrush and comb
   - small empty pitcher or cup
   - larger pitcher of water (105°F)—use if additional water is needed
3. Place a large, empty basin on the floor under the spout of the shampoo tray.
4. Arrange on the bedside stand, within easy reach (Figure 24-20A).
   - large pitcher of water (105°F)

continues

PROCEDURE 66

continued

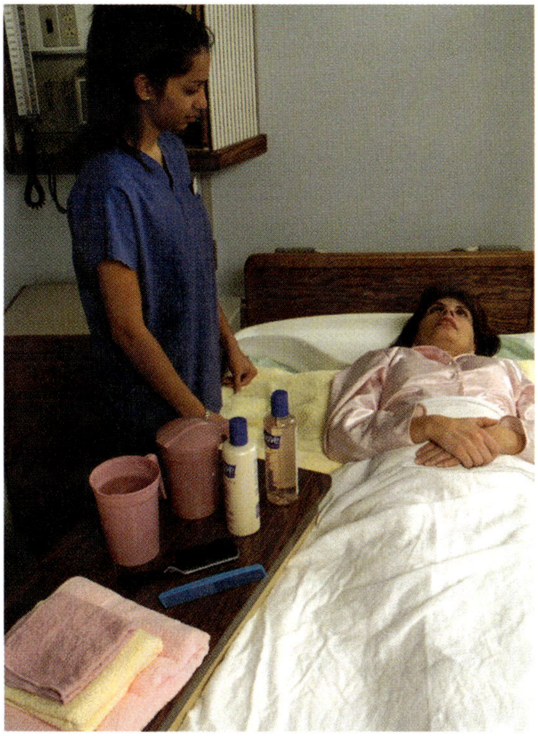

FIGURE 24-20A Assemble equipment.

- washcloth
- 2 bath towels
- shampoo
- small pitcher of water (105°F)

5. Replace the top bedding with a bath blanket.
6. Ask the patient to move to the side of the bed nearest you. Assist as needed.
7. Replace the pillowcase with a waterproof covering.
8. Cover the head of the bed with a bed protector. Be sure it goes well under the patient's shoulders.
9. Loosen neck ties of the gown.
10. Place a towel under the patient's head and shoulders. Brush hair free of tangles, working snarls out carefully.
11. Bring the towel down around the patient's neck and shoulders and pin it. Position the pillow under shoulders so that the patient's head is tilted slightly backward.
12. Raise the bed to high horizontal position.

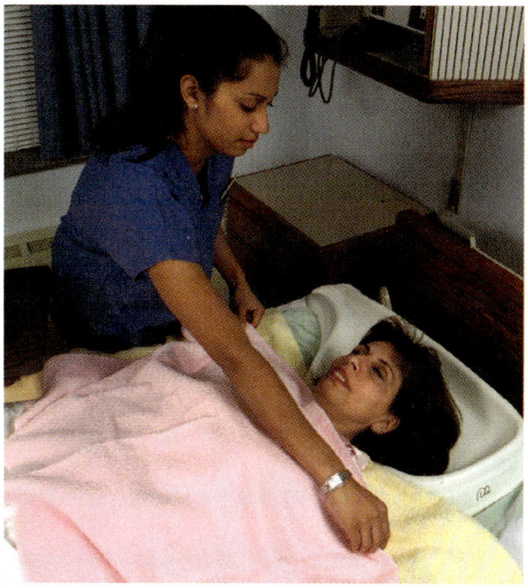

FIGURE 24-20B Position the patient's head on the shampoo tray. Protect the patient with a towel and the bed with a protector.

13. Raise the patient's head and position the shampoo tray (Figure 24-20B) so that the drain is over the edge of the bed directly above the basin.
14. Give the patient a washcloth to cover eyes (Figure 24-20C).

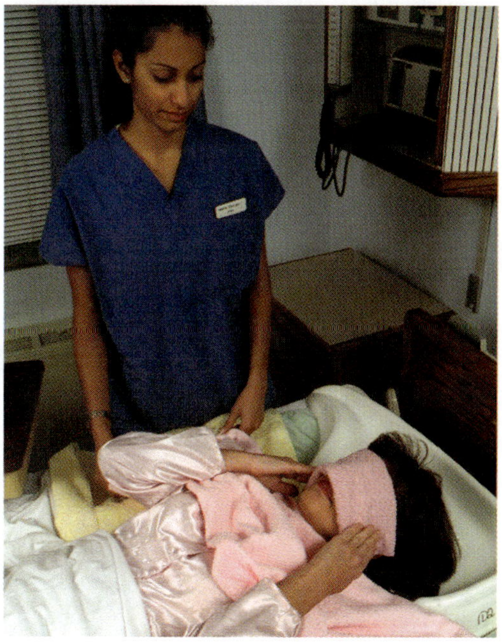

FIGURE 24-20C Give the patient a folded washcloth to protect her eyes.

continues

PROCEDURE 66

continued

15. Recheck the temperature of water in the basin.
16. Using the small pitcher (Figure 24-20D), pour a small amount of water over hair until thoroughly wet. Use one hand to help direct the flow away from the face and ears.
17. Apply a small amount of shampoo, working up a lather (Figure 24-20E). Work from scalp to hair ends.
18. Massage the scalp with your fingertips. Do not use your fingernails.
19. Rinse thoroughly, pouring from hairline to hair tips. Direct the flow into the drain. Use water from the pitcher if needed, but be sure to check the water temperature before use.
20. Repeat lathering and rinsing (steps 16–19).
21. Lift the patient's head. Remove the tray and bed protector. Adjust the pillow and slip a dry bath towel underneath the head.
22. Place the tray on the basin. Wrap hair in a towel. Be sure to dry face, neck, and ears as needed.
23. Dry hair with the towel. If available and not otherwise contraindicated, a portable hair dryer may be used to complete the drying process. Brushing the hair as you blow-dry helps the hair to dry. Be sure to keep the dryer moving and not too close to the hair.
24. Comb hair appropriately. Remove the protective pillow cover. Replace with a cloth cover.
25. Lower the bed to a comfortable working position.
26. Replace the bedding and remove the bath blanket.
27. Help the patient assume a comfortable position. Lower the bed to the lowest horizontal position. Leave the call bell within reach.
28. Allow the patient to rest undisturbed. The length of this procedure may tire the patient.
29. Empty the water from the collection basin.
30. Carry out procedure completion actions.

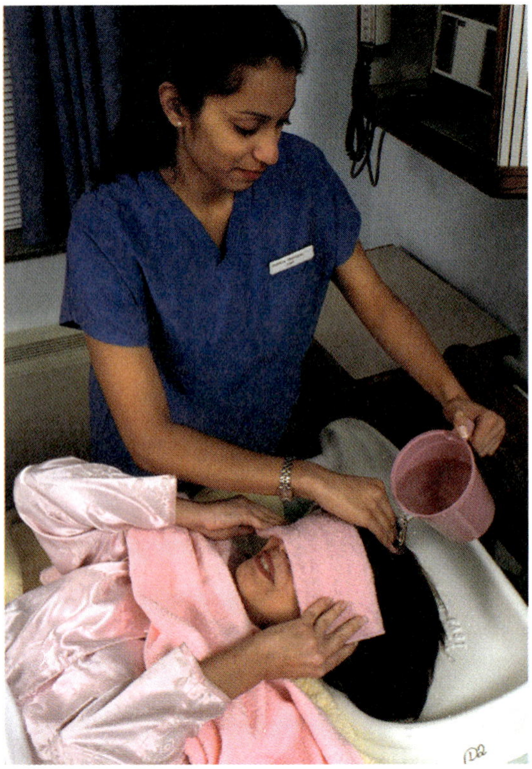

FIGURE 24-20D Wet the hair by slowly pouring warm water.

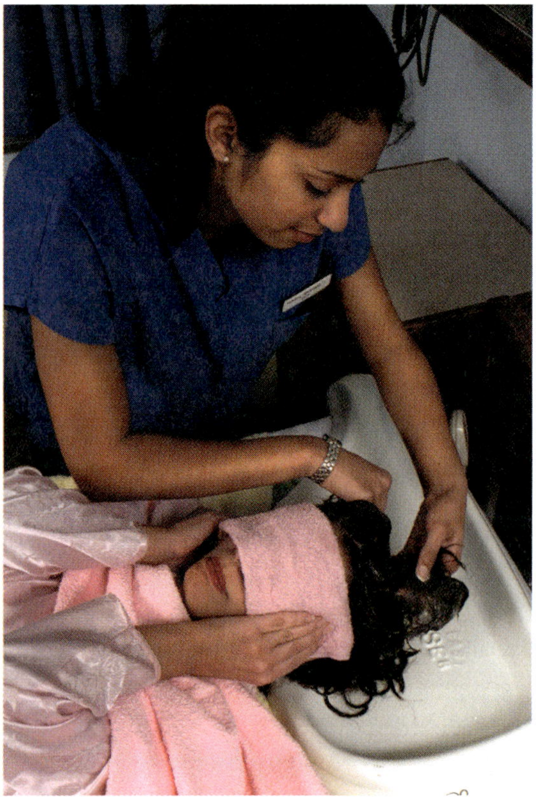

FIGURE 24-20E Apply shampoo and work into a lather, using your fingertips.

DRESSING A PATIENT

Patients in hospitals generally wear hospital gowns because they are in bed most of the time. However, some patients may prefer to wear their own nightgowns or pajamas and will need assistance in dressing. You may also need to assist patients to dress when they are discharged from the hospital. It is usually easier to help people dress while they are still in bed. (See Procedure 67.)

guidelines *for*

Dressing and Undressing Patients

The patient who requires help in dressing may wish to sit in a chair with clothing placed nearby. You can help by:

- Allowing the patient to choose the clothing to be put on.
- Encouraging the patient to participate in the dressing or undressing procedure as much as he or she is able.
- Being prepared to assist with shoes and stockings even for patients who can do much themselves. Bending over to adjust shoes and stockings can result in dizziness and loss of balance.
- Putting clothing on the affected or weakest side first if the patient has difficulty moving one side or is paralyzed.
- Removing clothing from unaffected or strongest side first if the patient has difficulty moving one side or is paralyzed.

PROCEDURE 67

DRESSING AND UNDRESSING THE PATIENT

1. Carry out beginning procedure actions.
2. Select appropriate clothing and arrange in order of application. Encourage the patient to participate in selection.
3. Cover the patient with a bath blanket and fanfold top bedclothes to the foot of the bed.
4. Elevate the head of the bed to sitting position.
5. Assist the patient to a comfortable sitting position.
6. Remove night clothing, keeping the patient covered with the bath blanket. Remove from strong side first and then from weaker side. Place night clothes in a laundry hamper or fold them to be taken home.
7. If the patient wears a bra, slip the straps over the patient's hands (weak side first), move the straps up her arms, and position them on her shoulders. Adjust the breasts in the bra cups. Then hook the bra in back (assist the patient to lean forward so the bra can be fastened).
8. For an undershirt, or any garment that slips on over the head:
   a. Gather the undershirt and place it over the patient's head (Figure 24-21A).

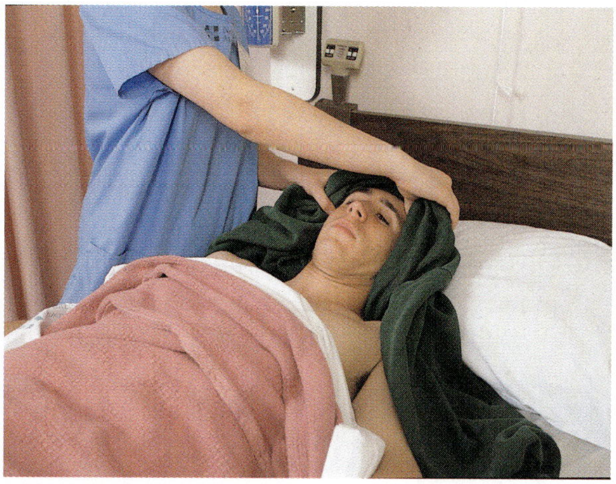

FIGURE 24-21A Gather the garment and pull it over the patient's head.

continues

PROCEDURE 67

continued

b. Grasp the patient's hand and guide it through the armhole by reaching into the armhole from the outside.
c. Repeat the procedure with the opposite arm.
d. Assist the patient to lean forward, and adjust the undershirt so it is smooth over the upper body.

9. Alternate procedure for slipover garments:

Note: *A garment must be large enough or made of stretchy fabric for this procedure.*

a. Place the garment front side down on the patient's lap, with the bottom opening facing the patient.
b. Put the patient's hands into the bottom of the garment and, one at a time, into the sleeve holes.
c. Pull the sleeves up as far as possible on the patient's arms and pull the hands through at the wrist if it is a long-sleeved garment. The garment should now be high on the patient's chest.
d. Gather up the back of the garment with your hand and slip the garment over the patient's head.
e. Smooth the garment down and position it comfortably about the patient's body. Adjust sleeves and shoulders as needed.

10. Shirts or dresses that fasten in the front:

a. Insert your hand through the sleeve of the garment and grasp the patient's hand. Draw the sleeve over your hand and the patient's.
b. Adjust the sleeve at the shoulder.
c. Assist the patient to sit forward. Arrange clothing across the patient's back.
d. Gather the sleeve on the opposite side by slipping your hand in from the outside.
e. Grasp the patient's wrist and pull the sleeve of the garment over your hand and the patient's hand. Draw the sleeve upward and adjust it at the shoulder.
f. Button, zip, or snap the garment.

11. Underwear or slacks:

a. Facing the foot of the bed, gather the patient's underwear from waist to leg hole.

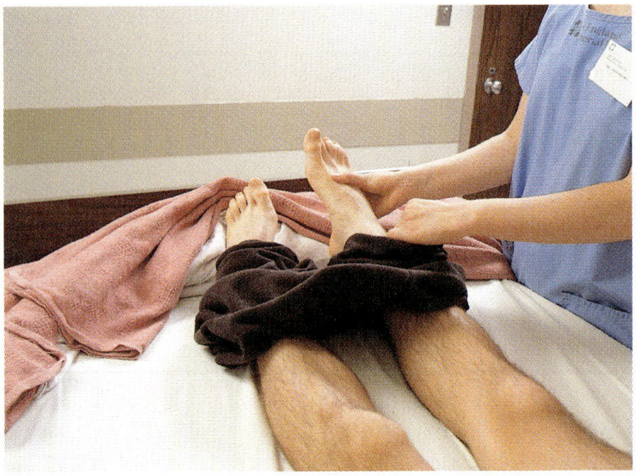

FIGURE 24-21B Slip pants over the feet and lower legs.

b. Slip the underwear over one foot at a time (Figure 24-21B). Pull underwear up legs as high as possible.
c. Assist the patient to raise the hips. Draw the garment over buttocks and up to waist. If patient cannot raise the buttocks, assist the patient to roll first to one side, as you pull up the garment, and then the other side (Figure 24-21C). Adjust the garment until comfortable.
d. Fasten the garment, if required.

12. Socks or knee-high (or thigh-high) stockings:

a. Roll a sock or stocking with heel in back and place it over the toes (Figure 24-21D).

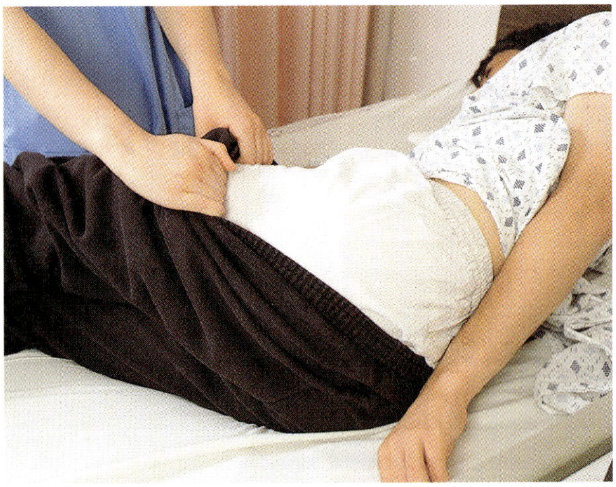

FIGURE 24-21C Have the patient roll onto the strong side first, then pull the pants over the upper hip. Then roll the patient to the other side and pull up pants. Adjust for comfort.

continues

PROCEDURE 67

continued

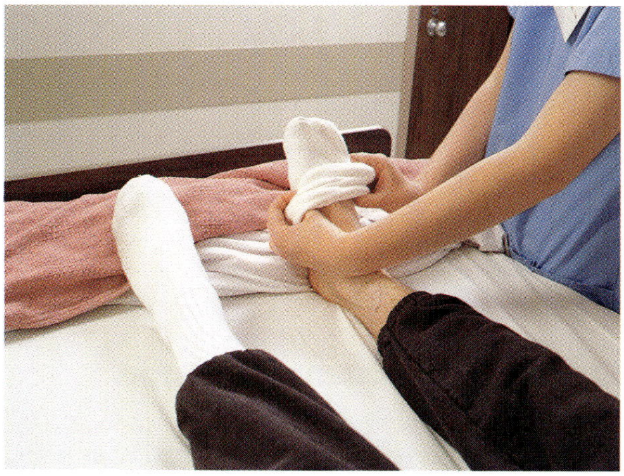

FIGURE 24-21D Adjust socks smoothly over the toes.

b. Draw the sock up over the foot and adjust until smooth. Pull stockings smoothly up to knee or thigh.

c. Repeat for other foot.

13. Pantyhose:

a. Gather pantyhose and adjust over toes and feet. Draw up legs as high as possible.

b. Draw over hips as described in step 11c. Adjust until comfortable at waist.

14. Shoes:

a. Slip shoe on, using a shoe horn if necessary. Open laces of shoes completely so the foot can easily slip into the shoe (Figure 24-21E).

b. Be sure the shoe is fastened securely (Velcro tabs or ties). If the shoes tie, be sure that the ends of the shoelaces do not drag on the floor. The shoes should be fastened tight enough to prevent them from slipping off the patient's feet but not so tight that circulation is impaired.

c. Shoes should be appropriate to the floor surface.

15. To undress, reverse order of steps.

16. Carry out procedure completion actions.

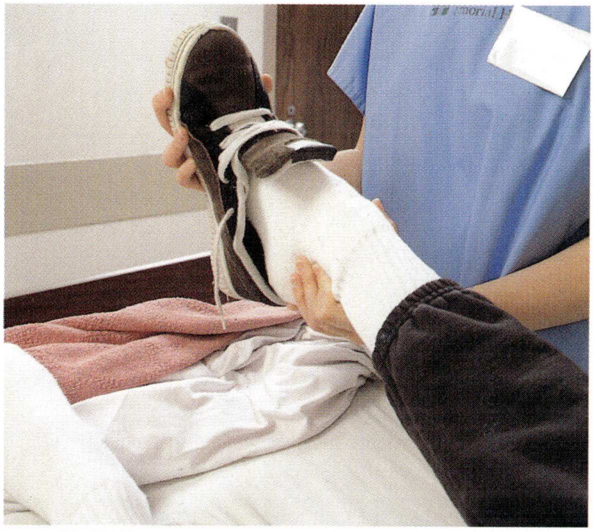

FIGURE 24-21E Open shoelaces completely so that the foot can easily slip into the shoe.

REVIEW

A. True/False.

Mark the following true or false by circling T or F.

1. T F The nursing assistant should carefully observe the patient during the bath procedure.
2. T F Perineal care is given with the patient positioned on a bedpan.
3. T F Range-of-motion exercises are often performed after the bath procedure begins.
4. T F The bath can be omitted if the patient is receiving an IV.
5. T F During the bed bath, only the part being bathed should be exposed.
6. T F Patients should be encouraged to use handrails when getting in and out of the bathtub.
7. T F Traction may be placed on drainage tubes as long as they are not disconnected.
8. T F Because soap is used during the bathing procedure, the tub need not be cleaned between patient uses.
9. T F The bathing procedure can provide the patient with mild exercise.

10. T F Disposable gloves should be worn during bathing if the patient has draining wounds.

B. Matching.

Match the words in Column II with the statements in Column I.

Column I	Column II
11. ____ External reproductive organs	a. axillae
12. ____ Area at base of nails	b. midriff
13. ____ Area under the arms	c. genitalia
	d. cuticle
	e. shampoo

C. Multiple Choice.

Select the one best answer for each of the following.

14. The room temperature during the bath procedure should be about
    - a. 62°F.
    - b. 68°F.
    - c. 70°F.
    - d. 78°F.
15. Patients needing special care during the bath period are those who
    - a. have drainage tubing.
    - b. are confused.
    - c. are paralyzed.
    - d. are independent.
16. Bath water temperature should be approximately
    - a. 105°F.
    - b. 90°F.
    - c. 100°F.
    - d. 115°F.
17. When giving hand and nail care, the hands should be soaked approximately
    - a. 1 hour.
    - b. ½ hour.
    - c. 20 minutes.
    - d. 5 minutes.
18. When a patient takes a bath, the bathroom door should
    - a. not be locked.
    - b. be left wide open for easier access.
    - c. be locked for privacy.
    - d. be left partially open.

D. Nursing Assistant Challenge.

Mr. Rodriguez is taking a shower before going home. He had bowel surgery four days ago. Answer the following about his care by selecting the correct word.

19. The person responsible for the cleanliness of the shower is the ________.
    (patient) (nursing assistant)
20. The patient ________ be assisted into and out of the shower.
    (should not) (should)
21. You can protect the patient from fatigue by ________ to the shower.
    (walking slowly) (transporting him by wheelchair)
22. If Mr. Rodriguez feels faint during his shower, you should turn the water ________.
    (to cold) (off)
23. To prevent chilling when Mr. Rodriguez felt weak, you should ________.
    (turn on the warm water) (wrap him in a bath blanket)

EXPLORING THE WEB

Description	Location
Bag bath	*http://www.bag-bath.com*
Infection control and bathing articles	*http://www.infectioncontroltoday.com*
Towel bath procedure	*http://www.dementiasolutions.com*
Ergonomics and Safety in Patient Bathing	*http://www.patientsafetycenter.com*
A Gentle Bathing Program Inservice	*http://www.dementiasolutions.com*
Procedure for Using the Arjo Bathing System	*http://www-nmcp.med.navy.mil/nursing/procman/Arjo_Bath_SOP.doc*
Skin Care Rituals That Do More Harm Than Good	*http://www.woundheal.com*
Using the Folding Bathtub for Bedfast Patients	*http://www.puntukas.it*

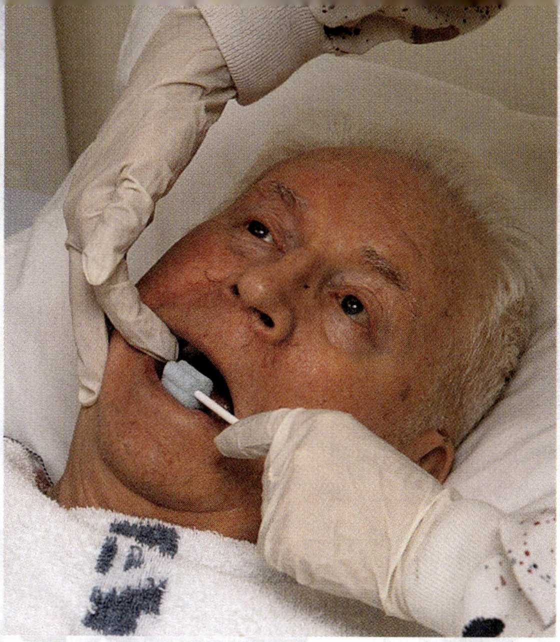

unit 25

General Comfort Measures

objectives

After completing this unit, you will be able to:

- Spell and define terms.
- Discuss the reasons for early morning and bedtime care.
- Identify patients who require frequent oral hygiene.
- List the purposes of oral hygiene.
- Explain nursing assistant responsibilities for a patient's dentures.
- State the purpose of backrubs.
- Describe safety precautions when shaving a patient.
- Describe the importance of hair care.
- Explain the use of comfort devices.
- Demonstrate the following procedures:
  - Procedure 68 Assisting with Routine Oral Hygiene
  - Procedure 69 Assisting with Special Oral Hygiene
  - Procedure 70 Assisting the Patient to Floss and Brush Teeth
  - Procedure 71 Caring for Dentures
  - Procedure 72 Backrub
  - Procedure 73 Shaving a Male Patient
  - Procedure 74 Daily Hair Care
  - Procedure 75 Giving and Receiving the Bedpan
  - Procedure 76 Giving and Receiving the Urinal
  - Procedure 77 Assisting with Use of the Bedside Commode

vocabulary

Learn the meaning and the correct spelling of the following words and phrases:

AM care	caries	footboard	oral hygiene
anticoagulants	dentures	foot drop	PM care
bridging	feces	halitosis	trochanter roll

INTRODUCTION

You can do many things for your patients that will add to their general comfort and feeling of well-being. This includes:

- Providing AM and PM care
- Giving oral hygiene care
- Giving backrubs
- Brushing hair
- Shaving
- Using pillows and special equipment to maintain comfortable positions

AM CARE AND PM CARE

Early morning (AM) care prepares the patient for a day of activities and PM care prepares the patient for a night of rest. Each provides an opportunity for the patient to meet elimination needs and to be refreshed. The nursing assistant has an opportunity to closely observe the patient's condition and to interrelate supportively with the patient.

Early Morning (AM) Care

Early morning or **AM care** helps to set the tone for the entire day. If the patient is refreshed and comfortable before eating breakfast, the day is off to a good start. The nursing assistant provides AM care by:

- Awakening the patient gently—never abruptly—by saying the patient's name (Figure 25-1). If necessary, gently touch the arm.
- Awakening the patient before breakfast.
- Giving the patient the opportunity to use the bathroom, if permitted, or to use the bedpan or urinal.
- Helping the patient to wash hands and face.

The patient is not awakened early if he or she is:

- Going to surgery
- Having tests that prohibit eating

Bedtime (PM Care)

The care given to the patient just before bedtime is similar to that given in the early morning. Bedtime care is called **PM care** (or HS care). The nursing assistant gives PM care:

- In a quiet, unrushed manner that will help prepare the patient for sleep (Figure 25-2)
- Before medication for sleep is given by the nurse

Other routine procedures that may be carried out during AM and PM care include:

- Measuring vital signs
- Giving a backrub
- Providing mouth and hair care
- Giving the patient the opportunity to use the bathroom, if permitted, or to use the bedpan or urinal.

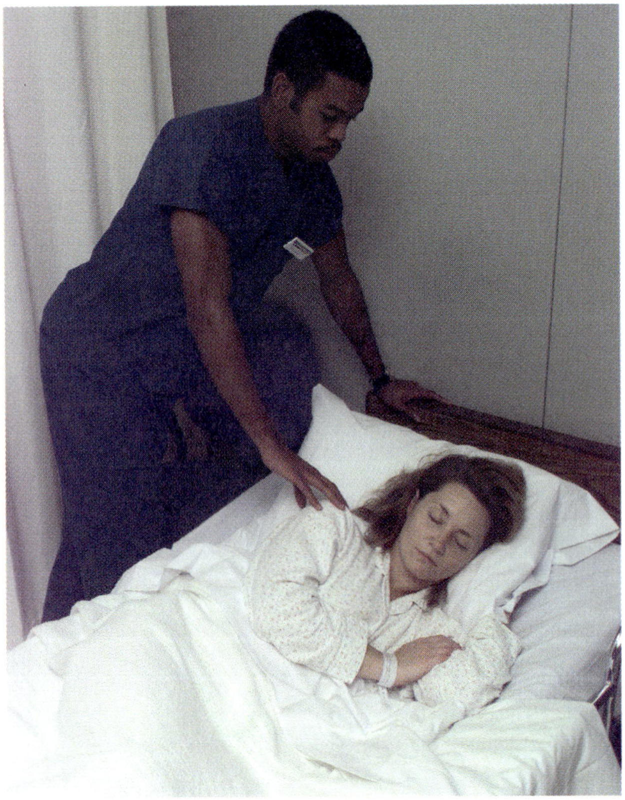

FIGURE 25-1 Early AM care. Wake the patient by saying the patient's name, then gently touching the arm, if necessary.

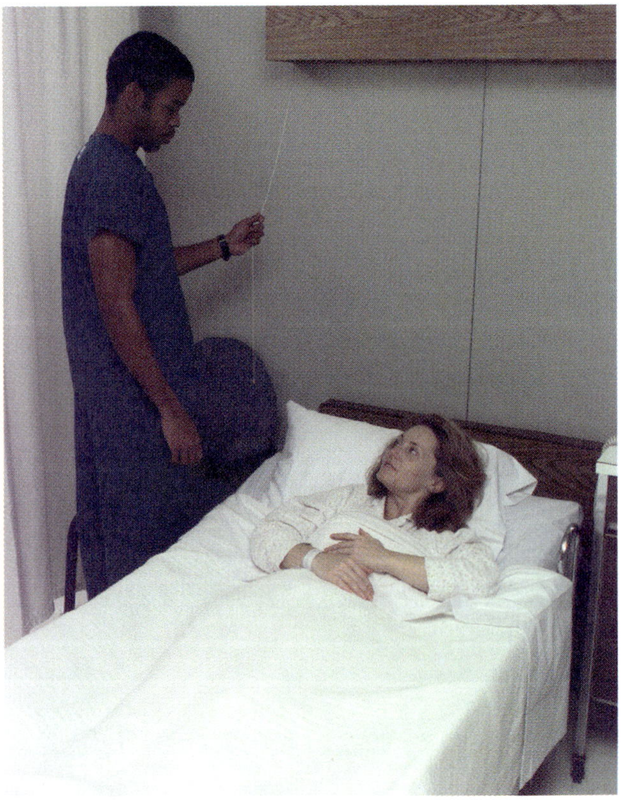

FIGURE 25-2 Turn off the light when the patient is settled and comfortable.

ORAL HYGIENE

Oral hygiene is the care of the mouth and teeth. (Refer to Procedures 68 to 70.)

- Routine oral hygiene (including brushing and flossing the teeth) should be performed at least three times a day.
- Patients should be encouraged to do as much as possible for themselves.
- *Special oral hygiene* is the cleansing of the mouth of the helpless patient using commercially prepared lemon and glycerine swabs, Toothettes®, and other preparations.

Patients requiring more frequent oral hygiene include those who are:

- unconscious
- vomiting
- experiencing a high temperature
- receiving certain medications
- dehydrated
- breathing through the mouth
- receiving oxygen
- receiving tube feeding
- dying

Proper cleansing of the teeth and mouth helps:

- prevent tooth decay (**caries**)
- eliminate bad breath (**halitosis**)
- contribute to the patient's comfort

INFECTION CONTROL *Alert*

Take care in storing the patient's toothbrush. Make sure it is covered or stored away from other items, such as the hairbrush.

INFECTION CONTROL *Alert*

Apply the principles of standard precautions when selecting protective equipment for assisting with dental procedures. Always wear gloves. If there is a chance of spraying or splashing of oral secretions, you will need a gown, gloves, mask, and face shield.

PROCEDURE 68

ASSISTING WITH ROUTINE ORAL HYGIENE

1. Carry out beginning procedure actions.
2. Assemble equipment:
   - disposable gloves and face mask
   - toothbrush
   - toothpaste
   - dental floss
   - mouthwash solution in cup
   - emesis basin
   - bath towel
   - straw
   - tissues
   - cup of fresh water
   - plastic bag
   - bed protector
3. Raise the head of the bed so that the patient may sit up, if his condition permits.
4. Lower the side rails and position the overbed table across the patient's lap.
5. Cover the table with a protector and place equipment on the table.
6. Place a bath towel over the patient's gown and bedcovers.
7. Be prepared to help as the patient brushes and flosses teeth.
8. Pour water over the toothbrush and put toothpaste on the brush.
9. Put on disposable gloves. A face mask may be used.

continues

PROCEDURE 68

continued

10. Brush teeth as follows (Figure 25-3):
    a. Insert the toothbrush into the mouth with bristles pointing downward.
    b. Turn the toothbrush with bristles toward teeth.
    c. Brush all tooth surfaces with a back-and-forth motion using short (tooth-wide) strokes.
    d. Use the "toe" end of the brush to clean the inner surfaces of the front teeth, using a gentle up-and-down motion.
    e. Brush the front of the tongue gently, if tolerated by the patient. Avoid the back of the tongue, as touching this area may cause gagging and coughing.
11. Give the patient water in a cup to rinse the mouth. Use a straw, if necessary. Turn the patient's head to one side, with the emesis basin near the chin, for return of fluid.
12. Repeat steps 10 and 11 as necessary.
13. To floss the patient's teeth:
    a. Select a piece of dental floss about 12 inches long. Wrap the end of the floss around your middle fingers, leaving the center area free (Figure 25-4).
    b. Ask the patient to open her mouth. Gently insert the floss between each tooth down to, but not into, the gum line.
    c. Ask the patient to rinse her mouth using the emesis basin.
14. Offer the patient mouthwash. Dilute the mouthwash if the patient wishes.

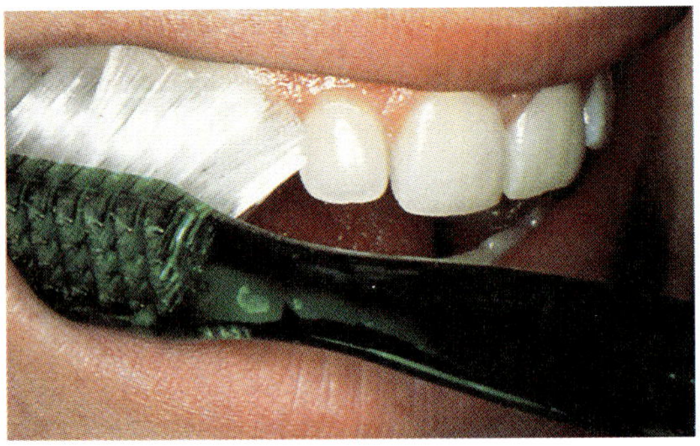

A. Place the head of the toothbrush beside the teeth, with the bristle tips at a 45-degree angle against the gum line. Move the brush back and forth in short (half-a-tooth-wide) strokes several times, using a gentle scrubbing motion. Brush the outer surfaces of each tooth, upper and lower, keeping the bristles angled against the gum line.

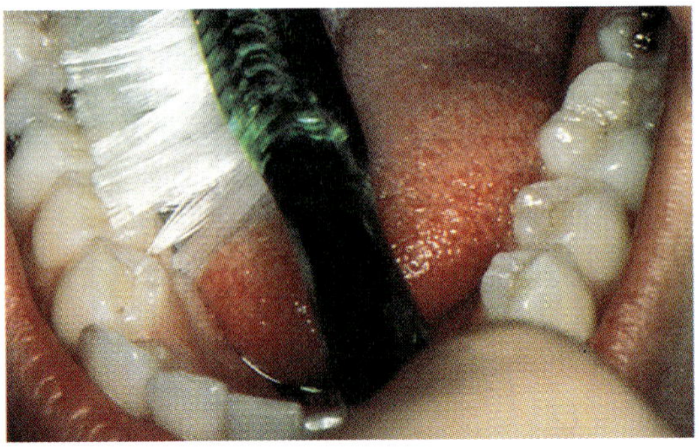

B. Use the same method on the inside surfaces of all the teeth, still using short back-and-forth strokes.

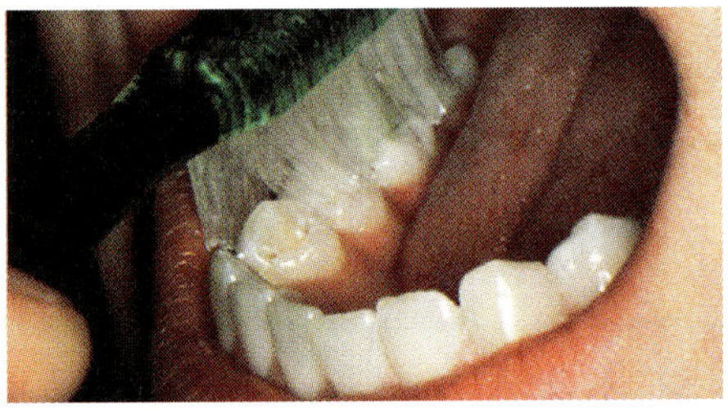

C. Scrub the chewing surfaces of the teeth.

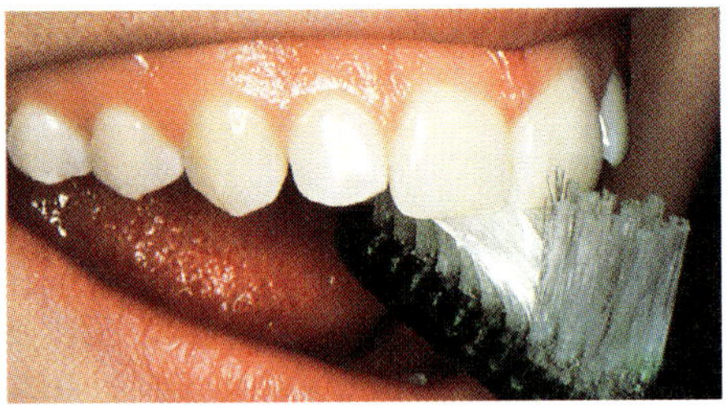

D. To clean the inside surfaces of the front teeth, tilt the brush vertically and make several gentle up-and-down strokes with the "toe" (the front part) of the brush.

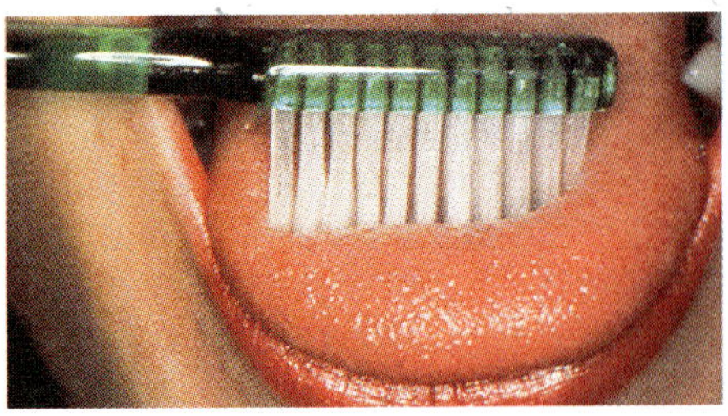

E. Brushing the patient's tongue will help freshen breath and clean the mouth by removing bacteria.

FIGURE 25-3 Brush teeth in the direction they grow and across the chewing surfaces. *(Toothbrushing photos and descriptions compliments of the American Dental Association)*

continues

PROCEDURE 68

continued

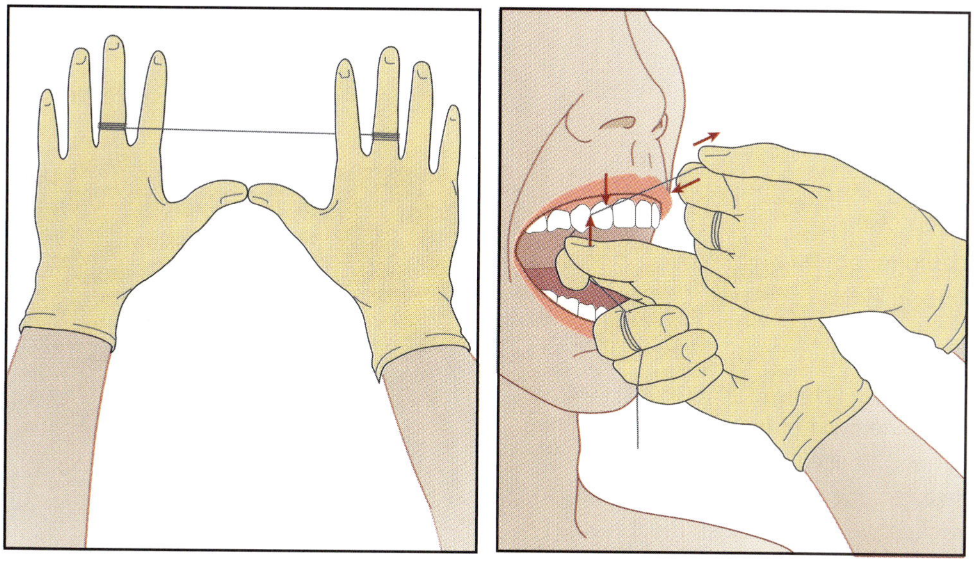

FIGURE 25-4 Floss is wrapped around the middle fingers (left). The proper method of using the floss to clean between the teeth (right).

15. Remove the basin. Wipe the patient's mouth and chin with tissue. Discard the tissue in a paper bag.
16. Remove the towel.
17. Rinse the toothbrush with water.
18. Remove and dispose of gloves and mask according to facility policy.
19. Carry out procedure completion actions.

CULTURE *Alert*

Many individuals have tongue piercings for fashion or cultural reasons. Many risks accompany this procedure. Inform the nurse promptly if a patient with a tongue piercing has pain, bleeding, increased flow of saliva, swelling, or signs of infection in the mouth. Swelling of the tongue can become severe, closing off the airway.

PROCEDURE 69

ASSISTING WITH SPECIAL ORAL HYGIENE

Note: *Special oral hygiene is provided when the patient cannot participate actively in such care.*

1. Carry out beginning procedure actions.
2. Assemble equipment:
   - disposable gloves
   - Toothettes® or lemon and glycerine applicators

continues

PROCEDURE 69

continued

- emesis basin
- 2 bath towels
- plastic bag
- premoistened applicators
- tissues
- tongue depressor
- water-based lubricant for lips
- laundry hamper

3. Put on gloves.
4. Cover pillow with a towel. If the patient is able to sit up, elevate the head of the bed. If the patient is unable, or not permitted to sit up, turn the patient's head to one side and slightly forward so any excess fluid will not run down the throat. Cover the patient's upper chest with a towel. Place an emesis basin under the patient's chin.
5. Gently pull down on the chin to open the mouth, or open the mouth gently with a tongue depressor.
6. Using moistened Toothettes®, wipe gums, teeth, tongue, and inside of mouth (Figure 25-5).
7. Discard used applicators in a plastic bag.
8. Using clean applicators, apply lubricant to the patient's lips. Place used applicators in a plastic bag.
9. Remove towels. Clean and replace equipment.
10. Remove and dispose of gloves properly. Wash your hands.
11. Carry out procedure completion actions.

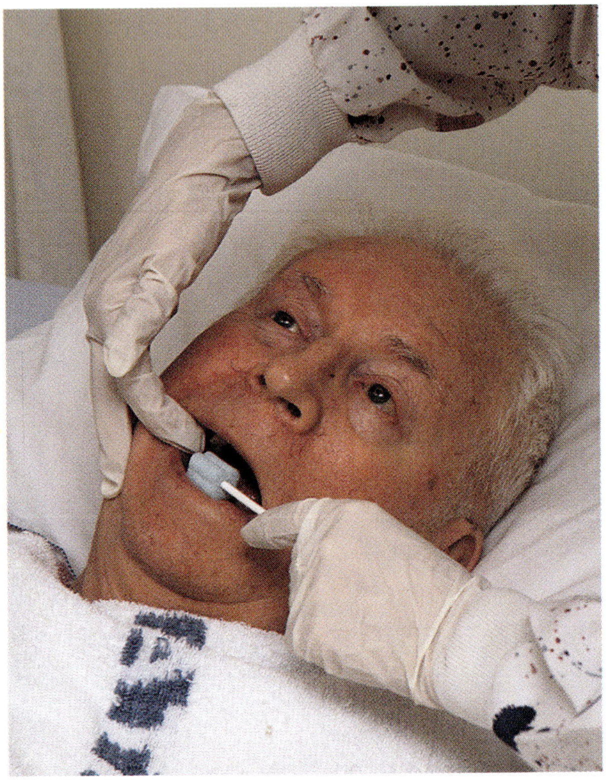

FIGURE 25-5 Using premoistened applicators, wipe gums, teeth, and tongue.

PROCEDURE 70

ASSISTING THE PATIENT TO FLOSS AND BRUSH TEETH

1. Carry out beginning procedure actions.
2. Assemble equipment:
   - disposable gloves
   - emesis basin
   - toothbrush
   - toothpaste
   - dental floss
   - glass of cool water
   - straw
   - mouthwash (if permitted)
   - hand towel
   - bed protector
   - plastic bag
   - laundry hamper

continues

PROCEDURE 70

continued

3. Elevate the head of the bed. Help the patient into a comfortable position.
4. Lower the side rails and position the overbed table across the patient's lap.
5. Cover the table with a plastic protector.
6. Place the emesis basin and a glass of water on the overbed table.
7. Place a towel across the patient's chest.
8. Be prepared to help as the patient flosses and brushes teeth. Remind the patient to clean the tongue and gums. Apply gloves and use standard precautions if you will be assisting with the procedure.
9. After the patient has flossed and brushed his teeth:
   a. Push the overbed table to the foot of the bed.
   b. Remove the emesis basin, clean it, and replace it according to facility policy.
   c. Rinse toothbrush.
   d. Remove the towels and put them with the soiled linen.
   e. Remove gloves and discard according to facility policy. Wash your hands.
10. Carry out procedure completion actions.

AGE-APPROPRIATE CARE *Alert*

Elderly patients may experience dry mouth and reduced saliva production. This commonly occurs as a side effect of medications. Related complaints are burning or sore throat, difficulty in swallowing, hoarseness, and dry nasal passages. Saliva is needed to help break down food for digestion. It also neutralizes acids in the mouth caused by plaque. Artificial saliva products are available, as are medicated oral rinses. The dentist may recommend that the patient use sugar-free gum or candy to increase saliva production. Inform the nurse if the patient experiences problems with saliva production.

DENTURES

Some patients have full sets of dentures. Other patients have partial plates that are removable, but attach by small metal clips to existing teeth. Partial plates should be given the same care as full dentures. **Dentures** are artificial teeth that are removable. They must be cleaned. The patient may feel embarrassed about wearing dentures and may dislike being seen after the dentures have been removed. Therefore, always provide privacy when dentures are to be removed and cleaned. (See Procedure 71.)

Denture Care

Denture care includes the following:

- Cleaning dentures daily under cool running water.
- Handling dentures carefully to prevent damage.
- Storing dentures in a safe place when they are out of the patient's mouth, such as in the drawer of the bedside stand in a container labeled with the patient's name (Figure 25-6).

SAFETY *Alert*

Remove dentures from a comatose patient to prevent accidental airway obstruction by the denture. Remove dentures from patients preoperatively to prevent potential damage to the dentures and accidental airway obstruction in surgery.

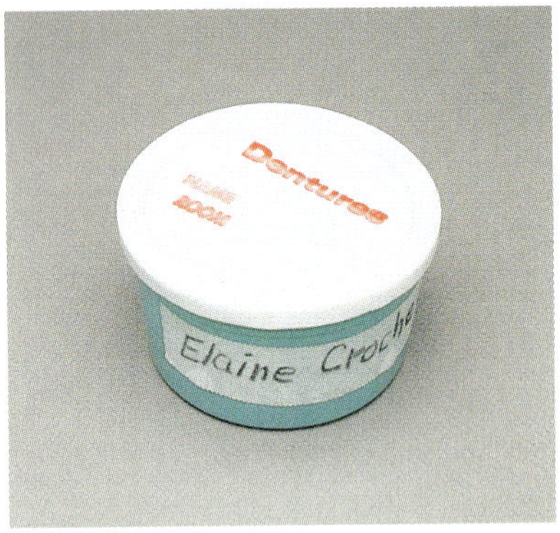

FIGURE 25-6 Dentures are stored in a cup labeled with the patient's name. The dentures are usually kept covered with water.

- Cleaning and checking the patient's mouth for signs of irritation.
- Checking the patient's lips for cracking and dryness.
- Applying cream, petroleum jelly, or glycerin to lips to avoid excessive dryness.

AGE-APPROPRIATE CARE *Alert*

Dentures are made to fit tightly in the patient's mouth. Natural aging changes in the bones and gums may cause the shape of the patient's mouth to change over time. If dentures are loose or ill-fitting, chances are that this is because of aging changes to the mouth. Loose dentures can cause sores in the mouth, and in the worst case can cause choking. Denture adhesives can be used temporarily to help keep dentures in place, but the patient will need to be referred to a dentist. Inform the nurse if the patient has problems with improperly fitting dentures.

PROCEDURE 71

CARING FOR DENTURES

1. Carry out beginning procedure actions.
2. Assemble equipment:
   - disposable gloves
   - tissues
   - emesis basin
   - tongue depressor
   - brush
   - toothpaste or tooth powder
   - mouthwash, if permitted
   - cup of water
   - straw
   - gauze squares
   - applicators
   - denture cup
3. Apply disposable gloves.
4. Allow the patient to clean the dentures if she is able to do so. If the patient cannot, give a tissue to the patient and ask her to remove the dentures. Assist if necessary.
   a. To remove upper dentures, grasp the dentures firmly, ease them downward and then forward, and remove them from the mouth (Figure 25-7).

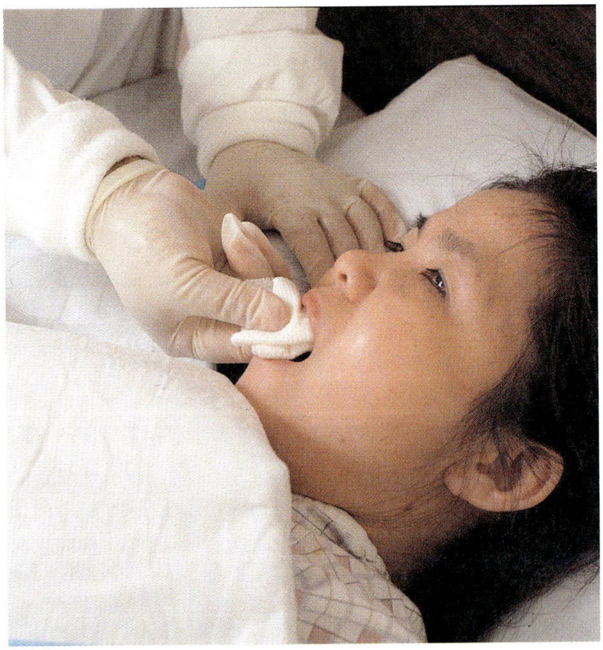

FIGURE 25-7 Grasp the upper dentures firmly with gauze-covered fingers, to prevent slipping. Ease them down and forward to remove.

   b. To remove lower dentures, grasp the dentures firmly, ease them upward and then forward, and remove them from the mouth.

continues

PROCEDURE 71

continued

5. Place the dentures in a denture cup padded with gauze squares. Take them to the bathroom or utility room.
6. Place a paper towel or washcloth in the bottom of the basin to protect the dentures (Figure 25-8). Fill the sink half full with cool water. The combination of water and towel protect the dentures from chipping or breaking if they are accidentally dropped in the sink.
7. Dentures may be soaked in a solution with a cleansing tablet before brushing, if desired.

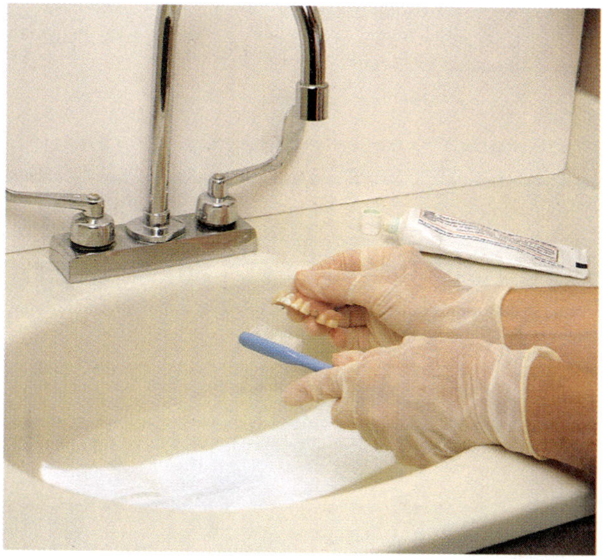

FIGURE 25-8 Brush dentures until all surfaces are clean.

8. Wet the dentures by rinsing under cool water.
9. Put toothpaste or tooth powder on a brush. Hold the dentures and brush until all surfaces are clean.
10. Rinse the dentures thoroughly under cool running water. Never use hot water. Rinse the denture cup.
11. Place fresh gauze squares in the denture cup with clean, cool water unless instructed otherwise.
12. Place the dentures in the gauze-lined cup and take them to the bedside.
13. Assist the patient to rinse her mouth with mouthwash, if permitted. Otherwise, use water. Hold the mouth open gently with a wooden tongue depressor. Clean the gums and tongue with applicators moistened with mouthwash, or use foam Toothettes.®

Note: *Carefully observe and report the condition of the teeth, mouth, tongue, lips, and dentures.*

14. Use a paper towel or gauze to hand wet dentures to the patient. If the patient is able, she can remove the dentures from the cup. Insert if necessary, upper denture first.
15. Clean and replace equipment according to facility policy.
16. Remove and dispose of gloves according to facility policy.
17. Carry out procedure completion actions.

BACKRUBS

When properly given, backrubs can be:

- stimulating to the patient's circulation.
- a major aid in preventing skin breakdown (*decubiti*).
- soothing.
- refreshing.

Keep your nails short to prevent injuring the patient. The backrub procedure provides a good opportunity for you to observe the condition of the patient's skin. (See Procedure 72.) Report all observations to the nurse. Look for:

- Reddened areas that do not blanch (whiten) when pressed
- Raw areas of skin
- Condition of skin over bony prominences

Unless contraindicated, the backrub is given:

- routinely as part of the bed bath or partial bath.
- following use of the bedpan.
- when changing the position of the helpless patient.

OSHA *Alert*

When giving a backrub, make sure the bed is elevated to a comfortable height for you. Stand with one foot slightly ahead of the other, with knees bent slightly. Use your arm and shoulder muscles to massage the back. Rock back and forth, using the strong muscles in your legs. Avoid bending from the waist.

- at bedtime.
- when it could be a comfort to the patient.

Long, smooth strokes are relaxing. Short, circular strokes tend to be more stimulating. Avoid massaging red areas over bony prominences.

The backrub is given with warmed lotion.

DIFFICULT *Situations*

For many years, backrubs were almost a sacred, routine part of nursing care. Over time, we have become much more dependent on technology. When we are busy or staffing is short, it seems as if there is no time to give backrubs. Yet, calming the agitated patient who cannot sleep is time-consuming; the pregnant mother with a backache may use the call signal frequently; the patient with spasticity just cannot get into a comfortable position. You may find that taking a few minutes to give a backrub will save you a great deal of time in caring for your patients. A good backrub is comforting and relaxing. Agitated patients often calm down. Uncomfortable patients become more comfortable and demand less attention. Do not omit this important part of nursing care that pays such large dividends in patient comfort and satisfaction. In the long run, it may even make your job easier.

PROCEDURE 72

BACKRUB

1. Carry out beginning procedure actions.
2. Assemble equipment:
   - disposable gloves
   - basin of water (105°F)
   - bath towel
   - soap and lotion
3. Put up the far side rail.
4. Place the lotion in a basin of water to warm (Figure 25-9).

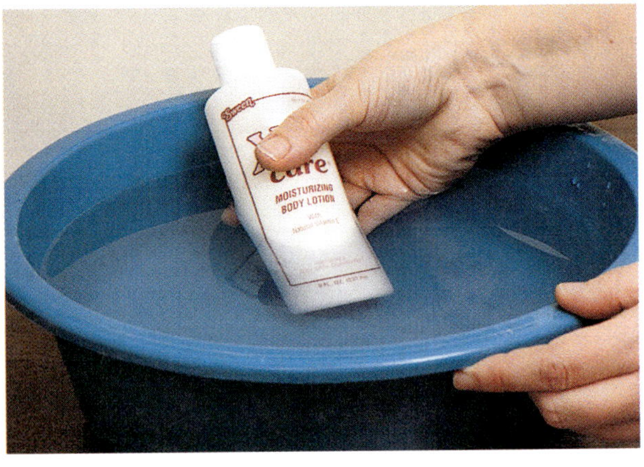

FIGURE 25-9 Warming the lotion in water for several minutes will make it more comfortable for the patient.

5. Put on disposable gloves if the patient has open lesions.
6. Turn the patient on the side with the back toward you.
7. Expose and wash the back; dry carefully. This step is not necessary if the backrub is given after a bath.
8. Pour a small amount of lotion into one hand and warm it in the palm of your hand. Cold lotion may be very uncomfortable to the patient.
9. Apply the lotion to the patient's skin and rub with gentle but firm strokes. Give special attention to all bony prominences (Figure 25-10). Do not rub red areas. Report these to the nurse, if noted.
10. Begin at the base of the spine:
    - With long, soothing strokes, rub up the center of the back, around the shoulders, and down the sides of the back and buttocks (Figure 25-11, *left*).

continues

PROCEDURE 72

continued

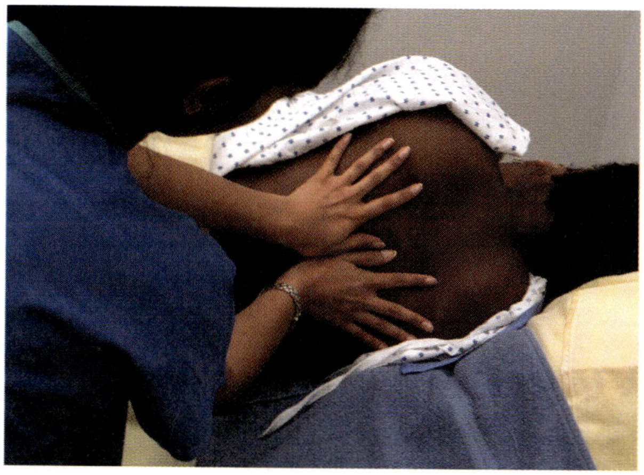

FIGURE 25-10 Use long, smooth, firm strokes to apply lotion.

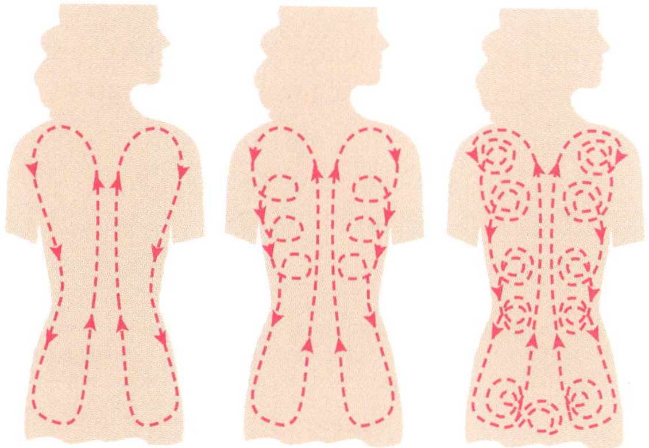

FIGURE 25-11 Strokes to be used during the backrub: soothing strokes (left), circular movement (middle), passive movement (right).

- Repeat the previous step four times, using long, soothing upward strokes and a circular motion on the downstroke (Figure 25-11, *middle*).
- Repeat, but on the downward stroke rub in small circular motions with the palm of your hand. Include areas over the coccyx (base of the spine) (Figure 25-11, *right*).
- Repeat long, soothing strokes on muscles for 3 to 5 minutes (Figure 25-11, *left*).
- Dry the area well.
- If redness on pressure areas is noted, report it to the nurse. Straighten and tighten the bottom sheet and draw sheet.

11. Change the patient's gown, if necessary.
12. Remove gloves if used. Discard according to facility policy and wash your hands.
13. Replace equipment.
14. Carry out procedure completion actions.

DAILY SHAVING

Daily shaving is part of the routine self-care of most men. It should not be neglected in a care facility. When patients are unable to shave themselves and a barber is not available, it is your responsibility. (See Procedure 73.)

Older women have an increase in the growth and coarseness of hairs on the chin and upper lip. Many women find this distressing. Tweezers can be used to remove some of the hairs, but a more permanent method is to have the hairs removed professionally with an electric needle. Some women may require a shave. In some facilities nursing assistants are not permitted to shave women patients. Be sure to check the policy of your facility.

OSHA *Alert*

Always wear gloves when shaving patients with a nonelectric razor, because of the high risk of contact with blood. Discard the razor in a puncture-resistant (sharps) container.

AGE-APPROPRIATE CARE *Alert*

Elderly women may grow facial hair as a result of hormonal changes during aging. Coarse hair is common on the chin. Most women prefer to have facial hair removed. Many women also prefer to have hair removed from their legs and underarms. Honor the patient's preferences. Know your facility policy for removing facial hair from female patients. Some facilities use depilatories. Although some facilities shave women, check with the nurse before performing this procedure because shaving may worsen the problem, causing the hair to become thicker and coarser.

guidelines *for*

Safety in Shaving

- Use the patient's own shaving equipment if possible. For safety, use an electric razor or rotary razor.
- If the patient is receiving **anticoagulants** (medications that thin the blood and increase the risk of bleeding), a special procedure may be required. For example, an electric razor provides the greatest safety. Check with the nurse for the proper procedure.
- If oxygen is being given, it may be possible to discontinue it during this procedure. Consult the nurse and follow hospital policy.

INFECTION CONTROL *Alert*

Shaving may be done with an electric razor, which is the patient's personal property. Such a razor is used for one patient only and cleaned according to manufacturer's directions after each use. This usually involves brushing the heads with a small brush designed for this purpose. All hair should be removed from the head of the razor. Some electric razors must be recharged periodically. Electric razors are expensive. Handle the razor carefully and avoid dropping it. If the electrical cord is frayed or worn, report to the nurse and remove the razor from use. If an electric razor is not available, use a disposable safety razor. Wearing gloves is usually not necessary when an electric razor is used.

PROCEDURE 73

SHAVING A MALE PATIENT

1. Carry out beginning procedure actions.
2. Assemble equipment:
   - disposable gloves
   - electric shaver or safety razor
   - shaving lather or preshave lotion for electric razor
   - basin of water (105°F)
   - face towels
   - mirror
   - washcloth
   - aftershave lotion
3. Raise the head of the bed. Place equipment on overbed table.
4. Put on gloves.
5. Place one face towel across patient's chest and one under head.
6. Moisten face and apply lather (or preshave lotion).
7. Starting in front of ear:
   a. Hold skin taut and bring razor down over cheek toward chin (Figure 25-12).
   b. Repeat until lather on cheek is removed and area has been shaved. Rinse frequently.
   c. Repeat on other cheek.
   d. Use firm, short strokes. Shave in direction of hair growth.
   e. Rinse razor frequently.

continues

PROCEDURE 73

continued

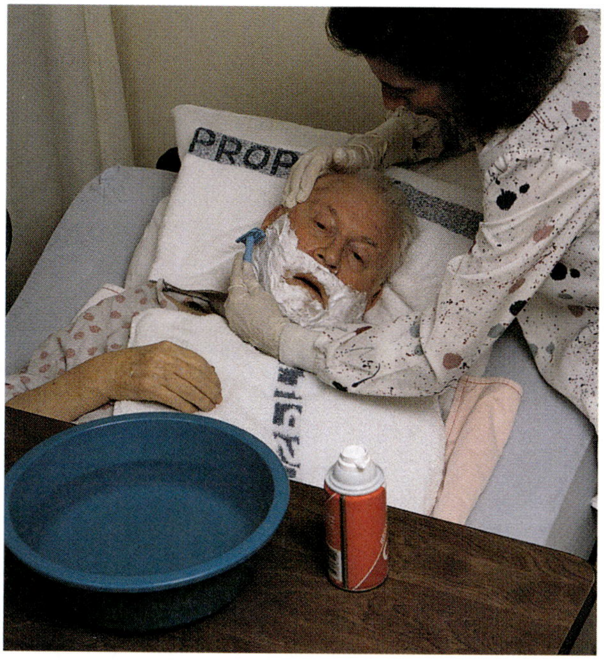

FIGURE 25-12 Shaving is part of the daily routine for most men.

8. Ask the patient to tighten his upper lip. Shave from the nose to the upper lip in short, downward strokes.
9. Ask the patient to tighten his chin. Shave the chin in downward strokes.
10. Assist the patient to tip his head back.
11. Lather the neck area and stroke up toward the chin. Rinse and repeat until all lather is removed.
12. Wash the patient's face and neck and dry thoroughly.
13. Apply aftershave lotion if desired.
14. If the skin is nicked, apply a small piece of tissue and hold pressure directly over the area. Then apply an antiseptic and bandage. Report the incident to the nurse.
15. Clean and replace equipment. Dispose of razor according to facility policy. Remove the head of an electric razor. Use a razor brush to remove clippings. Store the razor according to facility policy.
16. Remove and dispose of gloves according to facility policy.
17. Carry out procedure completion actions.

DAILY HAIR CARE

Daily care of the hair, for both male and female patients, is usually performed after the patient's bed bath. (See Procedure 74.)

The hair should be combed and brushed each morning. Tangles can be loosened by sectioning the hair with a comb or brush, working with one section at a time. Grasp the hair near the scalp to reduce pulling (Figure 25-13). Start combing or brushing tangles out starting at the ends and working toward the scalp. Braiding long hair after brushing can help reduce tangles. Tangles can be reduced in wiry, dry hair by using conditioner and keeping the hair short or in braids.

Tips: Avoid braiding a patient's hair tightly, because it can be uncomfortable. Secure the braids with hair ties. Avoid rubber bands, if possible. If the hair is very tangled, applying a small amount of alcohol or oil to the tangle will make it easier to remove.

Brushing the hair:

- stimulates circulation of the scalp.
- refreshes the patient.
- removes dust and lint.
- helps to keep the hair shiny and attractive.

If additional care is needed, a fluid dry cleaner to shampoo the hair is available. It leaves the hair soft and manageable and the hairstyle intact. This procedure is so simple that it

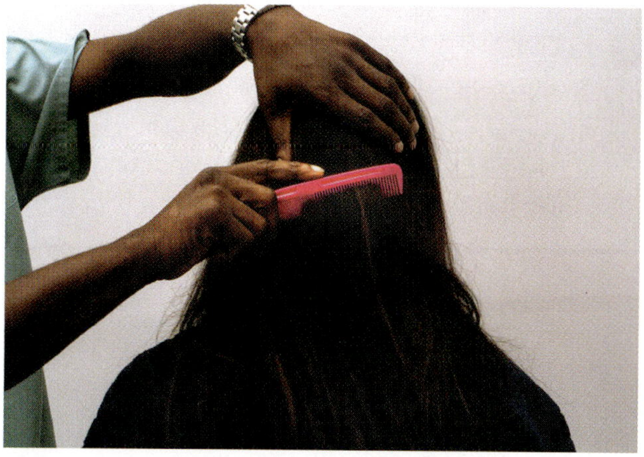

FIGURE 25-13 To remove tangles from long hair, divide the hair into sections. Work with one section at a time. Hold the hair near the scalp to reduce pulling and start combing at the end of the hair, working up toward the scalp.

is often used instead of the regular shampoo for patients who must remain in bed.

Sometimes, however, a shampoo may be advisable for the patient in bed. Approval for the procedure must be obtained from the doctor. Bed shampoos should be given every two weeks when the patient is bedbound for an extended period. (See Unit 24, Procedure 66.)

The following procedure assumes that the patient is a female. Hair care for a male is very similar, however, so the procedure can easily be adapted.

DIFFICULT *Situations*

Hair is important to everyone's self-esteem and appearance. Some diseases and medications cause hair loss. Some cause changes to the volume and texture of hair. Some medications cause hair to become dry and brittle. Patients who have problems with their hair may become anxious or angry because the appearance of the hair affects their self-esteem. If the patient is experiencing problems with hair, treat it gently. Use products such as baby shampoo and conditioner. Use tepid water. Pat the hair dry rather than rubbing it with a towel. Use a wide-toothed comb to style the hair gently. Avoid braids and rubber bands, which may worsen the problem. Assist the patient to wear a scarf or turban, if desired.

PROCEDURE 74

DAILY HAIR CARE

1. Carry out beginning procedure actions.
2. Assemble equipment:
   - towel
   - comb and brush
3. Ask the patient to move to the side of the bed nearest you; or the patient may sit in a chair if permitted. If the patient is sitting up, put a towel around her shoulders.
4. Cover the pillow with a towel.
5. Part or section the hair and comb with one hand between the scalp and the ends of the hair.
6. Brush carefully and thoroughly.
7. Have the patient turn so that you can comb and brush the hair on the back of her head. If the hair is tangled, work section by section to unsnarl it, beginning near the ends and working toward the scalp.
8. Complete brushing and arrange the hair attractively. Braid long hair to prevent repeated snarling. Allow the patient to choose the style, if able.
9. Clean and replace equipment according to facility policy.
10. Carry out procedure completion actions.

COMFORT DEVICES

The physician, nurse, or physical therapist orders comfort devices such as bed cradles, footboards, and pillows. They are designed to relieve pressure on specific areas or to help maintain body position.

Bed Cradle

A bed cradle (Figure 25-14) prevents the weight of the bedclothes from falling on some part of the body. It can be used therapeutically or as a comfort device. It is used:

- over fractured limbs

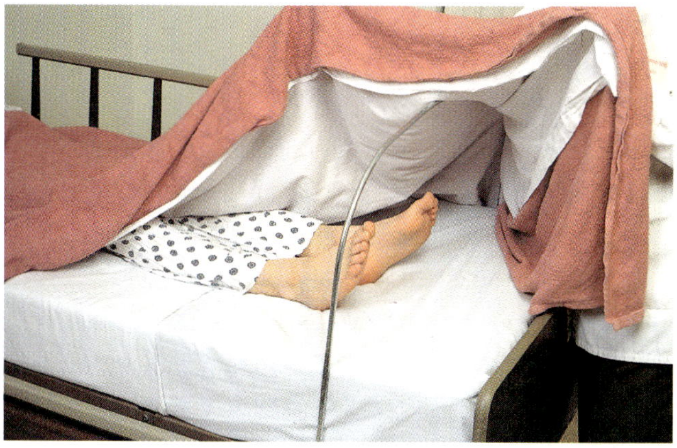

FIGURE 25-14 A bed cradle keeps the sheet and blanket from putting pressure on the feet.

- when there are burns
- to prevent skin lesions
- over widespread skin conditions, such as psoriasis or eczema
- to prevent contractures of the feet
- over a wet cast until it dries

Coverings that maintain some degree of warmth within the cradle may also be needed to keep the patient comfortable.

Care must be taken to position the limb within the cradle. It may be necessary to pad the cradle edges.

Footboard or Footrest

The **footboard** or footrest is a device placed between the mattress and bed to keep the feet at right angles to the legs (natural standing position). A footboard is always padded. It is used to prevent a type of contracture called **foot drop**. In foot drop, the muscle in the calf of the leg tends to tighten, causing the toes to point downward. Foot drop may happen when the patient must remain in bed over a long period of time. Even a brief period in bed is sufficient to cause a degree of foot drop that makes walking difficult when the patient does get out of bed.

If a footboard is not available, a pillow folded lengthwise may be placed against the foot of the bed to serve the same purpose. Some facilities use special tennis shoes or soft boots to prevent foot drop in patients who are at risk because they are bedfast.

Pillows and Bath Blankets

Pillows can be used as comfort devices and to maintain alignment when properly arranged. For directions on properly altering the patient's positions, refer to Unit 15.

The **trochanter roll** is used to prevent external rotation of the hip. Trochanter rolls should be used routinely for bedfast patients, to prevent deformities. Unless a specific medical condition, such as a hip fracture, is present, no special order is necessary.

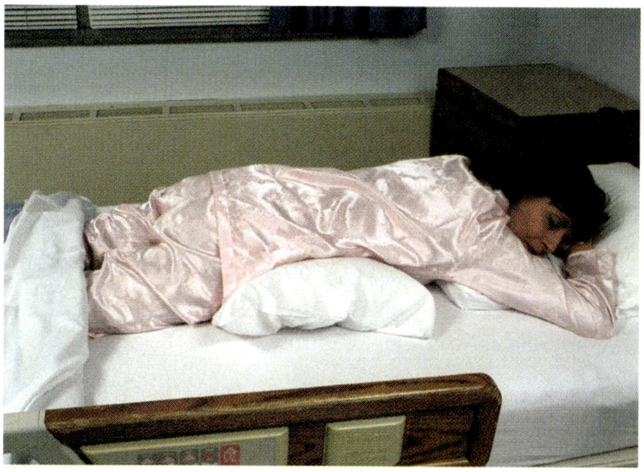

FIGURE 25-15 The patient is positioned on her abdomen and pillows are used to form a bridge, preventing pressure on her breasts.

A trochanter roll or support can be made as follows:

1. Fold a bath blanket lengthwise in thirds.
2. Position the patient in the center of the folded bath blanket. The blanket should extend from mid-thigh to above the waist.
3. Roll each side of the blanket under and toward the patient until the blanket roll is firmly against the patient. Then tuck the roll inward toward the bed and patient to maintain the patient's position.

Pillows are also used to relieve pressure in such a way that spaces are left for specific areas (Figure 25-15). This technique is called **bridging**. Bridging elevates an area of the body off the surface of the bed. It is useful for patients with healing pressure ulcers. Bridging is commonly used for the sacrum, hips, heels, and ankles. No special equipment is necessary. Facilities may use a combination of pillows, foam props, and bath blankets to support an area.

ELIMINATION NEEDS

Regular, periodic elimination of body wastes is essential for maintaining health. Patients who are confined to bed must rely on you to help them with this physical task. (See Procedures 75 to 77.) You should know that:

- The patient must regularly empty the bladder by urinating (voiding).
- A urinal (duct or bottle) is used by male patients when they need to urinate. A bedpan is used by female patients to void when they are confined to bed.
- A regular bowel movement (which is the discharge of solid waste from the body) is also important to a patient's health.
- The solid waste produced by the patient is called **feces** or *stool.*
- Both male and female patients use a bedpan for solid waste elimination when confined to bed.

- Many patients are somewhat sensitive about using a bedpan or urinal.
- Personal hygiene is exceedingly important in carrying out these procedures properly.
- Bedpans are very uncomfortable.

Four important points must be kept in mind. You must:

1. Wear disposable gloves.
2. Wash your hands immediately before and after the procedure. This will help prevent the transmission of any disease to others and to yourself.
3. Provide privacy for the patient. Obtain the proper bedpan according to patient needs.
4. As soon as possible, answer the light indicating that the patient is finished.

INFECTION CONTROL *Alert*

Make sure that bedpans and urinals are labeled with the patients' names for patients in rooms with two or more beds. After cleaning the bedpan or urinal, store it properly in the bedside stand or according to facility policy. Do not leave uncovered bedpans and urinals in the bathroom.

One-Glove Technique

Some facilities require health care providers to use the one-glove technique when removing bedpans, urinals, and other contaminated items. Gloves are worn on both hands when the contaminated item is removed. The bedpan or contaminated item is covered if it is to be carried to the bathroom or into the hallway. A glove is then removed from one hand. Do not put the glove on an environmental surface. The gloved hand carries the glove that you removed and the contaminated item. The ungloved hand is used to open doors and turn on faucets. By using this method, you avoid contaminating the environment with your gloves.

PROCEDURE 75

GIVING AND RECEIVING THE BEDPAN

1. Carry out beginning procedure actions.
2. Assemble equipment:
   - disposable gloves
   - bedpan and cover
   - basin
   - washcloth
   - bath blanket
   - paper towels/protector
   - toilet tissue
   - soap
   - towel
3. Lower the head of the bed, if necessary.
4. Put on gloves.
5. Take the bedpan and toilet tissue from the bedside stand.
   - Place a protector on the chair. Place the bedpan (Figure 25-16) on it.
   - Never place a bedpan on the bedside stand or overbed table.

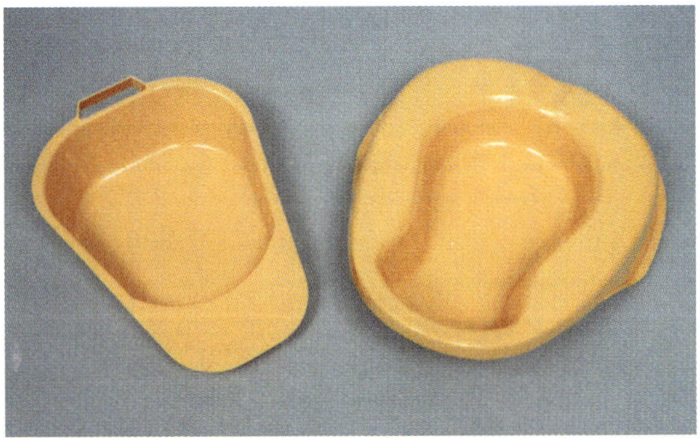

FIGURE 25-16 Orthopedic (fracture) bedpan (left) and regular bedpan (right).

   - Put the remainder of the articles on the bedside table.
6. Place the bedpan cover at the foot of the bed.
   - The bedpan may be warmed by running warm water into it and then emptying and drying it.
   - Plastic bedpans may be comfortable without warming.

continues

PROCEDURE 75

continued

Note: *Never carry or allow a used bedpan to sit uncovered. If a bedpan cover is not available, cover the bedpan with a towel, bed protector, pillowcase, or paper towels.*

7. Cover the patient with a bath blanket. Fold the top bedcovers back at a right angle. Raise the patient's gown. If the patient is thin or has a pressure sore, consult the nurse for the appropriate action. The nursing care plan may have specific instructions for such cases. For example, it may be necessary to pad the bedpan with a folded towel or to take some other action.
8. Ask the patient to flex the knees and rest weight on the heels, if able.
9. Help the patient to raise the buttocks by:
   - Putting one hand under the small of the patient's back and lifting gently and slowly with that hand.
   - With the other hand, place the bedpan under the patient's hips.
   - If the patient is unable to raise the buttocks, two assistants may be needed to lift the patient.
   - The pan may also be placed by rolling the patient to one side, positioning the bedpan against the buttocks, and rolling the patient back onto the pan (Figure 25-17). Check to be sure the bedpan is positioned properly.
   - Alternatively, if a trapeze is in place over the bed, place the bedpan under the patient as the patient lifts self using the trapeze (Figure 25-18).
   - The patient's buttocks should rest on the rounded shelf of the regular bedpan.
   - The narrow end should face the foot of the bed.
10. Replace the top bedcovers. Raise the head of the bed to a comfortable height. Remove gloves and dispose of properly.
11. Make sure the toilet paper and signal cord are within easy reach of the patient. Leave the patient alone unless contraindicated in the nursing care plan.
12. Wash your hands.

Note: *If a specimen is to be taken, instruct the patient that toilet tissue is not to be placed in the bedpan. In this case, the nursing assistant will clean the patient and provide perineal care.*

13. Watch for the patient's signal.

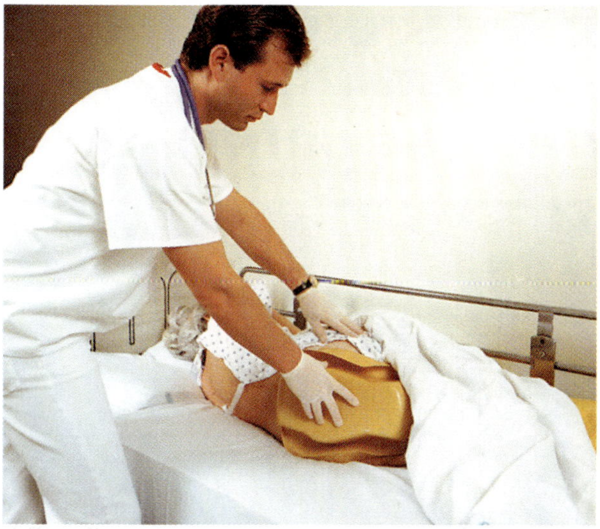

FIGURE 25-17 Roll the patient away from you while supporting the patient with one hand on the patient's hip. Place the bedpan with the other hand, then roll the patient back onto the bedpan.

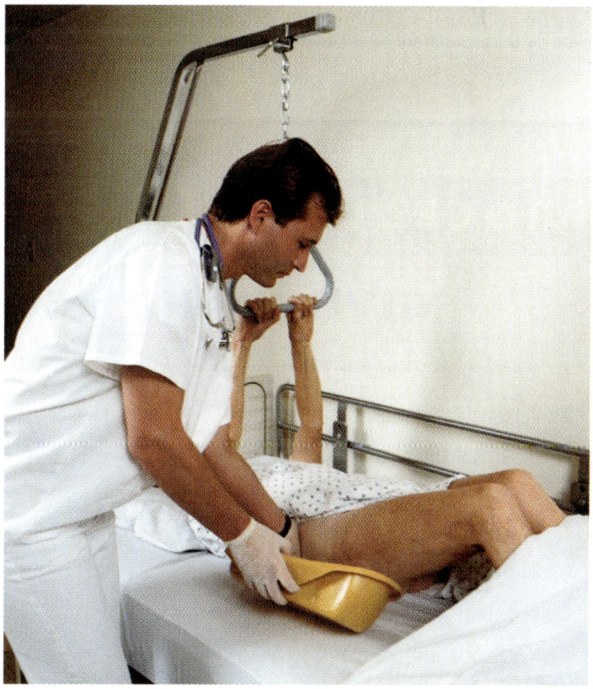

FIGURE 25-18 The patient assists by lifting with the trapeze as the nursing assistant places the bedpan under the patient. Note that the nursing assistant supports the patient's back with his hand.

continues

PROCEDURE 75

continued

14. Answer the patient's call signal immediately. Wash your hands and put on disposable gloves. Fill the basin with warm water (105°F) and place it next to soap, washcloth, and towel on the overbed table.
15. Fold the top bedcovers back so that the patient remains covered only with the bath blanket.
16. Remove the bedpan from under the patient.
    - Ask the patient to flex the knees and rest weight on the heels. Place one hand under the small of the back and lift gently to help raise the buttocks off the bedpan. Take the bedpan with the other hand. Cover it and place it on the chair.
    - If the patient is unable to raise the buttocks, two assistants may be needed to lift. Otherwise, roll the patient off the pan to the side and remove the pan. Lift and move carefully. Hold the pan firmly with one hand.
    - Many patients have difficulty cleaning adequately after using the bedpan. You may need to clean and dry the patient yourself.
17. Assist the patient to a clean area of the bed, if necessary. Provide perineal care.
    - Discard used toilet tissue in the bedpan unless a specimen is to be collected.
    - Cover the bedpan again.
    - Cleanse the patient with warm water and soap, if necessary.
18. Replace the bedclothes, changing linen or protective pads as necessary.
19. Cover the patient with top bedding and remove the bath blanket.
20. Encourage the patient to wash hands and freshen up after the procedure.
21. Take the bedpan to the bathroom or utility room and observe its contents. Measure, if required.
22. Empty the bedpan.
23. Turn on the faucet, using a paper towel. Rinse the bedpan with cold water and disinfectant. Rinse, dry, and return the bedpan to storage in the patient's bedside stand.
24. Remove gloves and dispose of them properly. Wash your hands.
25. Carry out procedure completion actions.

PROCEDURE 76

GIVING AND RECEIVING THE URINAL

1. Carry out beginning procedure actions.
2. Assemble equipment:
    - urinal (Figure 25-19)
    - basin
    - soap
    - washcloth
    - towel
    - disposable gloves
3. Put on gloves. Lift the top bedcovers and place the urinal under the covers so the patient can grasp the handle. Instruct the patient to place his penis in the urinal opening. If he cannot do this,

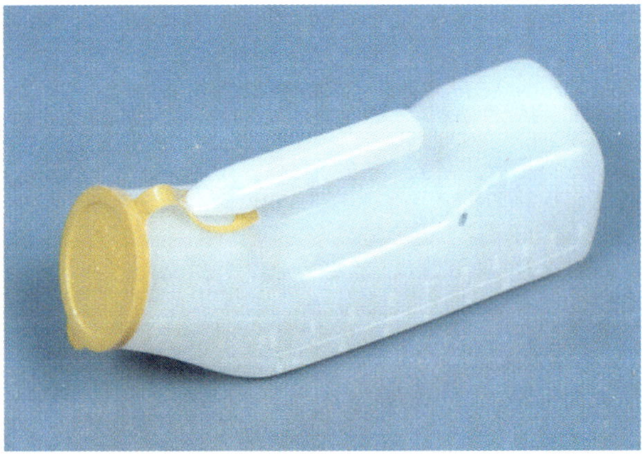

FIGURE 25-19 Male urinal with lid.

continues

PROCEDURE 76

continued

you must position the urinal and ensure that the penis is placed in the opening.

4. Remove gloves and dispose of them properly. Wash your hands. Make sure the signal cord is within easy reach of the patient. Leave the patient alone if possible. Watch for his signal.
5. Answer the patient's signal immediately. Wash your hands. Use a paper towel to turn on the faucet. Fill a basin with warm water (105°F), and place it next to soap, washcloth, and towel so the patient can wash and dry his hands.
6. Put on gloves. Ask the patient to hand the urinal to you. Cover it. Rearrange the bedclothes if necessary.
7. Take the urinal to the bathroom or utility room and observe the contents. Measure, if required. Do not empty the urinal if you observe anything unusual (such as blood). Rather, save the contents of the urinal for the nurse's inspection.
8. Empty the urinal. Use a paper towel to turn on the faucet and another towel to turn the faucet off. Rinse the urinal with cold water and clean it with warm soapy water. Rinse, dry, and cover the urinal. Remove gloves and dispose of them properly. Wash your hands.
9. Place the urinal inside the patient's bedside table. Clean and replace other articles.
10. Carry out procedure completion actions.

PROCEDURE 77

ASSISTING WITH USE OF THE BEDSIDE COMMODE

1. Carry out beginning procedure actions.
2. Assemble equipment:
   - disposable gloves
   - portable commode
   - toilet tissue
   - basin
   - washcloth
   - soap
   - towel
   - bath blanket
3. Position the commode beside the bed, facing the head. Lock the commode wheels and open the lid. Be sure a receptacle is in place under the seat.
4. If the bed and side rails are elevated, lower the side rail nearest you and lower the bed to the lowest horizontal position. Lock bed wheels.
5. Put on gloves.
6. Assist the patient to a sitting position. Swing the patient's legs over the edge of the bed.
7. Assist the patient to put on a robe. Put slippers on the patient. Assist the patient to stand. If needed, use a transfer belt.
8. Support the patient with hands on either side of the chest. Remember to use proper body mechanics. Pivot the patient to the right and lower her to the commode.
9. Cover the patient's legs with a bath blanket.
10. Leave the call bell and toilet tissue within reach.
11. Remove gloves and discard according to facility policy.
12. When the patient signals, return promptly. Wash your hands and put on gloves. Fill a basin with water at 105°F. Bring the basin to the bedside along with soap, a towel, and a washcloth.
13. Remove bath blanket. Assist the patient to stand.

continues

PROCEDURE 77

continued

14. Cleanse the anus or perineum if the patient is unable to do so.
15. Allow the patient to wash and dry her hands. Remove gloves and dispose of according to facility policy. Wash your hands.
16. Assist the patient to return to bed. Adjust bedding and pillows for comfort.
17. Leave the signal cord within easy reach.
18. Put on gloves.
19. Remove the receptacle from the commode and cover it. Close the commode lid.
20. Take the receptacle to the bathroom. Note its contents and measure if required.
21. Empty and clean the receptacle per facility policy. Replace it in the commode. Remove and dispose of gloves properly.
22. Put the commode in its proper place.
23. Carry out procedure completion actions.

REVIEW

A. True/False.

Mark the following true or false by circling T or F.

1. T F Dentures should be stored in an antiseptic solution.
2. T F Backrubs are routinely given as part of the bath procedure.
3. T F A padded footboard is used to prevent foot drop.
4. T F Routine oral hygiene should be carried out once daily.
5. T F Proper oral hygiene helps prevent tooth decay.
6. T F When not in the patient's mouth, dentures should be left on the bedside stand.
7. T F Patients should never be awakened abruptly.
8. T F When giving PM care, the bottom sheet should be tightened and the top linen straightened.
9. T F Disposable gloves should be used by a nursing assistant who is giving oral care.
10. T F The unconscious patient needs no oral care because he is not eating.

B. Matching.

Choose the correct word from Column II to match the phrases in Column I.

Column I	Column II
11. E bad breath	a. oral hygiene
12. A mouth care	b. caries
13. ____ tooth cavities	c. dentures
14. ____ means of relieving pressure	d. bridging
15. C artificial teeth	e. halitosis
	f. foot drop

C. Completion.

Complete the statements in items 16–20 by writing in the correct word from the following list.

arm	name
breakfast	PM care
down	removed
early AM care	surgery
hand	

16. After PM care, the bed should be left with the backrest ______.
17. PM Care should be completed before sleep medication is given.
18. The best way to awaken a patient is to place your hand on the patient's arm and say his name
19. Patients are not wakened early if they are going to have Surgery
20. Early morning care awakens the patient before AM Care

D. Multiple Choice.

Select the one best answer for each of the following.

21. Which of the following patients should be given special mouth care?
- **a.** One who can brush her own teeth
- **b.** One who is drinking water ad lib
- **c.** One who has a broken leg
- **d.** One who has a high fever

22. To warm lotion before giving a backrub,
- **a.** hold it under running water.
- **b.** soak it in a basin of warm water.
- **c.** let the patient hold the bottle for a few minutes.
- **d.** microwave the bottle for 15 seconds.

23. The best way to support a patient in a side-lying position is to
- **a.** use a footboard to keep the feet aligned.
- **b.** place a pillow doubled under the head.
- **c.** place two pillows lengthwise between the legs.
- **d.** double a pillow lengthwise behind the back.

24. When brushing a patient's teeth, the best technique includes
- **a.** inserting the toothbrush with the bristles down.
- **b.** brushing in a circular motion.
- **c.** inserting the toothbrush with bristles facing the teeth.
- **d.** brushing the teeth in a downward motion only.

25. Backrubs are given
- **a.** routinely as part of the pericare procedure.
- **b.** before use of the bedpan.
- **c.** routinely every two hours.
- **d.** only for patients with red areas.

E. Nursing Assistant Challenge.

Your patient, Mrs. Ubanan, has a history of heavy smoking and breathes through her mouth. She has plastic dentures and her care plan indicates that she needs assistance with denture care. Complete the following statements regarding this patient.

26. State two reasons why special oral hygiene has been ordered for Mrs. Ubanan.
- **a.** ____________________
- **b.** ____________________

27. Where are the dentures stored when not in use? ____________

28. Should the dentures be kept dry or wet? ______

29. Should you wear gloves when removing her dentures? ______

30. Will you clean the dentures in cool or hot water? ______

EXPLORING THE WEB

Description	Location
Infection control and patient hygiene	*http://www.infectioncontroltoday.com*
American Dental Association	*http://www.ada.org*
Patient Hygiene PowerPoint Slides	*http://www.sonser4.nur.uth.tmc.edu*

section 8

Principles of Nutrition and Fluid Balance

UNIT 26

Nutritional Needs and Diet Modifications

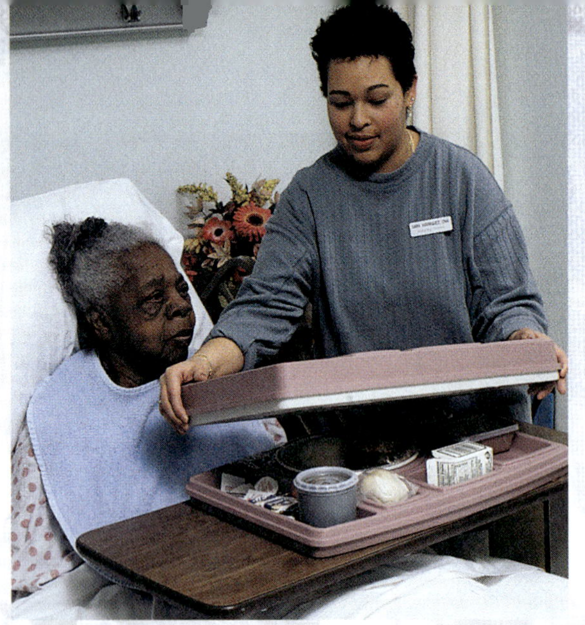

unit 26

Nutritional Needs and Diet Modifications

objectives

After completing this unit, you will be able to:

- Spell and define terms.
- Define normal nutrition.
- List the essential nutrients.
- Name the five food groups and list the foods included in each group.
- State the liquids/foods allowed on the four basic facility diets.
- Describe the purposes of the following diets:
  - clear liquid
  - full liquid
  - soft
- State the purpose of calorie counts and food intake studies.
- Define dysphagia and explain the risks of this condition.
- Describe general care for the patient with dysphagia and swallowing problems.
- State the purposes of therapeutic diets.
- List types of alternative nutrition.
- Describe the nursing assistant actions when patients are unable to drink fluids independently.
- Demonstrate the following procedures:
  - Procedure 78 Assisting the Patient Who Can Feed Self
  - Procedure 79 Feeding the Dependent Patient

vocabulary

Learn the meaning and the correct spelling of the following words and phrases:

amino acids
aspiration
carbohydrates
cellulose
clear liquid diet
defecation
dehydration
diaphoresis
digestion
diuresis
dysphagia
edema
emesis
enteral feeding
essential nutrients
exchange list
excrete
fats
fluid balance
force fluids
full liquid diet
gastrostomy feeding
graduate
hyperalimentation
intake and output (I&O)
intravenous infusion (IV)
mechanical soft
mechanically altered
minerals
nasogastric feeding (NG feeding)
nutrients
nutrition
protein
pureed diet
push fluids
soft diet
supplement
therapeutic diets
total parenteral nutrition (TPN)
vitamins

INTRODUCTION

Nutrition is the entire process by which the body takes in food for growth and repair and uses it to maintain health. The signs of good nutrition include:

- Shiny hair
- Clear skin and eyes
- A well-developed body
- An alert expression
- A pleasant disposition
- Healthy sleep patterns
- Appropriate appetite
- Regular bowel habits
- Body weight appropriate to height

NORMAL NUTRITION

Food is normally taken into the body through the mouth. The mouth is the beginning of the digestive tract. **Digestion** is the process of breaking down foods into simple substances that can be used by the body cells for nourishment. These substances are called **essential nutrients**.

ESSENTIAL NUTRIENTS

To be well nourished, we must eat foods that:

- supply heat and energy.
- build and repair body tissue.
- regulate body functions.

These foods are called **nutrients**. The six nutrients essential to maintain health are:

- Proteins
- Carbohydrates
- Fats
- Minerals
- Vitamins
- Water

Protein

Protein is an essential nutrient. It is the basic material of every body cell. It is the only nutrient that can make new cells and rebuild tissue. The foods that contain the greatest amount of protein come from animals. They include:

- Meat
- Poultry
- Eggs
- Milk
- Cheese

Proteins are made of small building blocks called **amino acids**. The body can manufacture some of the amino acids, but not all of them.

- *Complete proteins* are proteins that contain all the amino acids the body cannot manufacture. Examples of complete proteins are meat, fish, eggs, and poultry.
- *Incomplete proteins*, although still important, do not contain all the essential amino acids. Essential amino acids are those that must be obtained through foods. Examples of incomplete proteins are corn, soybeans, peas, and nuts.

Carbohydrates and Fats

Carbohydrates and **fats** are called energy foods because the body uses them to produce heat and energy. When a person eats more energy foods than the body needs, the remainder is stored as fat. Foods that contain the greatest amount of carbohydrates come from plants. They include:

- Fruits
- Vegetables
- Foods that are made from grains, such as breads, cereals, and pasta products

Carbohydrate foods also supply the body with fiber or roughage (**cellulose**). Cellulose is important in maintaining bowel regularity.

Fats come from both plants and animals. Examples of foods that are rich in fat include:

- Pork
- Butter
- Nuts
- Egg yolk
- Cheese

Vitamins and Minerals

Vitamins and minerals are present in a wide variety of foods. The best way to be sure that you are getting enough vitamins and minerals is to include a variety of foods in your daily diet.

Vitamins are substances that regulate body processes. They help to:

- build strong teeth and bones.
- promote growth.
- aid normal body functioning.
- strengthen resistance to disease.

You probably know the vitamins by their letter names:

- Vitamin A
- B-complex vitamins
- Vitamin C
- Vitamin D
- Vitamin E
- Vitamin K

Fat-soluble vitamins do not dissolve easily in water. They can be stored in the body. Vitamins A, D, E, and K are fat-soluble vitamins.

Vitamins B and C are water soluble. Water-soluble vitamins dissolve in water, so they can be lost in the cooking process.

In general, these vitamins are not stored in large amounts in the body. Deficiencies in water-soluble vitamins are more common.

Minerals help to build body tissues, especially the bones and teeth. They also regulate the chemistry of body fluids such as the blood and digestive juices. Minerals needed in the daily diet include:

- Calcium
- Phosphorus
- Iodine
- Iron
- Copper
- Potassium

THE FIVE FOOD GROUPS

The U.S. Department of Agriculture revised the recommendations for a balanced food intake. The guidelines now include:

- Eat a variety of foods.
- Maintain a healthy body weight.
- Select foods low in fat, saturated fat, and cholesterol.
- Select plenty of vegetables, fruits, and grain products.
- Use sugar in moderation.
- Use salt and sodium in moderation.
- Drink alcoholic beverages in moderation, if at all.

Food Guide Pyramid

Figure 26-1 shows the five food groups. Although the pyramid has six levels, the items in the small triangle do not fit in any of the major food categories. The sixth level at the top of the food pyramid is not considered a food group. The guide to daily food choices recommends:

- 6–11 servings daily from the bread, cereal, rice, and pasta group
- 2–4 servings from the fruit group
- 3–5 servings from the vegetable group
- 2–3 servings from the milk, yogurt, and cheese group
- 2–3 servings from the meat, poultry, fish, dry beans, eggs, and nuts group
- Use fats, oils, and sweets sparingly

The food pyramid shape represents the need for the foods at the bottom (grain foods) and gives equal importance to fruit and vegetables. Persons eating the lowest number of servings from each group will take in about 1,600 calories daily if low-fat foods are chosen. This may be adequate for most older women and some older men. Younger and more active people need more calories and can obtain them by choosing the larger number of servings.

Average servings of foods include:

- One medium-size fruit or its equivalent
- ½ cup cooked fruit or vegetable
- 2–3 ounces of meat
- ½ to 1 ounce of pasta/bread

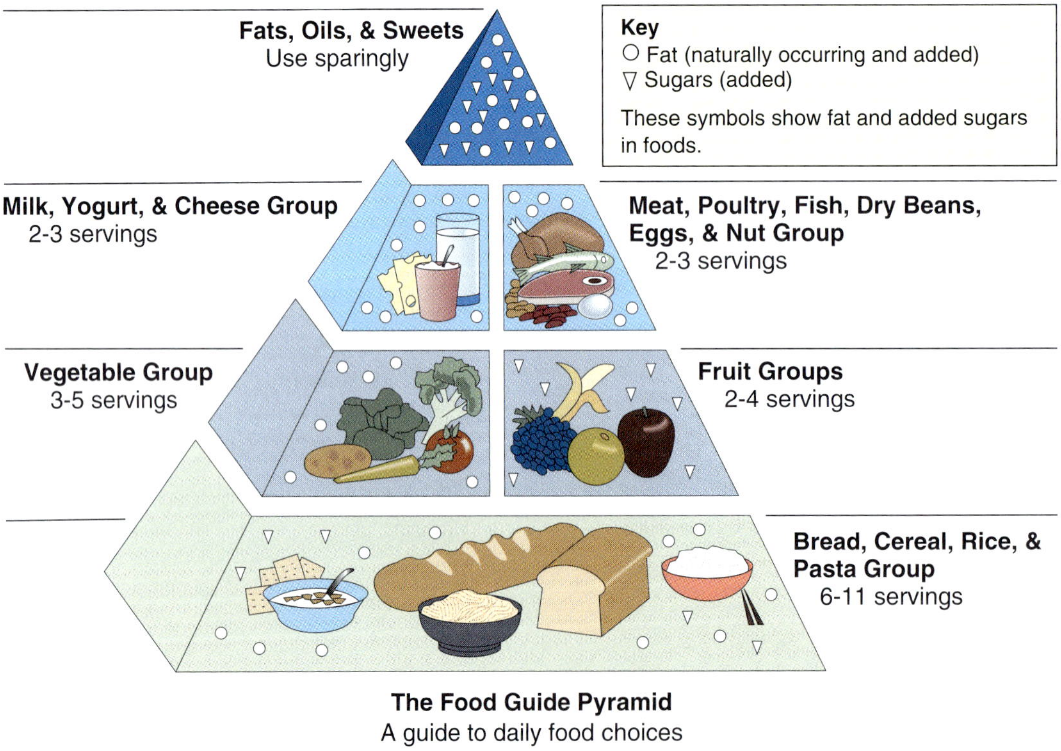

FIGURE 26-1 The USDA Food Guide Pyramid. *(Courtesy of US Department of Agriculture)*

Table 26-1 shows average servings for selected foods.

The food guide pyramid emphasizes foods from the five major food groups shown in the three lower sections of the pyramid. Each of these food groups provides some, but not all, of the nutrients you need each day. Foods in one group cannot replace those in another. No one food group is more important than another. For good health, you need them all.

Vegetable Group

- Select three to five servings. Include:
  - Dark green or yellow vegetables
  - Tomatoes
  - Leafy, green, and yellow vegetables

TABLE 26-1 AVERAGE SERVINGS FOR SELECTED FOODS

Food	Serving Size
Fruit	
Apple	1 medium
Banana	1 medium
Peach	1 medium
Apricots	2–3
Figs	2–3
Canned—	
Grapefruit	½ can
Pineapple	2 slices
Peaches	½ cup
Juice	6 ounces
Vegetables	
Fresh	3–4 ounces
Cooked	½ cup
Milk	8 ounces
Eggs	1 medium
Meat, Fish, Poultry	2½–3 ounces, cooked
Cereal (dried)	½ cup, uncooked
Bread	1 slice
Pasta	½ cup, cooked

- Use vegetables raw, cooked, frozen, or canned.
- This group provides vitamin A, vitamin C, B-complex vitamins, calcium, and iron.
- Leafy green vegetables furnish riboflavin and niacin, which are both B vitamins.

Three to Five Servings Daily

asparagus	mustard greens
beans	okra
broccoli	onions
brussels sprouts	parsley
cabbage	parsnips
carrots	peas (green)
cauliflower	peppers
celery	potatoes
corn	pumpkin
cucumber	radishes
eggplant	rutabaga
escarole	spinach
kale	squash
leeks	sweet potatoes
lettuce	tomatoes
other greens	turnips
mushrooms	

Fruit Group

- Select two to four servings daily.
- Use foods in this group raw, cooked, frozen, canned, or dried.
- When eaten in fairly large amounts, foods in this group provide thiamine, vitamins A and C, calcium, and phosphorus.

Two to Four Servings Daily

apples	kumquats
apricots	lemons
artichokes	limes
avocados	oranges
bananas	peaches
berries	pears
cantaloupe	persimmons
cherries	pineapple
cranberries	plums
currants	prunes
dates	raisins
figs	rhubarb
fruit juice	strawberries
grapefruit	tangerines
grapes	watermelon

Milk, Yogurt, Cheese Group

- This group provides calcium, phosphorus, riboflavin, protein, vitamin A, and fat.
- People need varying amounts of the nutrients in dairy foods at different periods of their lives.
  - Children should have three or four glasses of milk daily.
  - Teenagers need four or more glasses.
  - Adults should drink two or more glasses.
  - Pregnant women should drink at least one quart of milk, or the nutritional equivalent, daily.
  - Nursing mothers should increase the amount of milk in their diet to 1½ quarts daily.
- Daily calcium requirement for postmenopausal women is 1,500 mg.
- Cheese, ice cream, and other milk-made foods can be substituted for part of the milk requirement. (This increases fat and sodium content.)

The following dairy foods contain calcium equal to that in one cup of milk and may be substituted for milk:

Milk Substitutes

1½ ounces cheddar-type cheese
2 ounces cream cheese
2 cups cottage cheese
1½ cups ice cream
1 cup plain, lowfat yogurt
½ ice cream or ice milk
½ cup frozen yogurt

Milk is available in the following forms:

whole milk
skim milk
evaporated milk
condensed milk
buttermilk
dried milk

Grain Group

- Select six to eleven servings daily.
- This group provides carbohydrates, thiamine, niacin, iron, and roughage (fiber).

Six to Eleven Servings Daily

breads: whole wheat, dark rye, enriched cornmeal, whole grain enriched, or oatmeal

rolls or biscuits made with whole wheat or enriched flour

flour: enriched, whole wheat, other whole grain

grits, enriched cereals: whole wheat, rolled oats, brown rice, converted rice, other cereals, if whole grain or restored

noodles, spaghetti, macaroni

Meat Group

- Select two to three servings daily.
- Alternate dried beans, peas, or nuts. These are incomplete protein foods.
- This group provides protein, some fat, iron, phosphorus, and B-complex vitamins.
- Choose low-fat items.
- Remove skin from poultry and trim fat from meat.

Two to Three Servings Daily

beef	lunch meats, such as bologna
eggs	dried beans
lamb	dried peas
game	lentils
veal	nuts
pork (except bacon and fatback)	peanuts
poultry: chicken, duck, goose, turkey	peanut butter
fish, shellfish	soybeans
	soya flour and grits

Fats, Oils, and Sweets

The small triangle at the top of the food pyramid represents food items that should be consumed in very limited quantities, such as fats, sweets, and oils. Examples of foods in this category are salad dressings, cream, butter, margarine, sugars, soft drinks, candies, and sweet desserts. These foods are usually very high in calories, but have little nutritional value. Most people should use them sparingly. Some fat or sugar symbols are shown in the food groups to remind you that some food choices in these food groups can also be high in fat or added sugars. When choosing foods, consider both the fats and sugars in your choices from the food groups, as well as the fats, oils, and sweets from the pyramid tip.

Fats. As a rule, foods that come from animals (milk and meat groups) are naturally higher in fat than foods that come from plants. Many lowfat dairy and lean meat choices are available, and foods can be prepared in ways that lower fat. Fruits, vegetables, and grain products are naturally low in fat. However, fat may be used in food preparation or at the table, such as for french-fried potatoes, buttered vegetables, or croissants, making them higher-fat choices.

Added Sugars. The triangular symbols on the chart represent sugars added to foods in processing or at the table, not natural sugars. The added sugars provide calories with few vitamins and minerals. Most of the added sugars in the typical American diet come from foods in the pyramid tip: soft drinks, candy, jams, jellies, syrups, and table sugar that we add to foods like coffee or cereal.

Fat and Sugar Tips

- Select lower-fat foods from the food groups most often.

- Limit fats and sugars added to foods in cooking or at the table, such as butter, margarine, gravy, salad dressing, sugar, and jelly.
- Select fewer high-sugar foods, such as candy, sweet desserts, and soft drinks.

BASIC FACILITY DIETS

The food you will serve to patients in the health care facility will be prepared by the dietary department (Figure 26-2). It includes the essential nutrients. The way in which it is prepared and its consistency will depend on the individual patient's condition and needs. Sometimes very strict dietary control is needed.

The trays will usually be delivered to the patient floors in large food containers. Each tray will be labeled with the patient's name and type of diet. You will:

- Prepare the patient for the meal.
- Check the tray card for the patient's name.
- Check the tray card against the patient's armband.
- Check the items on the tray to make sure they are allowed on the patient's diet.
- Serve the tray to the patient.
- Assist with feeding as necessary.

Health care facilities usually have many types of diets. Four common diets are:

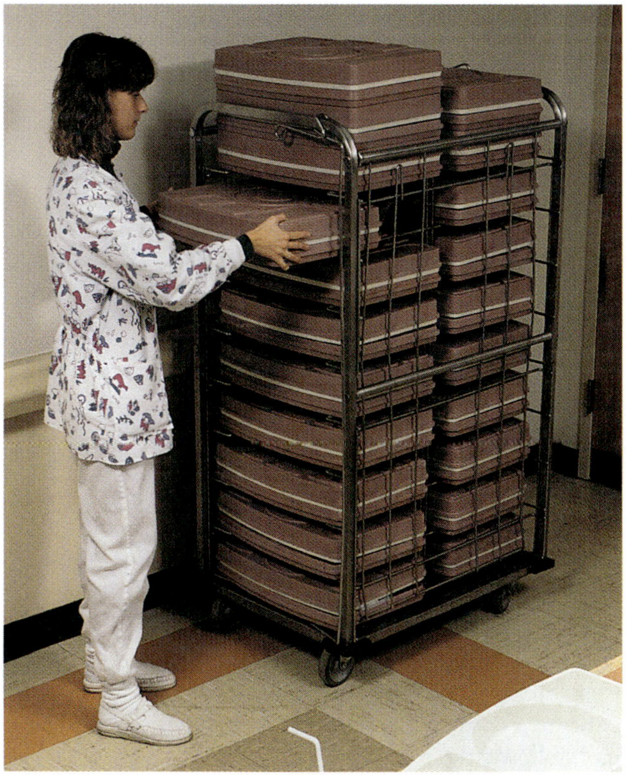

FIGURE 26-2 Patient diets are prepared in the dietary department and transported to the units in containers designed to maintain the temperature.

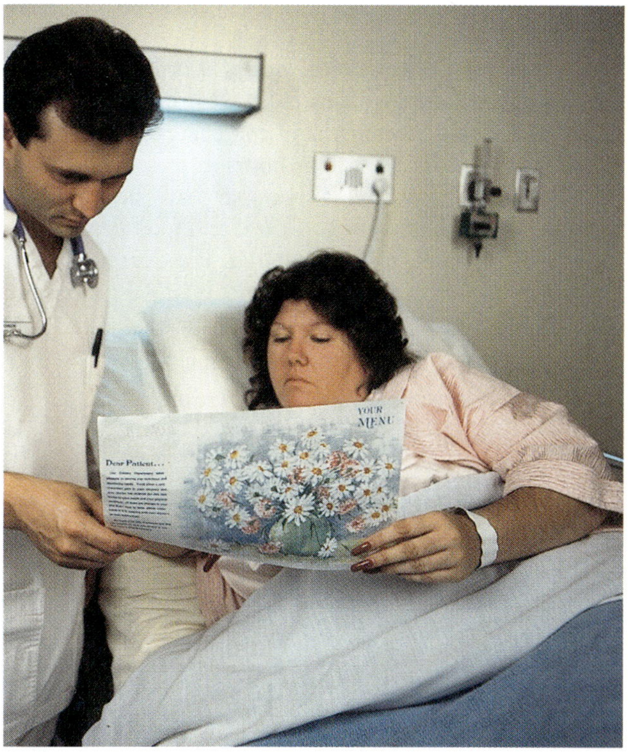

FIGURE 26-3 Patients on a house diet can select foods from a menu.

- Regular or house, sometimes called a general diet (Figure 26-3)
- Full liquid
- Clear liquid
- Soft

The progression of diets a patient is allowed following surgery is as follows:

1. Ice chips/sip of water
2. Clear liquids
3. Full liquids
4. Soft diet
5. Regular diet

In addition, the dietary department prepares special or **therapeutic** (treatment) **diets**. Therapeutic diets are discussed later in this unit.

Regular Diet

The regular-select or house diet is a normal or full diet based on the five food groups. The regular diet:

- Includes a great variety of foods.
- Excludes only very rich foods: pastries, heavy cakes, fried foods, and highly seasoned foods, which might be difficult for inactive people to digest.
- Has a lower caloric count, because an inactive person does not require as many calories as an active person.

In many health care facilities, patients may select foods from a menu.

Liquid Diets

Clear Liquid Diet. A **clear liquid diet** is a temporary diet because it is an inadequate diet. It is made up primarily of water and carbohydrates for energy. Feedings are given every two, three, or four hours as prescribed by the physician. It replaces fluids that may have been lost by vomiting or diarrhea. When a clear liquid food item is held up to the light, you can see through it. The clear liquid diet consists of liquids that do not irritate, cause gas formation, or encourage bowel movements (**defecation**).

Foods allowed on the clear liquid diet include:

- Tea, coffee with sugar but without cream
- Strained fruit or vegetable juice with gelatin (occasionally)
- Fat-free meat broths
- Ginger ale (usually), 7Up®, Coke®, strained grape or apple juice
- Gelatin (occasionally)
- Popsicles

Full Liquid Diet. The **full liquid diet** does supply nourishment and may be used for longer periods of time than the clear liquid diet. Six to eight ounces are usually given every two to three hours.

The full liquid diet is given to:

- Those with acute infections
- Patients who have difficulty chewing
- Those who have conditions involving the digestive tract

The diet includes all of the foods allowed on the clear liquid diet, in addition to the following:

- Strained cereal (gruel)
- Strained soups
- Sherbet
- Gelatin
- Eggnog
- Malted milk
- Milk and cream
- Plain ice cream
- Strained vegetables and fruit juices
- Junket
- Solids that liquefy at room temperature
- Yogurt

Soft Diet

The **soft diet** usually follows the full liquid diet. Although this diet nourishes the body, between-meal feedings are sometimes given to increase the calorie count. Foods allowed on the soft diet are:

- Low-residue, which are almost completely used by the body
- Mildly flavored, slightly seasoned, or unseasoned
- Prepared in a form that requires little digestion

The diet includes liquids and semisolid foods that have a soft texture and are easily digested. It is given to patients who:

- Have infections and fevers
- Have difficulty chewing
- Have conditions involving the digestive tract
- Are on a progressive postoperative dietary regime

The following foods are usually allowed on the soft diet:

- Soups
- Cream cheese and cottage cheese
- Crackers, toast
- Fish
- White meat of chicken or turkey (boiled or stewed)
- Fruit juices
- Cooked fruit (sieved)
- Tea, coffee
- Milk, cream, butter
- Cooked cereals
- Eggs (not fried)
- Beef and lamb (scraped or finely ground)
- Cooked vegetables (mashed or sieved)
- Angel food or sponge cake
- Small amounts of sugar
- Gelatin, custard
- Pudding
- Plain ice cream

Foods to be avoided include:

- Coarse cereals
- Spices
- Gas-forming foods (onions, cabbage, beans)
- Rich pastries and desserts
- Foods high in roughage/fiber
- Fried foods
- Raw fruits and vegetables
- Corn
- Pork (except bacon)

SPECIAL DIETS

Special diets are planned to meet specific patient needs. Patients may need special diets because of religious preferences or health needs.

Religious Restrictions

Religious practice requires changes in diet for some patients. For example, persons of the conservative Jewish faith follow strict food laws.

- There are strict prohibitions against shellfish and nonkosher meats such as pork.
- Certain fishes, such as tuna and salmon, are permitted.

- Foods may not be prepared with utensils that have been used for nonkosher food preparation.
- There are strict rules regarding the sequence in which milk products and meat may be consumed.

Some other faith restrictions are summarized in Table 26-2.

Therapeutic Diets

Standard diets can be changed to conform to special dietary requirements. For example, an order might be written for a low-sodium soft diet when a patient has ill-fitting dentures and heart disease. These therapeutic diets are planned and prepared according to a patient's individual health problems.

Commonly prescribed therapeutic diets include the diabetic diet, sodium-restricted diet, and low-fat diet.

The Diabetic Diet

Diet is an integral part of the therapy of the patient with diabetes mellitus. The diet is nutritionally adequate. It provides enough energy in the form of calories for a 24-hour period. Sometimes a proper diet is all that is needed to control the disease. Usually, however, the food intake is balanced by the administration of insulin or hypoglycemic drugs.

It is important for you to accurately evaluate and report the patient's intake. Foods and liquids have a major impact on diabetes management. Illness increases the need for insulin because the liver releases more glucose in response to the stress. Dehydration is a particularly serious problem for the diabetic. This can occur when not enough foods and fluids are taken in. Insulin administration may depend on your observations. Not all physicians prescribe dietary intake in the same way.

TABLE 26-2 RELIGIOUS DIETARY PRACTICES

	Restricted Food						
Faith	**Coffee**	**Tea**	**Alcohol**	**Pork/Pork Products**	**Caffeine-Containing Foods**	**Dairy Products**	**All Meats**
Christian Science	•	•	•				
Roman Catholic							1 hour before communion, Ash Wednesday, Good Friday
Latter Day Saints (Mormons)	•	•	•		•		
Seventh Day Adventist	•	•	•	•	•		
Some Baptist	•	•	•				
Greek Orthodox (on fast days)						•	Fasting from meat and dairy products on Wed./Fri. during Lent and other holy days
Jewish Orthodox				• Also shellfish		Certain holy days	Forbids the serving of milk and milk products with meat; regulates food preparation; forbids cooking on the Sabbath
Moslem, Islamic			•	•			Fasting during Ramadan during day, feasting at night
Hindu							Some are vegetarians
Buddhist							Meat must be blessed and killed in special ways; some sects are vegetarians

- Some physicians prescribe a very carefully balanced diet and insulin to maintain the level of blood sugar (glucose) within normal limits. All foods must be measured and repeated injections of insulin are required.
- Other physicians are much more liberal in their approach. They permit an unmeasured diet, limiting only sugar and high-sugar foods. This diet is known as a no-concentrated-sweets diet. It may be balanced by insulin or hypoglycemic drugs.
- Many physicians treat diabetes with an approach that is midway between the preceding two methods. They prescribe the American Dietetic Association diets with specific calorie levels, such as the 1,200-calorie diet or the 1,500-calorie diet. The dietitian teaches the patient about the diet and acts as a major resource for health care providers. The diet is balanced by insulin or hypoglycemic drugs.

The Exchange List. The **exchange list** method of balancing the diabetic diet:

- is based on standard household measurements, to make it easier to measure.
- excludes sugar or high-sugar-content foods, to prevent rapid swings in blood sugar.
- divides foods into six groups.
- allows equivalent exchanges to be made within a group but not from group to group.

The six groups are:

- Milk exchanges
- Vegetable exchange: Group A, Group B
- Fruit exchange
- Bread exchange
- Meat exchange
- Fat exchange

Sodium-Restricted Diet

Sodium-restricted diets may be ordered for patients with chronic renal failure and cardiovascular disease. Sodium-restricted diets are some of the most difficult diets to follow. The average American consumes 2 to 6 grams of sodium in food each day. Table salt is a major source of sodium in the diet.

The physician may order several different levels of sodium restriction. These are listed in Table 26-3, in order of most to least salt content.

Processing may add significant amounts of sodium to foods. Food preservatives such as sodium citrate and sodium benzoate are added to many processed foods. This factor is considered in planning and selecting foods for the sodium-restricted diet. It is important to carefully read the labels for the contents of all commercially prepared foods.

Some foods naturally contain relatively large amounts of sodium. These foods may be restricted for this diet. They include:

TABLE 26-3 SODIUM-RESTRICTED DIETS

Type of Low-Sodium Diet	Amount of Sodium
No added salt (limited salt used in cooking, no salt added at meals)	3 to 4 grams daily
2 grams sodium	2 grams daily
1 gram sodium	1 gram daily
500-mg sodium	1/2 gram daily

- Meat
- Fish
- Poultry
- Milk and milk products
- Eggs

Avoid:

- Pork, ham
- Breads
- Potato chips, pretzels, and similar snacks
- Saltine crackers
- Pop (soda)
- Pickles
- Processed meats
- Canned foods, such as vegetables and soups

Some foods are naturally low in sodium. They can be used more liberally. They are:

- Some cereals, such as shredded wheat
- Vegetables
- Fruits

Calorie-Restricted Diet

As long as activity remains constant, a person must take in approximately 500 calories a day less than usual (3,500 calories deficit per week) to lose one pound.

Calorie-restricted diets are prescribed for patients who are overweight. These diets are planned to meet general nutritional needs. They take into consideration the patient's energy output, general nutritional state, and weight goal.

In planning the calorie-restricted diet, the dietitian tries to create a realistic balance between fats, proteins, and carbohydrates. This type of diet encourages the patient to develop better, more consistent eating habits. Exact amounts of the three nutrients are not uniformly prescribed, but they may be balanced as follows:

- Proteins, 20%
- Fats, 25–35%
- Carbohydrates, 45–65%

Some physicians use a factor of 10 calories multiplied by the desired weight in calculating the daily calorie requirements. For example:

- Desired weight 120 lb. × 10 = 1,200 calories per day
- Desired weight 160 lb. × 10 = 1,600 calories per day

Low-Fat/Low-Cholesterol Diet

Low-fat/low-cholesterol diets are prescribed for patients who suffer from vascular, heart, liver, or gallbladder disease, and for those who have difficulty with fat metabolism. Fats are limited and calories are balanced by increasing proteins and carbohydrates. Foods are baked, roasted, or broiled, and the skin is removed from chicken. Low-fat foods include:

- Low-fat cottage cheese (no other allowed)
- Skim milk, buttermilk, yogurt
- Lean meats, fish, chicken
- Vegetables and fruits
- Jams, jellies, ices
- Cereals, pasta, bread, potatoes, rice
- Carbonated beverages, tea, coffee

Mechanically Altered Diets

Any diet may be **mechanically altered**. This means that the consistency and texture are modified, making the food easier to chew and swallow. The **mechanical soft** diet is commonly served to patients who have no teeth, or those with serious dental problems. Meats and hard foods are ground to the consistency of hamburger. Soft items, such as bread, are not ground. The **pureed diet** (Figure 26-4) is blended with gravy or liquid until it is the consistency of pudding. This diet is used for patients who have difficulty swallowing. Pureed foods should not be watery. Properly prepared food items will support a plastic spoon in the upright position.

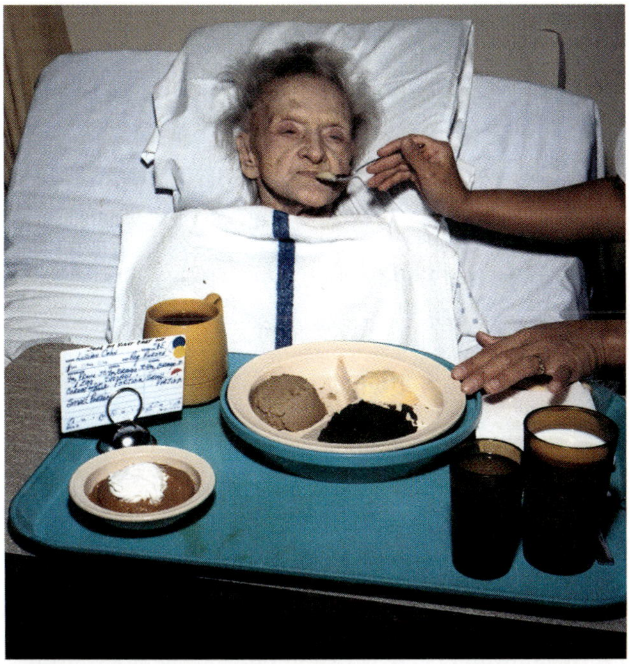

FIGURE 26-4 The pureed diet is given to patients who have difficulty swallowing.

SUPPLEMENTS AND NOURISHMENTS

Many patients receive a nutritional **supplement** or between-meal nourishments. Supplements are ordered by the physician and have a definite therapeutic value. Patients who have wounds may receive supplements high in protein to facilitate healing. These supplements may be liquid or in any form that is easy to eat and digest. It is essential that the patient consume the entire serving. Between-meal nourishments are snacks served to patients to provide the required nutrient daily intake or to prevent between-meal hunger.

Serving between-meal snacks and supplements is an important function of the nursing assistant (Figure 26-5). Between-meal nourishments are usually served:

- Midmorning—between 9:30 and 10:00 AM
- Midafternoon—between 2:30 and 3:00 PM
- At bedtime—between 8:00 and 10:00 PM

Snacks served include:

- Milk
- Juices

DIFFICULT *Situations*

Liquid nutritional supplements are very filling, which is why they are usually served between meals and not with meals. Most patients prefer them cold. If the beverage is warm, the patient may not accept it. Because some of these products are milk-based, serving them warm can also be an infection control hazard. When serving supplements and nourishments, make sure the patient is able to consume the beverage independently. Do not just set it on the table and walk out. Pour the beverage into a cup, if that is what the patient prefers. Provide a straw. If the patient cannot consume the product independently, assist him or her. Document the percentage consumed on the proper form. Record the amount if the patient is on intake and output. Inform the nurse if the patient expresses a preference or dislike for a certain product or flavor.

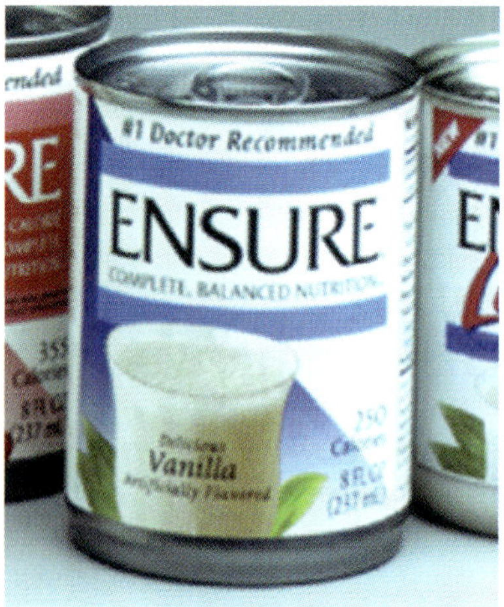

FIGURE 26-5 Supplements and nourishments are an important, planned part of the diet. They are usually given to patients who have had undesirable weight loss, and are served between meals. *(Photo used with permission of Ross Products Division, Abbott Laboratories, Columbus, Ohio)*

- Gelatin
- Custard
- Ice cream
- Sherbet
- High-protein drinks
- Fruits

To serve nourishments:

- Wash your hands.
- Check the nourishment list of each patient for any limitations or special dietary instructions.
- Allow patients to choose from the available nourishments whenever possible.
- Assist those who are unable to take their nourishment alone.
- Remember to pick up used glasses and dishes after the patient has finished and return them to the proper area.
- Notice what the patient was or was not able to take.
- Record on intake and output (I&O) sheet if required.

CALORIE COUNTS AND FOOD INTAKE STUDIES

The physician or dietitian may order special food intake studies for patients with special nutritional needs. The patient's food intake is carefully recorded for a period of time, usually three days. The food intake is analyzed for nutritional adequacy and number of calories consumed. The dietitian uses this information to plan a diet to meet the patient's special medical needs.

If the physician orders a food intake study, nursing personnel will notify the dietary department. A special food documentation form (Figure 26-6) is prepared and placed on the medical record or other designated location. The food intake study usually begins with the breakfast meal on the day after the physician writes the order. Some facilities post a sign in the room or on the door to remind staff and visitors that a study is in progress. In some facilities, each food item is weighed or measured. At the end of each meal, you will accurately record the patient's food intake on the form. Facility policies vary on how food intake is documented, but this is usually done by recording an accurate percentage of each individual meal item consumed. You will also accurately document intake of all snacks, liquid nutritional beverages, and food items brought from home by visitors.

At the end of the study period, the form is returned to the dietitian or dietetic technician. He or she uses the information to calculate the amount of protein, carbohydrates, fat, and calories the patient consumed each day. In some facilities, nutrient, vitamin, and mineral intake are also calculated. The dietitian uses this information to adjust the patient's diet and nutritional plan of care. The results of the study and the dietitian's recommendations are communicated to the physician, who may order extra vitamin or mineral supplements necessary for the patient's medical condition. Completing a food intake or calorie count study requires a team effort, good communication, and accurate documentation.

DYSPHAGIA

Some patients have **dysphagia**, or difficulty swallowing food and liquids. This condition may occur in patients who have:

- had a stroke
- neurological diseases
- cancer of the head, neck, or esophagus
- undergone radiation therapy to the head or neck
- dementia

People who take medications that cause sedation or reduce saliva production are also at risk of dysphagia. Signs and symptoms of dysphagia are:

- taking a long time before beginning to swallow
- swallowing three or four times with each bite of food
- frequent throat clearing or coughing
- lack of a gag reflex or weak cough
- difficulty controlling liquids and secretions in the mouth
- wet, gurgling voice
- refusing to eat, spitting food out, or pocketing food in cheeks
- unintentional weight loss
- tightness in the throat or chest
- feeling as if food is sticking in the esophagus or sternal area

If you observe any of these signs or symptoms, inform the nurse. Patients with dysphagia are at high risk of developing malnutrition and dehydration. Consultation with a speech language pathologist and diagnostic tests for dysphagia may be necessary.

Diet ____________________

CALORIE/PROTEIN SUMMARY

PATIENT ______________________________ ROOM # ____________

DAY 1					DAY 2					DAY 3				
DATE ___/___/___					DATE ___/___/___					DATE ___/___/___				
	% 0–25	% 25–50	% 50–75	% 75–100		% 0–25	% 25–50	% 50–75	% 75–100		% 0–25	% 25–50	% 50–75	% 75–100
Breakfast					**Breakfast**					**Breakfast**				
Meat					Meat					Meat				
Milk					Milk					Milk				
Fruit					Fruit					Fruit				
Starch					Starch					Starch				
Fat					Fat					Fat				
Other					Other					Other				
AM Supp.					AM Supp.					AM Supp.				
Noon Meal					**Noon Meal**					**Noon Meal**				
Meat					Meat					Meat				
Milk					Milk					Milk				
Juice					Juice					Juice				
Starch					Starch					Starch				
Vegetable					Vegetable					Vegetable				
Bread					Bread					Bread				
Fat					Fat					Fat				
Dessert					Dessert					Dessert				
Other					Other					Other				
PM Supp.					PM Supp.					PM Supp.				
Evening Meal					**Evening Meal**					**Evening Meal**				
Meat					Meat					Meat				
Milk					Milk					Milk				
Juice					Juice					Juice				
Starch					Starch					Starch				
Vegetable					Vegetable					Vegetable				
Bread					Bread					Bread				
Fat					Fat					Fat				
Dessert					Dessert					Dessert				
Other					Other					Other				
PM Supp.					PM Supp.					PM Supp.				
Total Kcal					**Total Kcal**					**Total Kcal**				
Total Pro					**Total Pro**					**Total Pro**				
Avg. for 3 days Kcal:								**Avg. Protein for 3 days:**						

PLEASE RETURN COMPLETED FORM TO NUTRITION CARE MANAGER

FIGURE 26-6 The calorie count provides an accurate picture of the patient's calorie and nutrient intake over a three-day period. The information is used to adjust the patient's diet and nutritional plan of care.

Dysphagia is treated with swallowing exercises, practice of proper swallowing techniques, and alteration of the consistency of food and beverages. The dietitian works closely with the speech language pathologist to ensure that the food is the proper consistency to meet the patient's needs and reduce the risk of aspiration. The goal is to keep the look, taste, and food consistency as close to normal as possible, considering the patient's safety needs. Extra gravies or sauces may be added to some foods. Adults may be resistant to eating pureed food because it resembles baby food. Molds and special methods of preparation are used to enhance the appearance of pureed foods, making them more acceptable to the patient. You may be instructed to monitor the patient's food and fluid intake accurately. Inform the nurse if the patient has special dietary requests. The physician may order frequent weight monitoring.

Patients with dysphagia will use special approaches to eating and drinking to prevent aspiration and ensure proper intake. The speech therapist works closely with these patients. Liquids are usually the most difficult to swallow. The speech professional may recommend using food thickeners (Figure 26-7) to slow the movement of fluid through the esophagus. Thickeners are nonprescription, powdered products that are mixed into beverages and some foods to make swallowing easier and prevent aspiration. The consistency of the liquid depends on the amount of powder added. It is important to add exactly the amount that has been ordered. Thickeners do not change the taste of food or liquids, but they may change the intensity, making it taste stronger. Prethickened liquids are also available.

The care plan will specify the type and amount of thickener to use to achieve the necessary texture. For example, the therapist may recommend that liquids be mixed to the consistency of peach juice, nectar, honey, or pudding. Add the thickener immediately before serving the product. Follow the therapist's directions exactly. When adding thickeners:

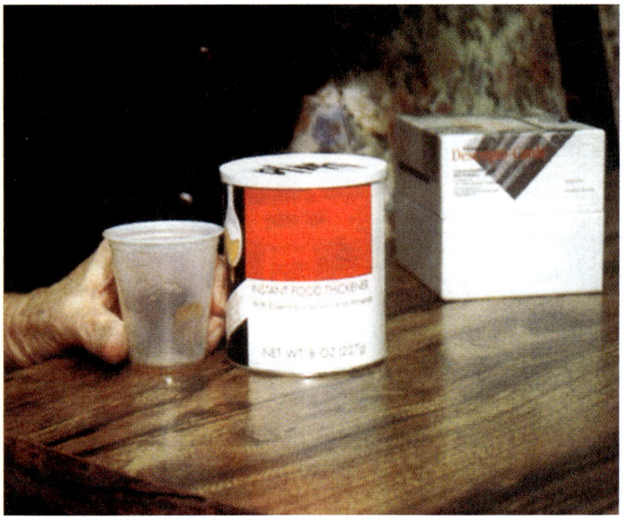

FIGURE 26-7 Food thickener is used to change the texture and consistency of liquids to prevent choking.

- Use the correct product
- Use the correct amount
- Follow the manufacturer's directions
- Stir the thickener well
- Follow the speech therapist's instructions and plan of care for positioning and feeding

FLUID BALANCE

Fluid balance is the balance between liquid intake and liquid output. Because two-thirds of the body's weight is water, there must be a balance between the amount of fluid taken into the body and the amount lost under normal conditions. Generally, we do not need to concern ourselves about this balance. It usually takes care of itself.

The metric system is used for fluid measurements: milliliters (mL) or cubic centimeters (cc). A mL and a cc are the same amount. Table 26-4 provides a comparison of U.S. customary and metric measurements.

Intake

We take in approximately 2½ quarts (2,500 mL) of fluid daily:

- In liquids such as water, tea, and soft drinks.
- In foods such as fruits and vegetables.
- Artificially, such as by intravenous infusions or gavage.

Most adult patients need to consume an average 600 to 800 mL of fluid during each eight-hour shift. Because patients may sleep during most of the night shift, additional fluids must be provided during waking hours to keep

TABLE 26-4 COMPARISON OF U.S. CUSTOMARY AND METRIC MEASUREMENTS

U.S. Customary Units	Metric Units
1 minim	0.06 milliliter (mL)
16 minims	1 mL
1 ounce	30 mL
1 pint	500 mL
1 quart	1,000 mL (1 liter)
2.2 pounds	1 kilogram (kg)
1 inch	2.5 centimeters (cm)
1 foot	30 cm

the body in balance. Excessive fluid retention is called **edema**. Inadequate fluid intake results in **dehydration**, or the lack of sufficient fluid in body tissues. Some disease conditions may change the amounts of fluid the patient is allowed to have.

Output

Typical output equals about 2½ quarts daily in the form of:

- Urine, 1½ quarts (1,500 mL)
- Perspiration
- Moisture from the lungs
- Moisture from the bowel

Excessive fluid loss results in dehydration. This can occur through:

- Diarrhea
- Vomiting
- Excessive urine output (**diuresis**)
- Excessive perspiration (**diaphoresis**)
- Wound drainage or blood loss

Recording Intake and Output

An accurate recording of **intake and output** (**I&O**), or fluid taken in and given off by the body, is basic to the care of many patients. Intake and output records are kept when specifically ordered by the physician and when patients:

- are dehydrated.
- receive intravenous infusion.
- have recently had surgery.
- have a urinary catheter.
- are perspiring profusely or vomiting.
- have specific diagnoses such as congestive heart failure or renal disease that require accurate monitoring of I&O.

Fluid intake may have to be encouraged in some patients. This is called **push fluids** or **force fluids**. In some situations (as in kidney disease), fluid intake may have to be restricted.

Fluid intake and output is calculated by measuring and recording the fluids the patient takes in and the fluids the patient **excretes** (eliminates from the body) (Table 26-5). Because the fluids taken in by the patient cannot actually be measured, an estimate is made and recorded. This is done by:

- Knowing what the liquid container holds when full.

Note: Sizes of containers vary. Learn the fluid content of the containers used at your facility. Remember that there are 30 mL per ounce (240 mL ÷ 30 mL = 8 oz).

  - Coffee/tea cup, 8 oz = 240 mL
  - Water carafe, 16 oz = 480 mL
  - Foam cup, 8 oz = 240 mL
  - Water glass, 8 oz = 240 mL
  - Soup bowl, 6 oz = 180 mL
  - Jello, 1 serving = 130 mL
  - Ice chips, full 4 oz glass = 120 mL
- Estimating how much is gone from the container (what the patient drank), such as one-third of a glass of juice or half of a cup of coffee
- Converting this to mL. *Example:* A water glass holds 240 mL when filled. The patient drinks ¾ of the glass of water. ¾ × 240 = 180 mL. Intake for the glass of water is recorded as 180 mL. Fluids that are calculated and recorded include all liquids, such as water, juices, soda, coffee, tea, milk, and soup. Also included are foods that melt at room temperature: ice cream, sherbet, and gelatin.

TABLE 26-5 COMPUTING INTAKE AND OUTPUT

Intake	
IV	1,500 mL
By mouth	2,000 mL
Total	3,500 mL
Output	
Urine	1,500 mL
Vomitus	500 mL
Drainage	600 mL
Total	2,600 mL

Note: Containers may vary from one facility to the next. Each facility should have a chart available that tells you what each size of glass, cup, and bowl holds when full.

Fluids taken by mouth, through intravenous infusion, or through gastric feeding are all recorded separately (Figure 26-8). At the end of each 8-hour shift and the end of 24 hours, the figures are totaled.

Fluid output amount is obtained by measuring all fluids excreted from the body. This includes urine, **emesis** (vomitus), and drainage from body cavities, such as gastric drainage. A container called a **graduate** is marked in mL or cc. The substance is poured into the graduate to determine the amount of output. Urine and any other excretions are recorded separately.

Note: Standard precautions must be followed when measuring any body excretion. Gloves are required for measuring all forms of output (Figure 26-9).

Date	Time	Method of Adm.	Solution	Intake Amounts Rec'd	Time	Output Urine Amount	Others: Kind	Others: Amount
7/16	0700	PO	water	120 mL		500 mL		
	0830	PO	coffee	240 mL				
			or. ju.	120 mL				
	1030	PO	cran.ju.	120 mL				
	1100					300 mL		
	1230	PO	tea	240 mL				
	1400	PO	water	150 mL				
Shift Totals	1500			990 mL		800 mL		
	1530	PO	gelatin	120 mL				
	1700	PO	tea	120 mL				
			soup	180 mL				
	2000					512 mL		
	2045						vomitus	500 mL
	2205						vomitus	90 mL
Shift Totals	2300			420 mL		512 mL		590 mL
	2345						vomitus	80 mL
	0130	IV	D/W	500 mL				
	0315					400 mL		
Shift Totals	0700			500 mL		400 mL		80 mL
24 Hour Totals				1910 mL		1712 mL		670 mL vomitus

FIGURE 26-8 Sample intake and output record.

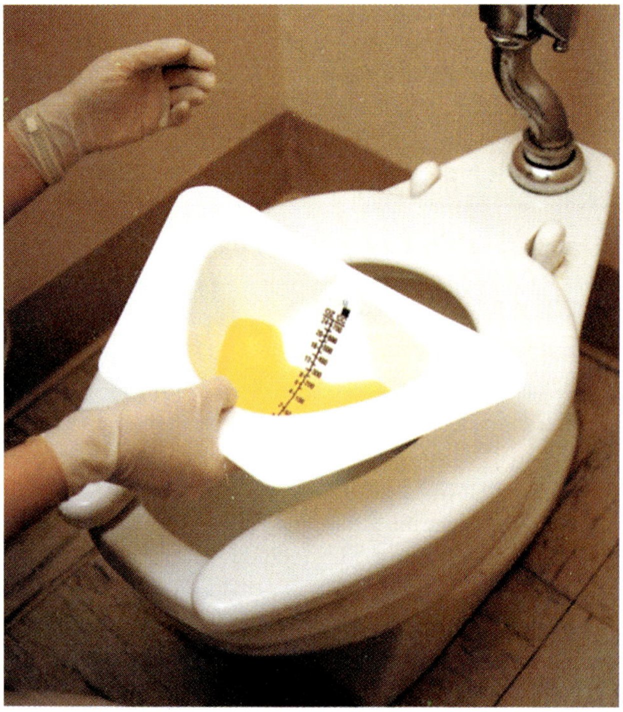

FIGURE 26-9 The specimen collection container is placed under the toilet seat when the patient eliminates. Wear gloves when measuring output, then clean and replace the collection device.

CHANGING WATER

It is important to provide fresh water for patients, because water is essential to life. In all cases, you should know whether a patient is allowed ice or tap water and if water is

INFECTION CONTROL *Alert*

Avoid contaminating the ice chest or ice scoop when filling pitchers and passing drinking water. Keep the ice scoop covered when not in use. Note that the handle is contaminated and should not touch the clean ice supply. Avoid filling the pitcher over the source of clean ice. (If ice hits the rim of the pitcher and drops back into the clean ice supply, it is contaminated.) Do not allow the scoop to touch the pitcher. Always keep water pitchers covered at the bedside. If more than one patient shares the room, make sure each pitcher and cup are labeled with a single patient's name.

to be especially encouraged. Even without an order to force fluids, you must encourage patients to take 6 to 8 glasses of fluids daily, unless the patient is NPO (nothing by mouth) or on restricted fluids. Give special attention to confused patients, patients who may not be able to reach a source of water, and the elderly. The need for adequate water intake cannot be overstressed. Because patients often do not drink enough water, sometimes the physician will leave orders that fluids are to be forced to a specific number of mL per day. *Forcing fluids* is an old term that is not quite accurate. Patients should never actually be forced to consume water or other beverages. When "force fluids" is ordered, encourage the patient to drink each time you are in the room. Offer to assist, if necessary. Some patients will not drink water. Find out what beverages the patient likes, and provide these, if possible.

Providing fresh water is one way to encourage the patient to increase intake of fluids. The procedure for providing fresh water varies greatly.

- In some hospitals, the water pitcher and glass are replaced with a new disposable set each time water is provided.
- In others, the pitcher and glass are washed, refilled, and returned to the patient's bedside table.

In all cases, be sure you know whether a patient is allowed ice or tap water.

FEEDING THE PATIENT

Eating should be an enjoyable experience. (See Procedures 78 and 79.) Prepare the patient for the meal tray before it arrives by:

- Offering the bedpan or helping the patient to the bathroom.
- Assisting the patient to wash hands and face.
- Assisting with oral hygiene, if needed.
- Raising the head of the bed, if permitted, or assisting the patient out of bed and into a chair, if permitted.
- Adjusting the in-bed patient's position with pillows.
- Clearing away anything that is unpleasant, such as the emesis basin and bedpan.
- Clearing the overbed table.
- Encouraging the patient to do as much as possible.

When you have served the tray and after you have washed your hands, assist the patient as needed by:

- Being unhurried and pleasant.
- Opening prepackaged items.
- Cutting meat.
- Pouring liquids.
- Buttering bread.
- Explaining the arrangement of the tray as if items were on the face of a clock (Figure 26-10) if the patient cannot see.

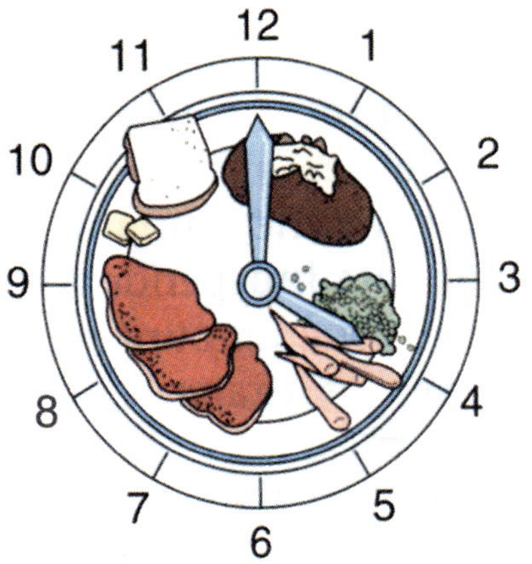

FIGURE 26-10 Describe the location of each food item compared with its position on the face of a clock.

There are times when you will be responsible for the entire feeding procedure.

Note: Carry some extra straws with you during meal times. It can save you steps.

INFECTION CONTROL *Alert*

Keep the soiled linen hamper and housekeeping cart separated from the food cart by *at least* one room's width (approximately 12 to 16 feet). Some facilities remove the linen hampers and housekeeping carts from the hallway when food is being served. Know and follow facility policies and state requirements. When passing trays, close the door to the food cart as soon as each tray is removed. This maintains food temperature (which prevents pathogen growth), and prevents environmental contamination of food items. Serve food promptly when it arrives on the unit. Maintaining proper food temperature is key to preventing foodborne infection. If a patient must be fed, leave the tray on the cart to maintain temperature until you are ready to feed the patient. Avoid placing used meal trays back on the food cart until all fresh trays have been served. Avoid placing lab specimens in the refrigerator with food and beverages. Store these biohazardous items separately in a refrigerator or cooler marked with a biohazard label.

PROCEDURE 78

ASSISTING THE PATIENT WHO CAN FEED SELF

1. Carry out beginning procedure actions.
2. Assemble equipment:
   - bedpan/urinal
   - disposable gloves
   - basin of warm water
   - towel
   - soap
   - washcloth
   - oral hygiene items
   - tray of food
3. Offer bedpan/urinal. (If used, follow Procedure 75 in Unit 25—"Giving and Receiving the Bedpan.") Use standard precautions if you anticipate contact with blood, body fluids, mucous membranes, or nonintact skin when assisting the patient with elimination or feeding.
4. If permitted, elevate the head of the bed or assist the patient out of bed.
5. Provide a washcloth to wash the patient's hands and face.
6. Assist with oral hygiene or assist with dentures.
7. Remove and discard personal protective equipment, if used, according to facility policy.
8. Clear the overbed table and position it in front of the patient. Remove unpleasant equipment from the sight.
9. Wash your hands. Obtain the meal tray from the dietary tray conveyor.
10. Check the diet with the dietary card and with the patient's identification band (Figure 26-11A).
11. Place the tray on the overbed table and arrange food in a convenient manner.
12. Assist in food preparation as needed (Figure 26-11B). Encourage the patient to do as much as possible.
13. Remove the tray as soon as the patient is finished. Make sure to note what the patient has and has not eaten.
14. Record fluids on intake record, if necessary. Record food intake.
15. Push the overbed table out of the way.
16. Carry out procedure completion actions.

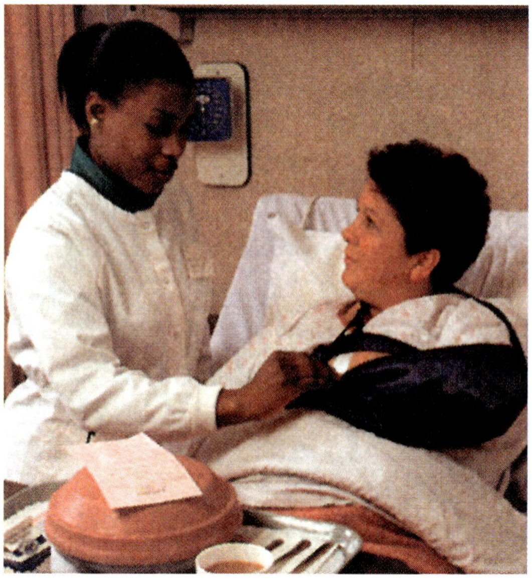

FIGURE 26-11A Check the patient's identification band against the tray card.

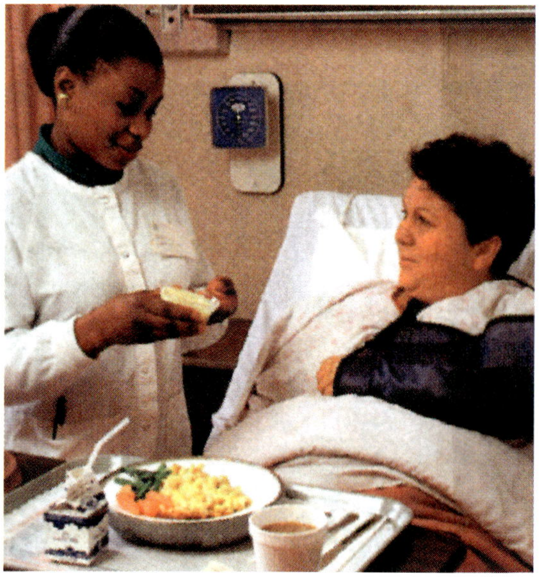

FIGURE 26-11B Assist with food preparation as needed.

PROCEDURE 79

FEEDING THE DEPENDENT PATIENT

1. Carry out beginning procedure actions.
2. Assemble equipment:
   - bedpan/urinal
   - basin
   - soap
   - towel
   - washcloth
   - clothing protector
   - oral hygiene items
   - tray of food
3. Offer the bedpan or urinal. (If used, follow Procedure 75 in Unit 25—"Giving and Receiving the Bedpan.") Follow standard precautions.
4. Provide oral hygiene, if desired.
5. Remove unnecessary articles from the overbed table.
6. Elevate the head of the bed with the patient's head bent slightly forward.
7. Place a towel or protector under the patient's chin (Figure 26-12A). Avoid calling this item a "bib," which is demeaning to adults.
8. Obtain the meal tray. Check the diet against the patient's identification band and dietary card.
9. Place the tray on the overbed table (Figure 26-12B).
10. Butter bread and cut meat. Do not pour a hot beverage until the patient is ready for it.
11. Use different drinking straws to give each fluid, or use a cup. Thick fluids are more easily controlled by using a straw. Use adaptive devices as indicated on the care plan.
12. Sit down while you are feeding the patient, so that you are at eye level.
13. Holding the spoon at a right angle:
    - Give solid foods from the point of the spoon (Figure 25-12C).
    - Alternate solids and liquids.
    - Ask the patient in what order she would like the food.
    - Describe or show the patient what kind of food you are giving.
    - If the patient has had a stroke, direct food to the unaffected side and check for food stored

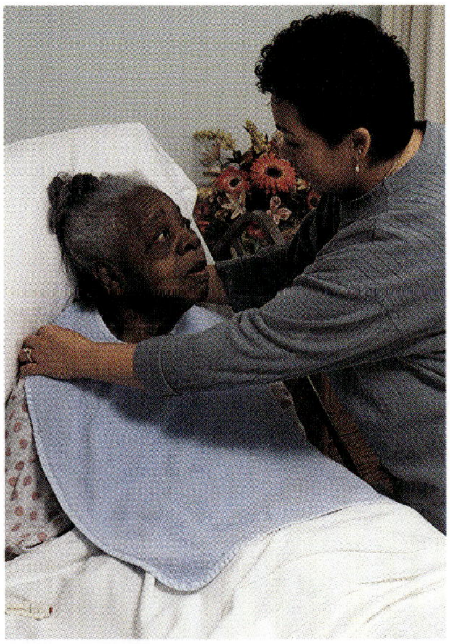

FIGURE 26-12A Place a towel or garment protector over the patient.

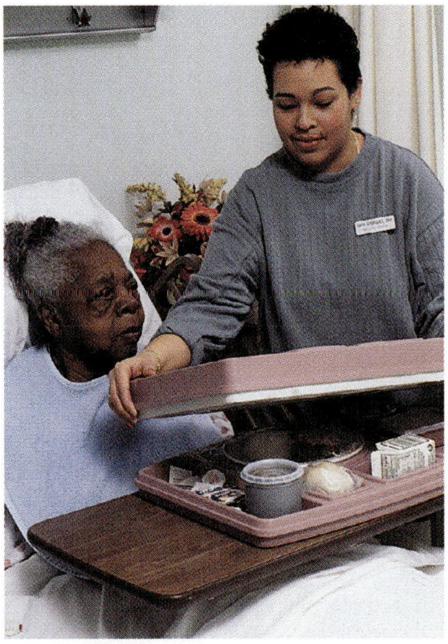

FIGURE 26-12B Uncover the food and arrange it on the overbed table.

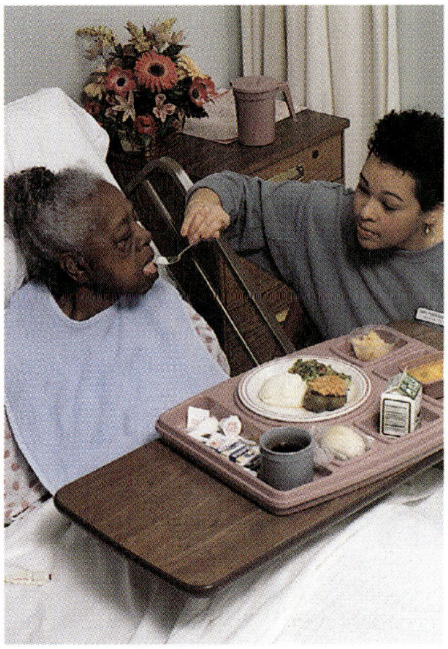

FIGURE 26-12C Give solid foods from the tip of the spoon.

continues

PROCEDURE 79

continued

in the affected side. Watch the patient's throat to check for swallowing.

- Test hot foods by dropping a small amount on the inside of your wrist before feeding them to the patient.
- Never blow on the patient's food to cool it.
- Never taste the patient's food.
- Do not hurry the meal.

14. Allow the patient to assist to the extent that he or she is able.
15. Use a napkin to wipe the patient's mouth as often as necessary.
16. Remove the tray as soon as the patient is finished. Record percentage of food eaten. Record fluid intake.
17. Carry out procedure completion actions.

Mealtime Assistance for Patients Who Have Swallowing Problems

Patients who have difficulty swallowing may require one-to-one assistance, prompting, or supervision at meals. The speech therapist will recommend special techniques and positions for improving swallowing and preventing aspiration. These will be listed on the care plan. The therapist may work closely with each staff member who may feed the patient. In general:

- Before serving food or beverages, make sure the patient is fully awake and alert.
- Position the patient as upright as possible.
- The head should face forward, with the neck flexed forward slightly.
- During the meal, reduce distractions.
- Limit conversation. The patient with dysphagia should not try to carry on a conversation while eating. Focus the patient on eating.
- Prompt or feed the patient slowly, offering small bites. Remind the patient to chew the food well.

The speech language pathologist may order other special positions and exercises, depending on the patient's medical condition and needs. The care plan will provide additional directions, such as reminding the patient to tuck the chin in when swallowing. In some types of dysphagia, this changes the position of the airway, further reducing the risk of aspiration. In other types, this technique increases the risk. Because dysphagia care is highly individualized, many staff members must work as a team to ensure that the patient's nutritional needs are safely met.

ALTERNATIVE NUTRITION

There may be situations in which the patient is unable to take in food in the usual way. This may occur if the patient:

- is unconscious.
- has a disease of the digestive tract.
- has persistent vomiting and cannot hold down food.
- is unable to swallow without **aspiration** (choking).

To maintain life, the body must meet its requirements for daily essential nutrients. This may be done by:

- administration of **total parenteral nutrition** (**TPN**) (also called **hyperalimentation**), which is a form of **intravenous infusion** (**IV**), or by
- **enteral feedings** (tubes inserted into digestive tract).

Total Parenteral Nutrition

TPN is a technique in which high-density (concentrated) nutrients are introduced into a large vein, such as the subclavian or the superior vena cava. This method of feeding is used for patients with diseases of the digestive tract. Caring for patients with TPN is discussed in Unit 35 (Subacute Care).

Enteral Feedings

Enteral feedings may be administered by a tube that is

- Inserted through the nose and into the stomach (**nasogastric** or **NG feeding**) (Figure 26-13).
- Inserted directly through the abdominal skin and into the stomach (**gastrostomy feeding**) (Figure 26-14).

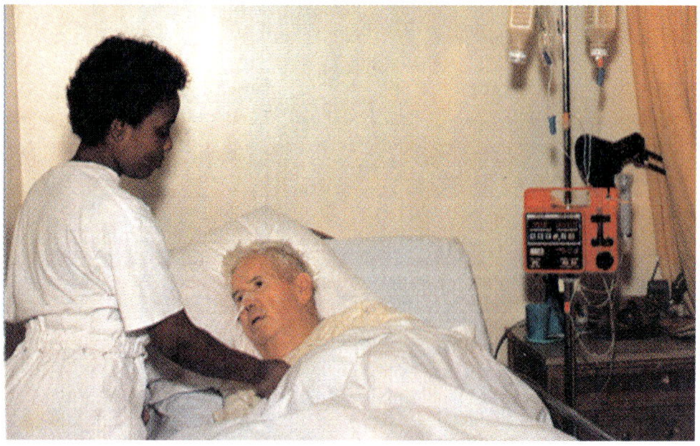

FIGURE 26-13 An NG tube is inserted through the patient's nose into the stomach.

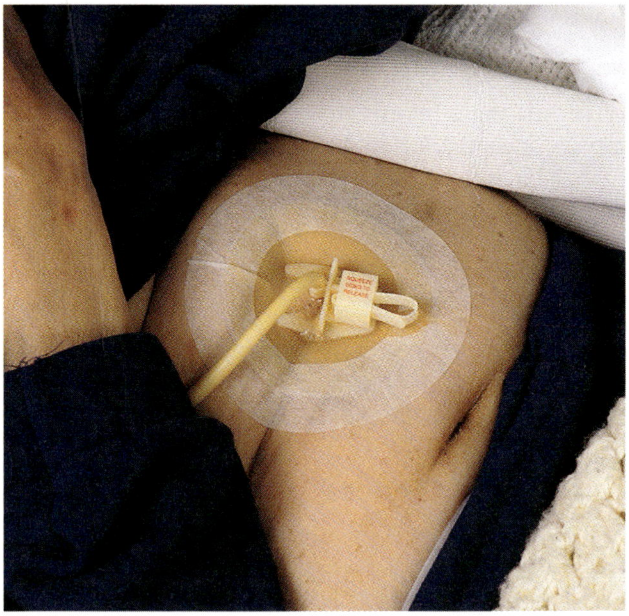

FIGURE 26-14 Gastrostomy tubes are surgically inserted through the abdominal skin into the stomach. This type of tube is used when long-term tube feeding is anticipated.

Many different types of tubes may be used for these feedings. The nurse or physician inserts the feeding tube. Specially prepared solutions contain all the nutrients required by the body. The feeding may be administered intermittently or it may run continuously. In either case, the container of solution is hung from an IV (intravenous) pole and is usually attached to a device that automatically controls the administration (Figure 26-15).

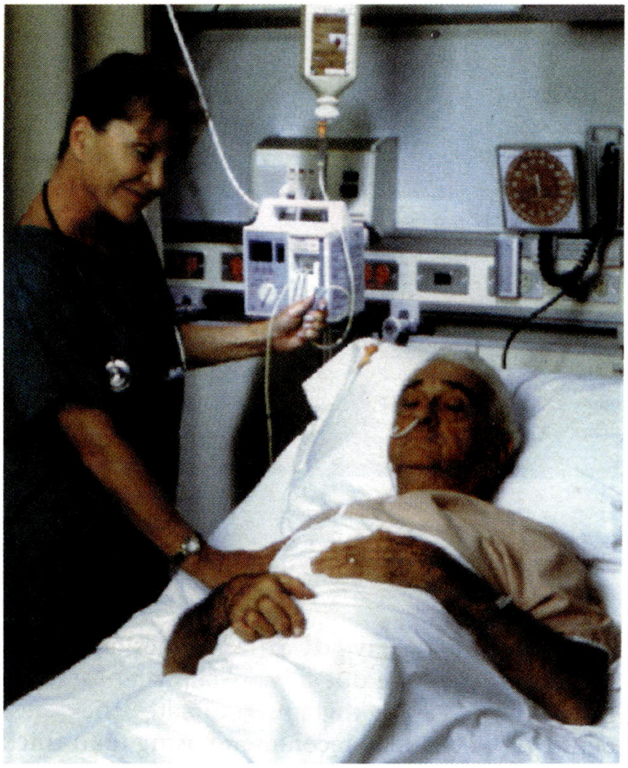

FIGURE 26-15 Enteral feedings are usually administered through a mechanical pump. *(Photo used with permission of Ross Products Division, Abbott Laboratories, Columbus, Ohio)*

SAFETY *Alert*

Most patients receiving tube feedings are NPO, but some are also permitted to have food or liquids orally. Verify the orders for that patient before giving food or fluids. When a patient receives a continuous tube feeding with a pump, the head must be elevated at all times. Keeping the head of the bed elevated when the tube feeding is infusing is critical to prevent accidental aspiration of formula into the lungs. Monitor the patient for signs of respiratory distress. If formula is aspirated into the lungs, the patient will begin coughing, choking, or gurgling, or will become cyanotic. If any of these occur, call for the nurse immediately. Monitor the skin on the hips and buttocks frequently, as this position increases pressure and the risk of skin breakdown. Move the patient in bed with an assistant. The elevation of the head of bed also increases the risk of skin damage from friction and shearing.

When caring for the patient with tube feedings, you need to:

- Keep the head of the bed elevated 45° to 60° during feeding and for 30 to 60 minutes after feeding.
- Check the taping of tubes. If tape is loose, or pulls, or is causing skin irritation, inform the nurse.

SAFETY *Alert*

Know the location of the tube at all times and avoid pulling on it. Avoid pulling on the tube when moving and transferring the patient. Serious complications can result if a feeding tube is dislodged. The skin around the feeding tube must be kept clean and dry. Sometimes the skin around a gastrostomy tube is covered with gauze. After the incision has healed, no dressing is necessary. If the patient has a nasogastric tube, it may be clipped to the gown or clothing to prevent pulling.

- Report any retching, nausea, or vomiting immediately.
- Check the tubing for kinks. Be sure the patient is not lying on the tubing.
- Provide frequent mouth hygiene. Patients with an NG tube will also need nasal care.
- Notify the nurse if a controlling device alarm sounds.

Adjusting to tube feeding formula can be difficult for the patient. The rate and strength of formula must be adjusted to meet the patient's needs. In some patients, the formula causes diarrhea. Inform the nurse if the patient's bowel activity increases, or if the patient experiences multiple loose or liquid stools. Keep the perineum clean and dry, and wash the patient well after each bowel activity.

REVIEW

A. True/False.

Mark the following true or false by circling T or F.

1. T F Vitamins are nutrients that help regulate body activities.

2. T F The exchange lists are used by patients on low-salt diets.

3. T F Fats are one of the six essential nutrients.

4. T F Ice cream would be served to a patient on a clear liquid diet.

5. T F Labels of canned foods must be checked when planning their use in low-sodium diets.

6. T F A gastrostomy tube introduces nutrients directly into the stomach.

7. T F Carbohydrate foods are used to make new body cells and build tissues.

8. T F Green leafy vegetables are a good source of calcium, iron, and B vitamins.

9. T F Complete protein foods like poultry contain all of the essential amino acids.

B. Matching.

Match the correct term from Column II with the words and phrases in Column I.

Column I	Column II
10. ____ difficulty swallowing	**a.** therapeutic
11. ____ roughage	**b.** mineral
12. ____ encourage liquid intake	**c.** dysphagia
13. ____ all the processes involved in taking in food and building and repairing the body	**d.** force fluids
14. ____ treatment	**e.** cellulose
15. ____ calcium	**f.** gastrostomy
	g. nutrition

C. Multiple Choice.

Select the one best answer for each of the following.

16. Feeding the patient through a nasogastric tube is known as a/an
- **a.** intravenous infusion.
- **b.** gastrostomy feeding.
- **c.** enteral feeding.
- **d.** hyperalimentation.

17. Which of the following is a water-soluble vitamin?
- **a.** Vitamin C
- **b.** Vitamin E
- **c.** Vitamin A
- **d.** Vitamin D

18. An example of a fat-soluble vitamin is
- **a.** vitamin C.
- **b.** vitamin B-complex.
- **c.** vitamin D.
- **d.** vitamin N.

19. An average serving of meat is
- **a.** 1 ounce.
- **b.** 2 to 3 ounces.
- **c.** 8 ounces.
- **d.** 16 ounces.

20. Which of the following is part of the meat group?
- **a.** Peas
- **b.** Rice
- **c.** Poultry
- **d.** Cottage cheese

21. Foods naturally high in sodium include
- **a.** milk.
- **b.** cereals.
- **c.** vegetables.
- **d.** fruits.

22. Supplemental nourishments might include
- **a.** hot fudge sundaes.
- **b.** mashed potatoes.
- **c.** scrambled eggs.
- **d.** high-protein drinks.

23. A serving of cooked vegetables would be approximately
- **a.** ½ cup.
- **b.** ¾ cup.
- **c.** 1 cup.
- **d.** 1½ cups.

24. It is especially important to report to the nurse that the patient only ate two-thirds of her meal when the patient is on a
- **a.** low-salt diet.
- **b.** calorie-restricted diet.
- **c.** diabetic diet.
- **d.** house diet.

D. Nursing Assistant Challenge.

Mrs. Gole is one of your assigned patients. She is 72 years old, is on a 1,500-calorie diabetic diet, and is a member of the Seventh Day Adventist Church. She also has Parkinson's disease with tremors of her hands, and occasionally has trouble swallowing. Mrs. Gole sometimes eats food brought in by family and friends that is not on the 1,500-calorie diet. Consider Mrs. Gole's care:

25. Discuss safety issues that you need to think about when Mrs. Gole is eating.

26. Are there conflicts between the ordered diet and the dietary restrictions of her church? If so, what are the conflicts and how might they be resolved?

27. Do you anticipate that Mrs. Gole will have any problems feeding herself? If so, what are those problems, and what can you do to help her eat independently?

28. Discuss the issues of residents' or patients' rights that may arise because of the conflict between the patient's desire to eat more food than ordered and foods different from what the physician has prescribed.

EXPLORING THE WEB

Description	Location
Basic nutrition	*http://www.delmarhealthcare.com/olcs/white/pnotes.asp* (see Chapter 18)
Carbohydrates	*http://www.delmarlearning.com/companions/content/0766835677/student/student4.asp*
Diet and weight control	*http://www.delmarlearning.com/companions/content/0766835677/student/student16.asp*
Diet during young and middle adulthood	*http://www.delmarlearning.com/companions/content/0766835677/student/student14.asp*
Digestion, absorption, and metabolism	*http://www.delmarlearning.com/companions/content/0766835677/student/student3.asp*
Food-related illness and allergies	*http://www.delmarlearning.com/companions/content/0766835677/student/student10.asp*
Lipids or fats	*http://www.delmarlearning.com/companions/content/0766835677/student/student5.asp*
Minerals	*http://www.delmarlearning.com/companions/content/0766835677/student/student8.asp*
Nutritional care of clients	*http://www.delmarlearning.com/companions/content/0766835677/student/student23.asp*
Planning a healthy diet	*http://www.delmarlearning.com/companions/content/0766835677/student/student2.asp*

continues

EXPLORING THE WEB *continued*

Description	Location
Proteins	*http://www.delmarlearning.com/companions/content/0766835677/student/student6.asp*
Relationship of food and health	*http://www.delmarlearning.com/companions/content/0766835677/student/student1.asp*
Vitamins	*http://www.delmarlearning.com/companions/content/0766835677/student/student7.asp*
Water	*http://www.delmarlearning.com/companions/content/0766835677/student/student9.asp*
American Diabetes Association	*http://www.diabetes.org*
American Dietetic Association	*http://www.eatright.org*
American Society on Parenteral and Enteral Nutrition	*http://www.nutritioncare.org*
Center on Nutrition	*http://navigator.tufts.edu*
Dysphagia Diet	*http://www.dysphagia-diet.com*
Dysphagia Information	*http://www.nidcd.nih.gov/health/pubs_vsl/dysph.htm*
Dysphagia Online	*http://www.dysphagiaonline.com*
Dysphagia Resource Center	*http://www.dysphagia.com*
Dysphagia Resource Society	*http://www.shs.uiuc.edu*
Education through Nutrition	*http://www.advancefornurses.com* (see past articles July 22, 2002)
Ethnic, Cultural, Special Audience Food Pyramids	*http://www.nal.usda.gov/fnic/etext/000023.html*
Food Guide Pyramid for Kids	*http://www.usda.gov/cnpp/KidsPyra*
Guide to Daily Food Choices	*http://www.nal.usda.gov:8001/py/pmap.htm*
Infusion Nurses Society	*http://www.ins1.org*
National Policy Center on Aging and Nutrition (also hydration information)	*http://www.fiu.edu*
Ross Laboratories	*http://www.ross.com*
Tufts University Nutrition Navigator	*http://navigator.tufts.edu*
United States Food and Drug Administration	*http://www.fda.gov*
Water Soluble Vitamins	*http://www.advancefornurses.com* (see past articles April 22, 2002)

section 9

Special Care Procedures

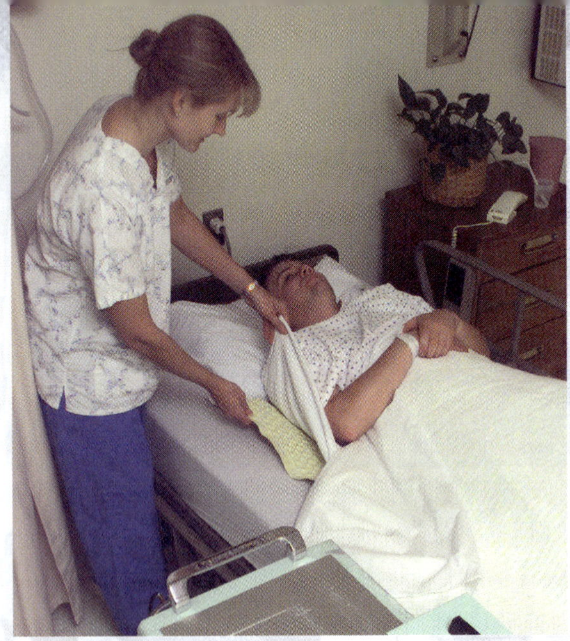

unit 27

Warm and Cold Applications

objectives

After completing this unit, you will be able to:

- Spell and define terms.
- List the physical conditions requiring the use of heat and cold.
- Name types of heat and cold applications.
- Describe the effects of local cold applications.
- Describe the effects of local heat applications.
- List safety concerns related to application of heat and cold.
- Demonstrate the following procedures:
  - Procedure 80 Applying an Ice Bag
  - Procedure 81 Applying a Disposable Cold Pack
  - Procedure 82 Applying an Aquamatic K-Pad®
  - Procedure 83 Performing a Warm Soak
  - Procedure 84 Applying a Warm Moist Compress
  - Procedure 85 Assisting with Application of a Hypothermia Blanket

vocabulary

Learn the meaning and the correct spelling of the following words and phrases:

Aquamatic K-Pad®
cold pack
diathermy
hemorrhage
hypothermia
hypothermia-hyperthermia blanket
ice bag
thermal blanket
vasoconstriction
vasodilation
warm soak
wet compress

INTRODUCTION

Heat and cold applications are used only on written orders from the physician or nurse, and only for a specific length of time. Some facilities allow only professional personnel to apply heat and cold. **Some states have laws against nursing assistants applying heat or cold in a home health setting.** In other facilities, nursing assistants who have been specially trained are permitted to carry out these procedures under the supervision of the nurse. Be sure you know and follow the policy of your facility and are adequately prepared and *supervised*.

THERAPY WITH HEAT AND COLD

The physician orders the use of heat or cold applications to:

- relieve pain.
- combat local infection, swelling, or inflammation.
- control bleeding (**hemorrhage**).
- reduce body temperature.

Local applications of heat and cold are made with:

- Ice bags.
- Electronically operated Aquamatic K-Pads®. K-Pads® come in many shapes and sizes. They can be used to apply dry heat. By using an attachment, they can also be used for cooling.
- Prepackaged, single-use units for the application of hot and cold. A single hit on the surface activates the contents, providing a controlled temperature.
- Gel packs that can be cooled or heated as needed.

General treatments of heat and cold consist of thermal mattresses known as **hypothermia-hyperthermia blankets**. These are widely used to:

- lower body temperature when there is fever.
- elevate body temperature in cases of hypothermia.

Applications of warm and cold may be either dry or moist. Moisture makes both heat and cold more penetrating. Therefore, moist heat or moist cold is more likely to cause injury. Extra care must be taken to protect the patient when moist treatments are used. Be sure you know:

- Exact method to be used
- Correct temperature and placement
- Proper length of time the warm or cold application is to be performed
- How often the area being treated is to be checked

Table 27-1 summarizes types of warm and cold applications.

Commercial Preparations

Easy-to-use commercial warm and cold packs are available for dry applications. For one type of pack, a single hit or blow to the pack before application activates it. The pack is discarded after one use. Reusable packs are also available, but infection control issues make them less desirable.

TABLE 27-1 WARM AND COLD APPLICATIONS

Dry Warm Applications	Dry Cold Applications
Aquamatic K-Pad®	Ice cap
Disposable warm pack	Ice bag
Electric heating pads	Disposable cold pack
Aquathermia blanket	Aquamatic K-Pad®
	Hypothermia blanket
Moist Warm Applications	**Moist Cold Applications**
Warm soaks	Compresses
Compresses	Soaks
Tub baths	Packs
Sitz baths	

guidelines *for*

Warm and Cold Treatments

You must be very watchful when applying cold or warm treatments. When assigned to this task, keep in mind the following:

- The age and condition of the patient. Give extra care to:
  - Young children
  - The aged
  - Patients with cognitive impairment
  - Patients who are uncooperative
  - Patients who are unconscious
  - Patients who are paralyzed

continues

guidelines *continued*

- Patients with tissue damage
- Patients with poor circulation

- Apply the principles of standard precautions if your hands will contact blood, moist body fluids (except sweat), secretions, excretions, nonintact skin, or mucous membranes.
- If the patient has a dressing covering the area to be treated, consult the nurse for directions.
- Check the temperature of the solution with a thermometer. You may need to add more liquid during the treatment to maintain the temperature. Avoid pouring hot or cold liquid directly over the patient.
- Remove all metal jewelry, buttons, or zippers that could conduct heat or cold and thereby injure the skin.
- Avoid using heat treatments with temperatures over 110°F. Temperatures greater than this can cause burns, particularly in infants and the elderly.
- Avoid using heat in the first 48 hours after an injury.
- Follow all safety rules to prevent spills and falls.
- An electric heating pad must not be used with moist dressings unless a rubber cover is placed over the pad. If the wires become damp, a short circuit may result. The patient must not lie on the pad, because severe burns can result. Sensitivity to heat varies, so patients receiving heat treatments must be checked frequently. Although heating pads are not used in health care facilities, they are used by individuals in homes.
- Heat is not applied to the head because it could make blood vessels in the area dilate, causing headache.
- Heat should not be applied to the abdomen if there is any chance that the patient has appendicitis, because it would increase the chance of the appendix rupturing.
- Check the skin under the application every 10 minutes, or according to facility policy. If the skin under a heat application appears red, or a dark area appears, stop the treatment. Notify the nurse immediately. Stop a cold application and notify your supervisor if the patient's skin appears cyanotic, pale, white, or bright red; if the patient complains of numbness; or if the patient is shivering. Cover the patient with a blanket.
- Rubber or plastic should never touch the patient's skin. Be sure all appliances are covered with cloth.
- Heat and cold applications are usually not left in place longer than 20 minutes, according to the purpose and type of treatment. Follow the care plan and the nurse's instructions.
- After the treatment, pat the skin dry. Make the patient comfortable. Clean and store used equipment. Remove gloves, if worn, and dispose of them according to facility policy. Wash your hands. Report to your supervisor that the procedure was completed and the patient's reaction to the treatment.

USE OF COLD APPLICATIONS

Applications of cold are given only with a physician's order. The application of cold:

- Constricts or decreases the size of blood vessels (**vasoconstriction**) and reduces swelling
- Decreases sensitivity to pain
- Reduces temperature
- Slows inflammation
- Reduces itching

Cautions

Remember, moisture intensifies the effect of cold just as it does heat. Caution must be used in the application of moist cold.

- Excessive cold can damage body tissues.
- Report color changes such as *blanching* (turning white) or *cyanosis* (becoming bluish).
- Report feelings of numbness or discomfort experienced by the patient.
- Stop the cold treatment if the patient starts to shiver. Cover the patient with a blanket and report immediately to the nurse. (See Procedures 80 and 81.)

Dry Cold Applications

There are several methods for applying therapeutic cold. Careful attention to the application is needed to prevent injury.

- Disposable **cold pack**—This single-use commercial pack can be stored until needed. Reusable commercial packs are also available (for both warm and cold

SAFETY *Alert*

Cold therapy should not be used for patients with:

- Deep vein thrombosis
- Peripheral vascular disease
- Open wound(s)
- Skin sensation impairment
- Severe cognitive impairment
- Cold intolerance, cold allergy
- Some medical conditions such as rheumatoid arthritis and Reynaud's phenomenon.

If a patient has any of these conditions, check with the nurse before applying a cold application.

applications). The pack remains effective for approximately 15 to 30 minutes. If the cold pack must be activated, follow the manufacturer's instructions exactly. When activating the pack, do not hold it in front of your face. If the pack leaks or bursts, the chemicals inside the pack may splash. Check the area being treated every 10 minutes. Discard the chemical cold pack after one use, or when the pack warms. Do not attempt to refreeze it.

- **Ice bag**—This reusable, waterproof, canvas or rubber container can be filled with ice to provide temporary local cold. An ice bag is never placed directly on the affected area because the weight of the bag will cause the patient discomfort.
- **Thermal blanket**—This is a large, fluid-filled blanket that is placed over or around the patient. The temperature of the fluid in the blanket may be raised or lowered. The blanket is used to lower or raise the patient's body temperature. However, it is most often used in care facilities to lower the body temperature. This process is called inducing **hypothermia**. A licensed professional usually monitors the use of this type of blanket.

Tips: Paper or styrofoam cups of ice are sometimes used to gently massage an injured area. To apply cold this way, hold the cup and make small, overlapping circles on the affected area for 20 minutes. An examination glove filled with ice and secured with a rubber band is also sometimes used as an alternate ice application.

Moist Cold Applications

- **Wet compresses** are moistened with a solution and placed on the affected area.
- A syringe may be used to add water to the compresses to keep them moist.
- The compresses can be kept cold by placing a covered ice bag against the affected area. Make sure the patient can tolerate the weight of the ice bag without increased pain.
- Each time the pad is removed and replaced, be careful to reposition the protective covering.

Follow facility policy for:

- method of applying the treatment.
- length of time the treatment is to be applied.
- how often the patient is to be checked for condition of the skin in the treatment area and general response to the treatment.
- signs that treatment should be discontinued.

PROCEDURE 80

APPLYING AN ICE BAG

1. Assemble equipment:
   - ice bag
   - cover (usually cotton, such as a towel, or cover specified by your facility)
   - paper towels
   - spoon or similar utensil
   - ice cubes or crushed ice
2. Prepare the ice bag as follows:
   a. Fill the ice bag with cold water and check for leaks.
   b. Empty the bag.
   c. If ice cubes are used, rinse them in water to remove sharp edges. The use of crushed ice makes the bag more flexible and is more comfortable for the patient.

continues

PROCEDURE 80

continued

d. Fill the ice bag half full, using an ice scooper, paper cup, or large spoon (Figure 27-1). Avoid making ice bags too heavy. Do not allow the scoop to touch the ice bag.

e. To remove air from the ice bag:
   - Rest the ice bag flat on a paper towel on a flat surface.
   - Put the top in place, but do not screw it on.
   - Press the bag until the air is removed (Figure 27-2).

f. Fasten the top securely.

g. Test for leakage.

h. Wipe the ice bag dry with paper towels. Place it in a cloth cover.

Note: *As an alternative, a gel pack stored in the freezer can be used for cold applications. These packs can be refrozen and reused if this is facility policy.*

3. Take the equipment to the bedside on a tray. Carry out beginning procedure actions.
4. Apply the ice bag to the affected part.

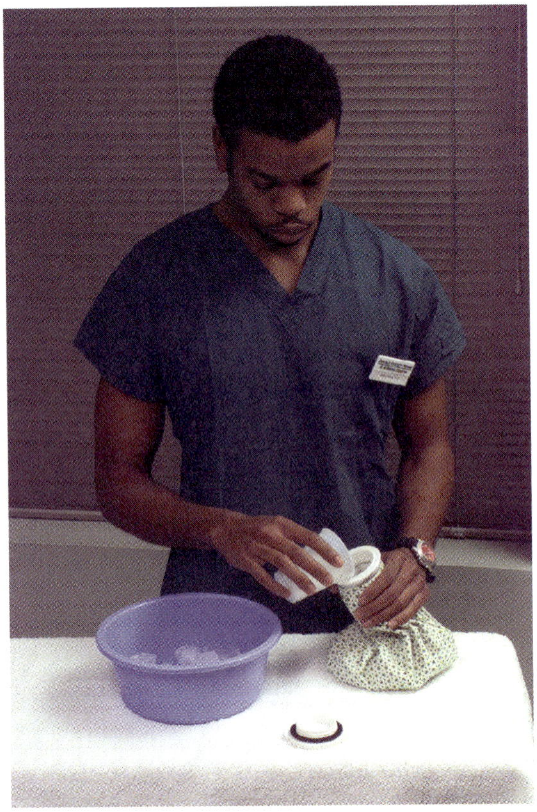

FIGURE 27-1 Fill the ice bag half full.

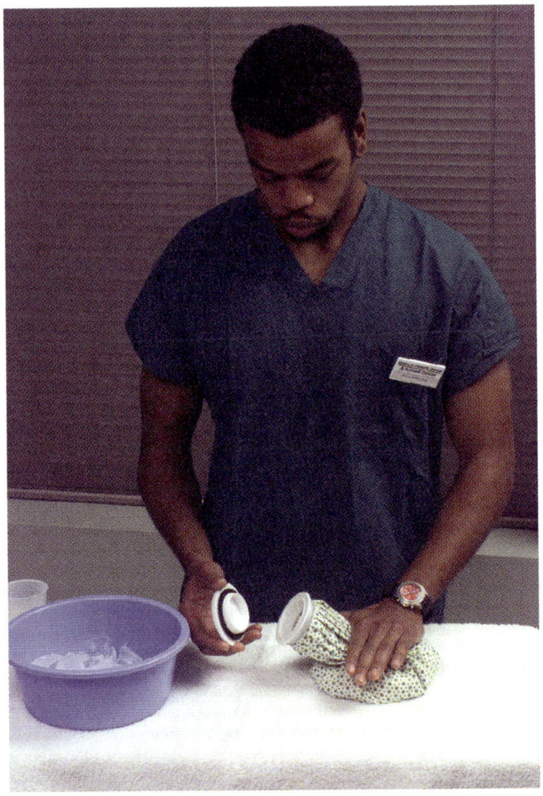

FIGURE 27-2 Place the ice bag on a flat surface, then press firmly to remove the air.

5. Refill the ice bag before all the ice has melted.
6. Check the skin area under the ice bag every 10 minutes. Report to supervising nurse immediately if skin is discolored or white or if the patient reports that the skin is numb.
7. Continue the cold application for the amount of time specified by your supervisor. If the patient feels cold, cover with a blanket, but do not cover the area being treated.
8. Carry out procedure completion actions.
9. When the treatment is complete, wash the bag with soap and water. Rinse and dry it completely, and then screw the top on. Wipe the bag with a disinfectant if this is your facility policy. Leave air in the ice bag to prevent the sides from sticking together.
10. If a reusable cold pack is used, wash it thoroughly with soap and water or wipe with a disinfectant, according to facility policy. Return the pack to the refrigerator. Discard a disposable pack.

PROCEDURE 81

APPLYING A DISPOSABLE COLD PACK

1. Carry out beginning procedure actions.
2. Assemble equipment:
   - disposable commercial cold pack
   - cloth covering (towel, warm water bag cover, or other cover specified by the facility)
   - tape or rolls of gauze
3. Expose the area to be treated. Note the condition of the area.
4. Place the cold pack in a cloth covering (Figure 27-3).
5. Strike or squeeze the cold pack to activate chemicals. (Follow manufacturer's instructions.)
6. Place the covered cold pack on the proper area and cover it with a towel (Figure 27-4). Note time of application.
7. Secure the cover with tape or gauze, if necessary, to hold it in place.
8. Leave the patient in a comfortable position, with the signal cord within easy reach.
9. Return to the bedside every 10 minutes. Check the area being treated for discoloration or numbness. If these signs and symptoms occur, discontinue treatment and report them to your supervisor.
10. If no adverse symptoms occur, remove the pack after 30 minutes, or after the amount of time given in your instructions. Note the condition of the area. Continuous treatment requires application of a fresh pack.
11. Remove the pack from the cover and discard according to facility policy. Return unused gauze and tape.
12. Put the cover in a laundry hamper.
13. Carry out procedure completion actions.

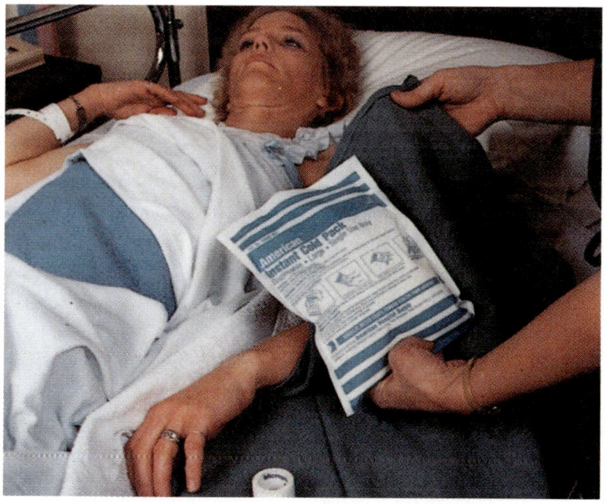

FIGURE 27-3 Cover the disposable cold pack with a cover before applying it to the patient.

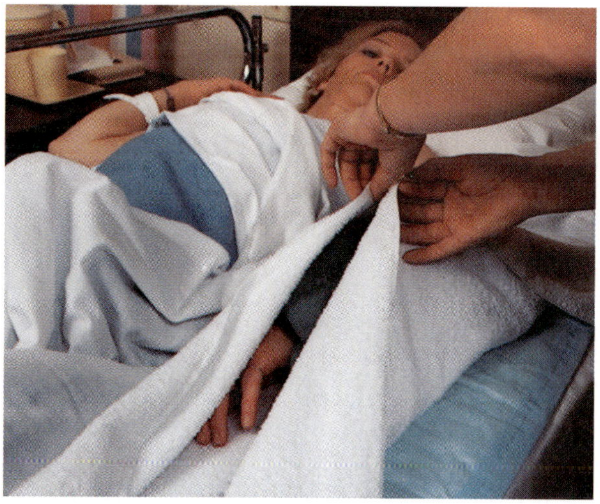

FIGURE 27-4 After positioning the cold pack, cover the application with a towel.

USE OF WARM APPLICATIONS

Warm applications are ordered to:

- relieve muscle spasms.
- reduce pain.
- reduce inflammation.
- promote healing.
- combat local infection.
- increase circulation.
- improve mobility before exercise periods.
- soothe the patient.

SAFETY Alert

The heat application should feel comfortably warm to the patient, not uncomfortably hot. If you will be applying a pack or pad, touch the device to your forearm to check the temperature before applying it. If the patient complains of burning, remove the application and consult the nurse.

The value of heat treatments (**diathermy**) is that heat dilates or increases the size of blood vessels (**vasodilation**). This brings more blood to the area to promote healing. Warmth is very soothing when there is pain.

There must be a specific order for a warm application. Some groups of people require extra care when they receive warm applications. (See Procedures 82 to 84.)

Cautions

Follow these cautions when working with patients:

- Constant warmth must be carefully monitored.
- Moisture intensifies the effect of warmth. Use extra caution.

SAFETY Alert

Heat therapy should not be used for patients with:

- Acute inflammation
- Dermatitis
- Deep vein thrombosis
- Peripheral vascular disease
- Open wound(s)
- Recent soft tissue injuries in which swelling or bleeding would be increased by heat
- Skin sensation impairment
- Severe cognitive impairment

Some physicians also recommend avoiding heat use with children and women during pregnancy. If a patient has any of these conditions, check with the nurse before applying a heat application.

- Hot packs are contraindicated for paralyzed areas or areas without sensation, acute edema or inflammation, infection, and hemophilia. They must be used with caution for patients with many medical conditions, including impaired circulation, sensory impairment, cancer, rashes, and open skin conditions. Take extra care with hot packs for very young and very old patients.
- Never allow a patient to lie on a constant heat unit, because heat may be trapped and build up to dangerous levels.
- Temperature of a constant heat unit should be between 95° and 100°F.
- Always use a bath thermometer to check solution temperatures.
- Always remove the body part being soaked before adding warm solution.
- Always stay with the patient during the treatment.
- Protect areas not being treated from excessive exposure.
- Warmth is not applied to the head because it could cause blood vessels in the area to dilate, resulting in headache.
- Rubber or plastic should never touch the patient's skin. Be sure all appliances are covered with cloth.

Dry Warm Applications

The **Aquamatic K-Pad®** is commonly used to provide dry warmth. It consists of a plastic pad with fluid-filled coils and a control unit that maintains a constant temperature of the fluid.

The fluid in the pad is distilled water that is supplied from a reservoir in the control unit. The control unit is placed on the bedside stand and is plugged into an electrical outlet. In most facilities, the temperature is preset by the central supply department. The temperature is usually set at 95° to 100°F.

Tips: When setting up the K-Pad® for the first time, check the pad for leaks. Tip it back and forth several times to eliminate air pockets, which cause hot spots. Place the control unit on the bedside stand so it is higher than the patient, so that water will run into the pad by gravity. Make sure the tubing is free of kinks.

Moist Warm Applications

SAFETY Alert

Moisture intensifies heat and you must use extra care.

For each of the warm treatments, follow facility policy for:

- method of applying the treatment.
- length of time the treatment is to be applied.
- how often the patient is to be checked for condition of the skin in the treatment area and general response to the treatment.
- signs that treatment should be discontinued.

Moist warm treatments include:

- **Warm soaks**—The patient, or the part of the patient's body that is being treated, is immersed in a tub filled with water at a specific temperature, usually 105°.
- Wet compresses—The same cautions apply to warm compresses as to cold compresses. They may be kept wet with a syringe and warm by covering them with an Aquamatic K-Pad®.

PROCEDURE 82

APPLYING AN AQUAMATIC K-PAD®

1. Carry out beginning procedure actions.
2. Assemble equipment:
   - K-Pad® and control unit
   - distilled water
   - covering for pad
3. Check the cord for frayed or damaged insulation. Also check that the tubing between the control unit and the pad is intact.
4. Place the control unit on the bedside stand (Figure 27-5).

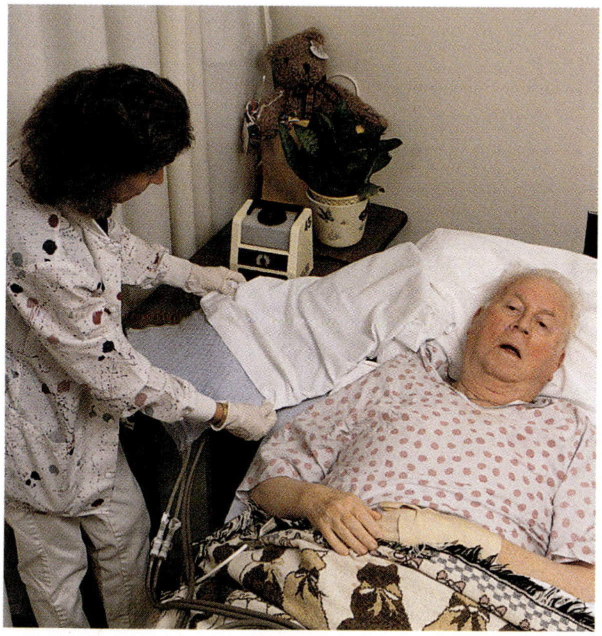

FIGURE 27-5 The control unit for the aquathermia pad maintains a constant temperature.

5. Remove the cover of the control unit and check the level of the distilled water. If it is low, fill the unit two-thirds full or to the fill line using distilled water. Tilt the unit back and forth gently to clear the tubing of air.
6. Screw the cover in place and loosen it one-quarter turn.
7. If the temperature was not preset, check with the nurse for the proper setting before turning on the unit. Remove the key after setting the temperature.
8. Plug in the unit.
9. Cover the pad with an appropriate cover, according to facility policy or as specified by the manufacturer of the unit. Do not use pins to hold the cover in place.
10. Expose the area on the patient to be treated. Place the covered pad on the patient and note the time.
    - Be sure the tubing between the control unit and the pad does not hang over the side of the bed. It should be coiled on the bed to promote the flow of liquid.
11. Following facility policy, periodically check the skin under the pad.
12. Check the level of the water in the control unit. Refill if necessary to the fill line.
13. Remove the pad after the prescribed amount of time.
14. Carry out procedure completion actions.

PROCEDURE 83

PERFORMING A WARM SOAK

1. Carry out beginning procedure actions.
2. Assemble equipment:
   - bath thermometer
   - soak basin
   - pitcher
   - large plastic sheet
   - bath towel
   - bath blanket
3. Bring equipment to the bedside.
4. Cover the patient with a bath blanket.
5. Fanfold bedding to the foot of the bed.
6. Expose the limb to be soaked.
7. Position the patient for comfort on the far side of the bed (opposite the part to be soaked). Be sure the side rail is up and secure.
8. Cover the bed with a plastic sheet and towel.
9. Fill the soak basin half full with water at the prescribed temperature (usually 105°F). Check the temperature with a bath thermometer.
10. Take the soak basin from the overbed table and position it on the bed protector.
11. Assist the patient to gradually place the limb in the basin (Figure 27-6). Cover the basin with a towel to help maintain temperature.
12. Check the temperature every 5 minutes. Use a pitcher to get additional water and add to the soak basin to maintain temperature. Remember to remove the patient's limb before adding water to the container.
13. Discontinue the procedure at the end of the prescribed time.

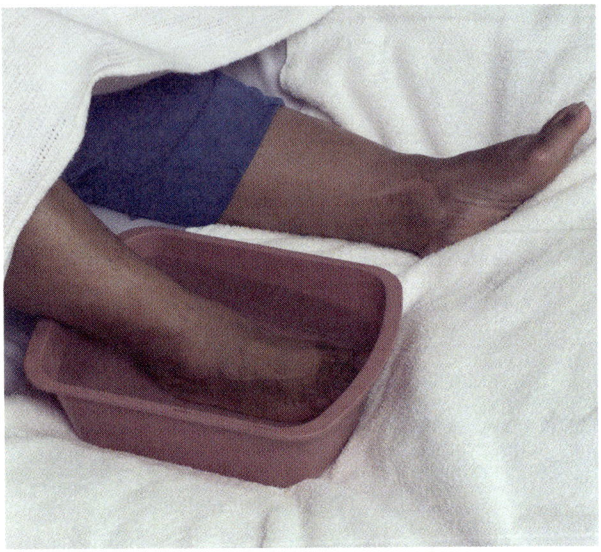

FIGURE 27-6 The patient is receiving warm soak therapy.

   a. Lift the patient's limb out of the basin.
   b. Slip the basin forward and allow the limb to rest on the bath towel.
   c. Place the basin on the overbed table. Gently pat the limb dry with a towel.
14. Remove the plastic sheet and towel.
15. Adjust bedding and remove the bath blanket. If the treatment is to be repeated, fold the bath blanket and place it in the bedside stand. Leave the unit tidy and the call bell within reach.
16. Lower the head of the bed and make the patient comfortable.
17. Take equipment to the utility room. Clean and store it according to facility policy.
18. Carry out procedure completion actions.

PROCEDURE 84

APPLYING A WARM MOIST COMPRESS

1. Carry out beginning procedure actions.
2. Assemble equipment:
   - disposable gloves
   - syringe
   - bed protector
   - compresses
   - bath thermometer
   - binder or towel
   - pins or bandage
   - basin with prescribed solution at temperature ordered
3. Bring equipment to the bedside.
4. Expose only the area to be treated.
5. Protect the bed and the patient's clothing with a bed protector (Figure 27-7A).
6. Put on disposable gloves.
7. Check the temperature of the solution. Moisten the compresses; remove excess liquid (Figure 27-7B). Apply to treatment area (Figure 27-7C).
8. Secure the compresses with a bandage or binder. The compress must be in contact with the patient's skin.
9. Help the patient to maintain a comfortable position throughout the treatment.
10. Unscreen the unit. Leave the unit neat and tidy, with the signal cord within easy reach.
11. Maintain proper temperature and moisture.
    - If the compresses are to be kept warm, a K-Pad® may be applied.
    - If the compresses are to be kept cool, an ice bag may be applied.
    - A syringe may be used to apply more solution to keep the compresses wet.
12. Remove the compresses when ordered. Change as ordered or once in 24 hours. Check skin several times each day.
13. Discard the compresses.
14. Remove and dispose of gloves according to facility policy.
15. Carry out procedure completion actions.

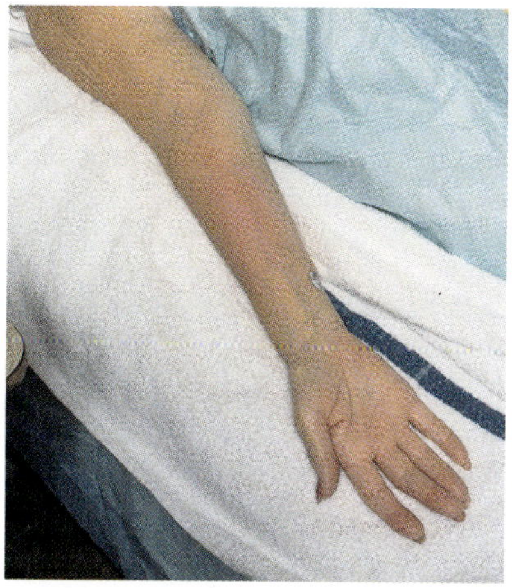

FIGURE 27-7A Protect the bed with a towel or underpad.

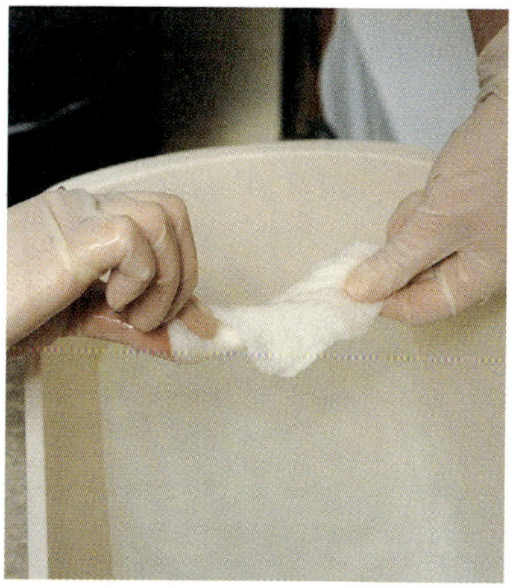

FIGURE 27-7B Dip the compress into a basin of warm (105°F) water. Grasp the edges, then squeeze out excess liquid.

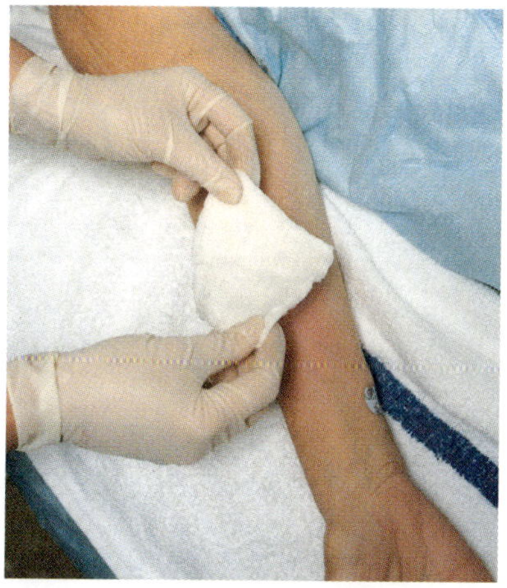

FIGURE 27-7C Open the compress and apply it to the inflamed area.

TEMPERATURE CONTROL MEASURES

Excessively high or low body temperatures are treated in acute care facilities by placing hypothermia-hyperthermia blankets (Figure 27-8) over and under the patient. These blankets are units filled with water. The blankets may be called *aquathermia blankets*. "Aqua" is the Latin term for *water*. The temperature of the water can be adjusted higher or lower depending on whether the patient's body temperature is to be raised or lowered.

Using the Aquathermia Blanket

The aquathermia blanket is operated either manually or automatically. For manual operation, the licensed nurse will set the blanket to a predetermined temperature, which is ordered by the physician. The blanket maintains this temperature regardless of changes in the patient's body temperature. When the unit is set for automatic operation, it monitors the patient's temperature through a rectal, skin, or esophageal probe. The probe is secured to the body with tape to prevent injury. The blanket temperature changes according to the patient's temperature. The goal is to maintain the patient's body temperature. An alarm will sound for abnormal temperature variations. Before using the blanket, check it for cracks, tears, or leaks in the system. Do not use it if there are cracks or an electrical malfunction.

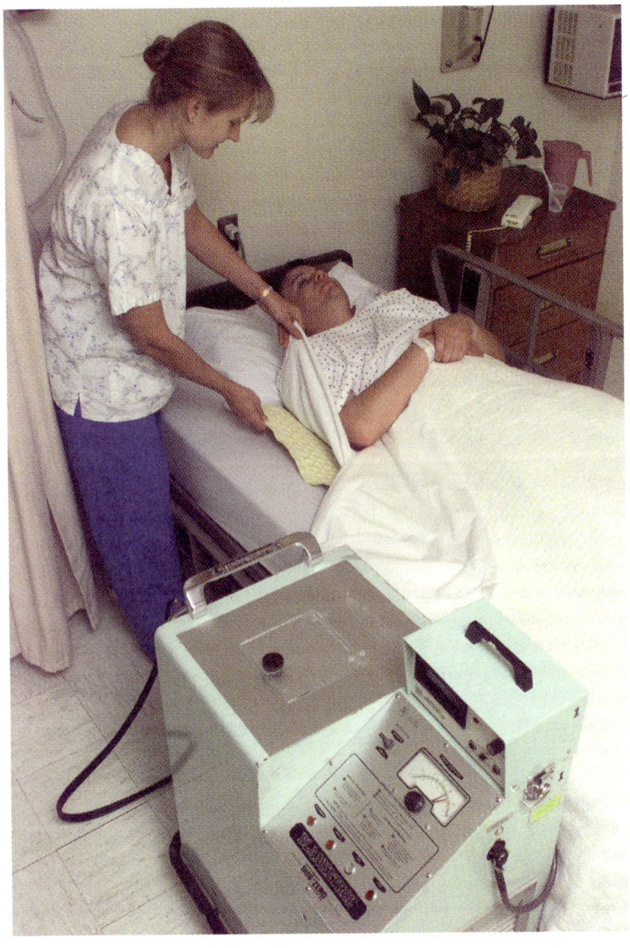

FIGURE 27-8 Hypothermia-hyperthermia blanket.

The patient should wear a hospital gown when the aquathermia blanket is used. Use a gown with tie closures. Snaps, pins, or other metal may cause injury to the skin. Before beginning the procedure, check and record the patient's baseline vital signs as a basis for comparison.

One or two aquathermia blankets may be used. The nurse may instruct you to place one under the patient, and to cover him or her with the other. The blankets must be covered with a disposable cover, sheet, or bath blanket to absorb perspiration and prevent complications. Avoid using pins to cover the blanket. These can puncture the unit or injure the patient's skin by creating hot or cold spots. Use tape or Velcro® fasteners, if necessary, to cover the unit.

The blanket should be set up and preheated or precooled before it is applied to the patient. Connect the blanket to the control unit by plugging in the tubing. The nurse will set the blanket for automatic or manual operation. He or she will also set the desired body temperature or blanket temperature and instruct you as to what temperature values are being used. Turn the device on, then add distilled water to the reservoir. Position the controls at the foot of the bed. After the blanket has reached the designated temperature, apply it to the patient. If the patient will be lying on a blanket, place a pillow or folded bath blanket under the patient's head.

The patient's head should not contact the blanket directly. The combination of heat or cold and the surface of the blanket promotes skin breakdown on the back of the head. The nurse may instruct you to apply lanolin or another designated product to the skin in exposed areas that contact the blanket directly. You may wrap the patient's hands and feet to prevent chilling, if desired.

Complications. Immediately notify the nurse if you observe any of these complications:

- Changes in skin color
- Cyanosis of the lips or nail beds
- Sudden changes in body temperature
- marked changes in pulse, respirations, and blood pressure
- respiratory distress
- pain
- changes in sensation
- edema
- shivering and chills
- urinary output below 50 mL/hour

Discontinuing Blanket Use. The nurse will inform you when to discontinue use of the blanket. Follow the manufacturer's directions for the type of blanket you are

SAFETY *Alert*

The nurse will instruct you on the frequency for monitoring vital signs when an aquathermia blanket is being used. The patient's temperature and the blanket temperature are usually monitored and documented every 15 to 30 minutes. Inform the nurse immediately if the patient's temperature drops more than one degree in 15 minutes. Continued temperature monitoring is necessary after the blanket is removed because the patient's temperature can continue to drop as much as 5 degrees after the procedure ends.

using. Turn the unit off. (Some types must remain plugged in for 30 to 60 minutes to dry condensation inside the unit.) Dry the patient's skin and assist him or her into a dry gown. Position the patient in a comfortable position. Remove the aquathermia blanket from the bed after the designated time. Continue checking vital signs and intake and output every 30 minutes for the first 2 hours, then hourly or as directed by the nurse. (See Procedure 85.)

Hypothermia

Hypothermia is a drop in core body temperature below 95°F (35°C) rectally. This can occur:

- when people are exposed to cold without adequate protection.
- in the elderly, when a person is exposed to external temperatures as warm as 60°F.
- when deliberately induced before surgery to slow body metabolism.

Indications of hypothermia to report include:

- Drop in body temperature
- Poor coordination and confusion
- Slurred speech
- Decreased respiratory and heart rates

Nursing Assistant Actions

- Report observations to the supervisor.
- Check the environmental temperature and adjust it.

AGE-APPROPRIATE CARE *Alert*

In children, temperatures tend to rise higher than in adults. This puts children at greater risk for seizures.

- Provide external warmth with a sweater or blanket.
- Reduce drafts with screens or curtains.
- If permitted, give something warm to drink.
- Check vital signs.

Hyperthermia

Hyperthermia is an elevation of core body temperature to 104°F (40°C) rectally or higher. This can occur:

- when a person is exposed to high external temperature.
- with serious injuries such as burns.
- when there is damage to the temperature control center in the brain.
- with infections.

Indications of hyperthermia to report include:

- Elevated body temperature
- Hot, flushed skin
- Faintness
- Headache
- Nausea
- Convulsions

Fever or *pyrexia* occurs when core body temperature rises to at least 101°F (rectally). Fever is often associated with infections, injury, surgery, and serious trauma. Indications of fever are the same as those for general hyperthermia.

Nursing Assistant Actions

- Report observations to the supervisor.
- Check environment temperature and adjust it.
- Reduce external warmth. Cover the patient only with a gown or sheet.
- If permitted, give cooling drink.
- Carry out cooling procedures as ordered. For example, give cooling baths or enemas.
- Check vital signs frequently.

PROCEDURE 85

ASSISTING WITH APPLICATION OF A HYPOTHERMIA BLANKET

Applying a hypothermia blanket and monitoring a patient who is receiving a hypothermia treatment is a professional nursing responsibility. The nurse will supervise the procedure and monitor the patient throughout the treatment. The nurse will check the specific gravity of the patient's urine, vital signs, and nervous system response. The nursing assistant may be asked to assist in setting up equipment, positioning the patient and the thermal blanket, observing the patient during the treatment, and keeping the patient comfortable. In addition, the nursing assistant may be asked to transport equipment to and from the central supply service.

1. Wash your hands, collect equipment, and take equipment to the bedside.
2. Assemble equipment:
   - disposable gloves
   - hypothermia-hyperthermia control unit
   - fluid for control unit
   - thermometer probes (rectal or skin)
   - adhesive tape
   - sphygmomanometer
   - stethoscope
   - hypothermia-hyperthermia blanket (disposable or reusable), one or two as ordered
   - bath blanket or sheet, one or two as ordered
   - lanolin-based skin cream
3. Follow manufacturer's directions for setting up equipment. Check equipment for safety. Be sure the control unit is grounded.
4. Connect the blanket(s) to the control unit and set the control.
5. Turn on the control unit and add liquid.
6. Allow the blanket(s) to precool as you prepare the patient.
7. Carry out beginning procedure actions.
8. Place the patient in a hospital-type gown with ties.
9. Measure vital signs and record.
10. Place the hypothermia-hyperthermia blanket on the bed and cover it with a sheet. Position the patient on the sheet-covered thermal blanket in the recumbent position, with the head on a pillow that does not touch the blanket.
11. Wash your hands. Put on gloves.
12. Insert a rectal thermometer probe into the patient's rectum (unless contraindicated) and tape it in place. (Alternatively, place a skin probe into an axilla and tape it in place.)
13. Plug the end of the probe into the proper jack on the control panel.
14. Place a second sheet over the patient and place a second thermal blanket over the sheet, if ordered.
15. Apply lanolin-based cream to the patient's skin where it contacts the blanket.
16. Remove gloves. Discard according to facility policy. Wash your hands.
17. Monitor vital signs, neurologic response, and intake and output every 5 minutes until the desired body temperature is reached, and then every 15 minutes, or as ordered.
18. Report color changes in skin or excessive shivering.
19. The blanket's texture increases the risk of skin breakdown. The patient should be repositioned every 30 minutes to 1 hour. Reapply skin cream as necessary. Change the gown and top sheet as often as necessary if the patient is actively perspiring. Put on gloves each time you care for patient. At the end of care, remove gloves, discard according to facility policy, and wash your hands.
20. At completion of the treatment, follow manufacturer's instructions for turning off the unit, disconnecting the blanket(s), and returning them to storage.
21. Put on gloves. Continue to monitor the patient as you remove the equipment.
22. Replace any damp bedding or garments and cover the patient. Continue to monitor the patient every 30 minutes until he or she has been stable for 2 hours.
23. Clean the thermometer probe and store it according to facility policy.
24. Remove gloves and discard according to facility policy.
25. Carry out procedure completion actions.

REVIEW

A. True/False.

Mark the following true or false by circling T or F.

1. T F Heat and cold treatments should be supervised by the nurse.

2. T F If a patient has a possible diagnosis of appendicitis, heat should not be applied to the abdomen.

3. T F The temperature of a warm soak solution should be approximately 100°F.

4. T F Special blankets used to alter the patient's temperature are called infrared blankets.

5. T F A patient who is unconscious must receive special attention during a heat treatment.

6. T F Hyperthermia is an elevation of core body temperature to below 95°F.

7. T F Heat is frequently applied to the head.

8. T F When charting an application of cold, always include the length of time of the application.

9. T F Aquamatic K-Pads® are usually set at 115°F.

B. Multiple Choice.

Select the one best answer for each of the following.

10. Heat affects the body by
- **a.** causing constriction.
- **b.** increasing blood supply to the area.
- **c.** reducing oxygen in tissues.
- **d.** increasing white blood cells.

11. Special care with heat and cold treatments must be taken when the patient is
- **a.** alert and oriented.
- **b.** very young.
- **c.** cooperative.
- **d.** ambulatory.

12. Dry cold is provided by
- **a.** compresses.
- **b.** a hyperthermia blanket.
- **c.** ice caps.
- **d.** soaks.

13. Cold affects the body by
- **a.** reducing pain sensations.
- **b.** stimulating life processes.
- **c.** promoting inflammation.
- **d.** promoting healing.

14. Moist cold is applied with
- **a.** ice bags.
- **b.** ice caps.
- **c.** ice collars.
- **d.** soaks.

15. When applying heat and cold treatments, the nursing assistant should
- **a.** always remain in the room for the duration of the treatment.
- **b.** check the temperature of the solution with an elbow.
- **c.** monitor the skin under the application every 30 minutes.
- **d.** remove jewelry, buttons, or zippers that may conduct heat or cold.

16. When caring for a patient who is using an aquathermia blanket, the nursing assistant should
- **a.** regulate blanket temperature at least every 15 minutes.
- **b.** give the patient plenty of iced liquids to drink to reduce fever.
- **c.** monitor the patient for cyanosis or changes in vital signs.
- **d.** turn the patient at least every 2 hours.

C. Matching.

Choose the correct word from Column II to match each blank in Column I.

Column I	Column II
17. ____ excessive blood loss	**a.** diathermy
18. ____ increase in size of blood vessel	**b.** vasoconstriction
19. ____ heat treatment	**c.** vasodilation
20. ____ decrease in size of blood vessel	**d.** hypothermia blanket
21. ____ used to lower body temperature	**e.** hemorrhage
	f. infrared

D. Nursing Assistant Challenge.

Peggy, 17 years of age, was admitted to your unit from the emergency room. She fractured an ankle and will require internal repair with screws and wire. You will care for her prior to surgery. The physician has ordered an ice bag for her ankle and her leg is to be elevated. Answer the following questions.

22. What are two reasons for applying the ice bag?

23. How full should the ice bag be filled?

24. Why should ice cubes be rinsed?

25. How should the metal cap be positioned when the ice bag is placed on the patient?

26. When should the ice bag be refilled?

27. How is the ice bag held in place?

28. What important observation should be reported immediately to the nurse?

EXPLORING THE WEB

Description	Location
Aquatic Therapy	*http://www.advancefornurses.com* (see past articles February 11, 2002)
Heat and Cold Therapy	*http://www.genufix.com*
Hot and Cold Therapies	*http://www.spineuniverse.com*
Managing Pain with Heat and Cold	*http://www.orthop.washington.edu*
	http://www.arthritis.org
Post Acute Pools	*http://www. advancefornurses.com* (see past articles September 9, 2002)
Principles of Heat and Cold: Clinical Application	*http://jan.ucc.nau.edu*
Use of Heat and Cold in Pain	*http://www.kasenterprises.com*
Using Heat and Cold	*http://www.silvercross.org*
Water World	*http://www.advancefornurses.com* (see past articles October 7, 2002)

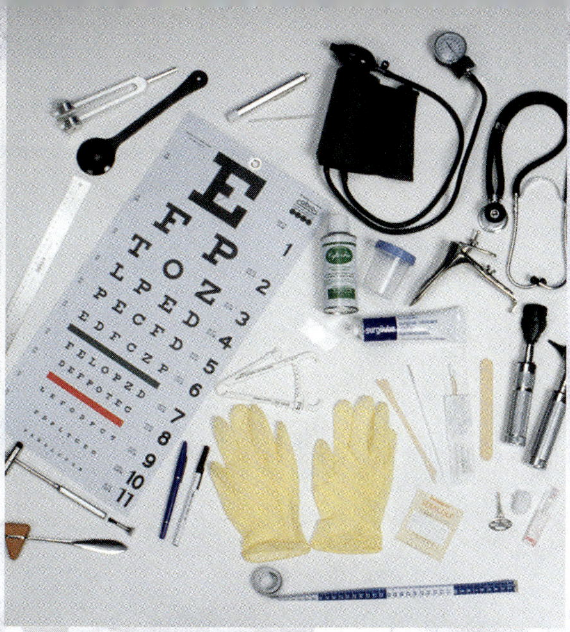

unit 28

Assisting with the Physical Examination

objectives

After completing this unit, you will be able to:

- Spell and define terms.
- Describe the responsibilities of the nursing assistant during the physical examination.
- Name the positions for the various physical examinations.
- Drape patient for the various positions.
- Name the basic instruments necessary for physical examinations.
- Demonstrate the following procedure:
  - Procedure 86 Assisting with a Physical Examination

vocabulary

Learn the meaning and the correct spelling of the following words and phrases:

- dorsal lithotomy position
- dorsal recumbent position
- knee-chest position
- ophthalmoscope
- otoscope
- percussion hammer
- speculum
- Trendelenburg position

INTRODUCTION

Physical examinations are done in the physician's office, in clinics, after the patient's admission to the facility, and in the patient's home. Remember to carry out each beginning procedure action and procedure completion action as you assist.

The physical examination helps the physician:

- evaluate the patient's current status.
- establish a diagnosis.
- determine the patient's progress and response to therapy.

Nursing physical assessments will be performed by the nurse in the facility after the patient is admitted. This information is used by the nurse to establish a nursing diagnosis.

Both of these procedures are carried out in a similar manner. The responsibilities of the nursing assistant include:

- providing for the comfort and privacy of the patient.
- trying to anticipate the examiner's needs.
- draping and positioning patients.
- using proper body mechanics and exposing only the part of the patient being examined.
- preparing equipment that might be needed.
- reassuring the patient.
- caring for and labeling specimens.
- handing equipment as needed.
- cleaning equipment after use.
- adjusting lighting.
- remaining available during the examination.
- assisting the patient after the examination.

Tips: Adjust the room temperature for comfort and make sure the room is free of drafts. Cover the examination table with a clean sheet or disposable paper. Instruct the patient to empty the bladder before beginning.

POSITIONING THE PATIENT

When the physical examination takes place on an examination table, extra attention must be given to safety. The examination table may be raised or lowered in sections and stirrups and shoulder braces applied to assist in positioning. Be sure you know how to properly operate the examination table before positioning a patient on it. In Figures 28-2 to 28-9, an examination table is shown.

Modifications

Some of the positions discussed here may be modified and used for other purposes. For example, they might be used to change the position of a patient who is confined to bed, or to perform specific procedures. Pillows must be used to support a patient who is to be kept in position for a period of time. Remember, the patient who "feels" covered and comfortable will be able to cooperate more fully. Providing privacy for the patient is one of your tasks (Figure 28-1).

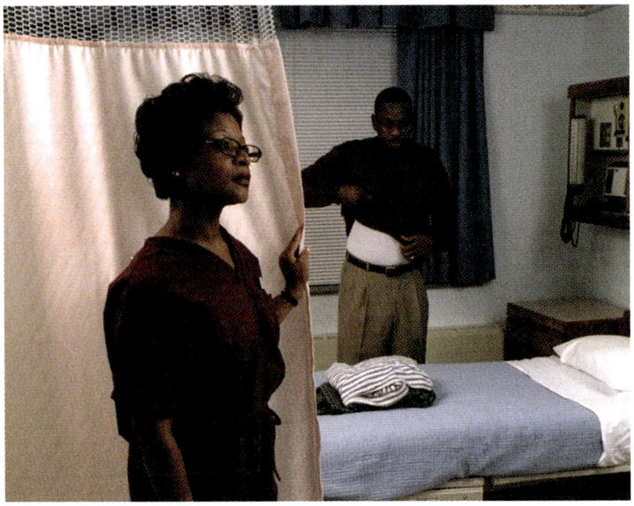

FIGURE 28-1 Provide privacy before the examination begins.

Dorsal Recumbent Position

The **dorsal recumbent position** is the basic examination position.

- Assist the patient to be flat on the back, with knees flexed and slightly separated. The feet should be flat on the bed or table (Figure 28-2).
- Place a small pillow under the patient's head.
- Loosen the gown at the neck.
- Cover the patient with a sheet.

Supine or Horizontal Recumbent Position

- Assist the patient to lie flat on the back. The legs are extended and slightly separated (Figure 28-3).
- Place a pillow under the patient's head.
- Cover the patient with a sheet.
- Loosen the gown at the neck.

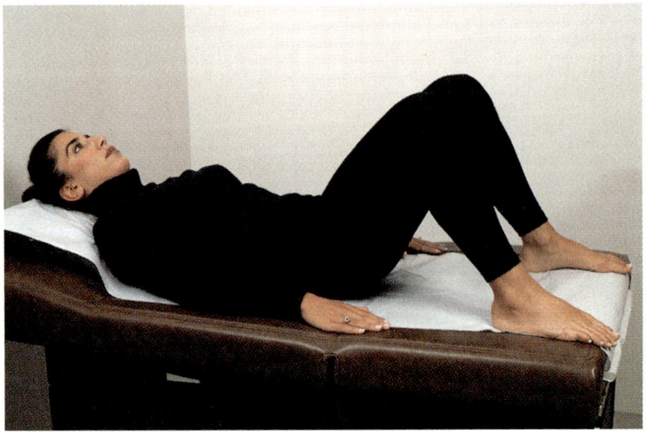

FIGURE 28-2 Dorsal recumbent position. (Draping has been omitted for clarity.)

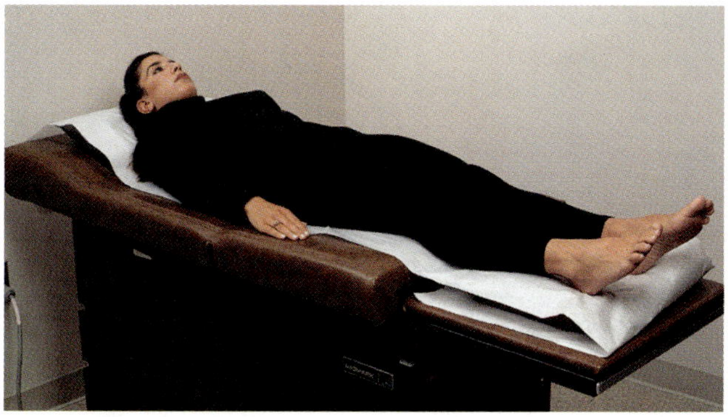

FIGURE 28-3 Supine or horizontal recumbent position.

Knee-Chest Position

The **knee-chest position** may be used to examine the rectal or vaginal areas and to relieve pain following childbirth. This is a difficult position to maintain, so never leave the patient alone. Position the patient in a prone position until the examiner is ready.

- Draping may be done with one or two sheets.
- Place a small pillow under the patient's head.
- Assist the patient to turn and lie on the abdomen with head turned to one side.
- Have the patient flex the arms and bring them up on either side of the head.
- Assist the patient to flex the knees and draw them up as far as possible toward the chest (Figure 28-4).

Prone Position

This position is used to examine the patient's back.

- Assist the patient to lie on the abdomen with head turned to one side.
- Place a small pillow under the patient's head.
- Arms may be extended at the patient's side or flexed and brought up on either side of the head (Figure 28-5).
- One sheet is used for draping.

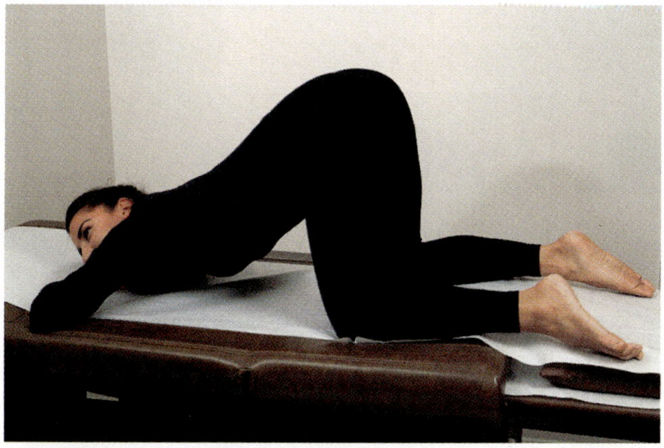

FIGURE 28-4 Knee-chest position.

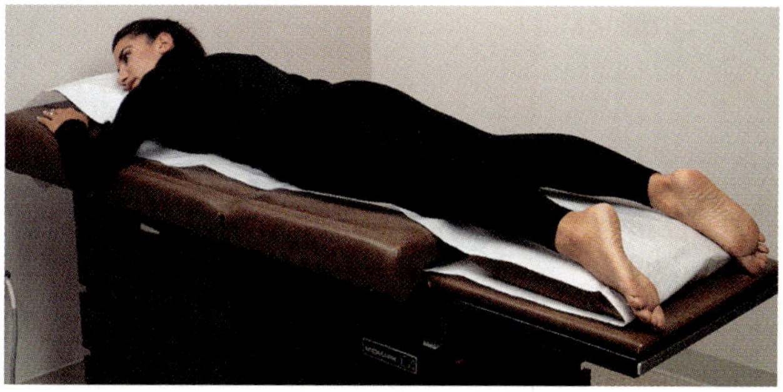

FIGURE 28-5 Prone position.

Sims' Position

This position is used for vaginal and rectal procedures, including enema administration.

- Assist the patient to turn on the left side, with the head turned to the same side and resting on a small pillow.
- Position the left arm extended behind the body.
- Flex the right arm and position it in front of the patient.
- The left leg is slightly bent, while the right leg is sharply flexed (Figure 28-6).
- One drape is usually adequate.

Semi-Fowler's Position

This is a common position for head and neck examinations of the in-bed patient.

- Assist patient to a semi-sitting position with backrest elevated at a 45-degree angle to the bed.
- The knees are supported in a slightly flexed position (Figure 28-7).

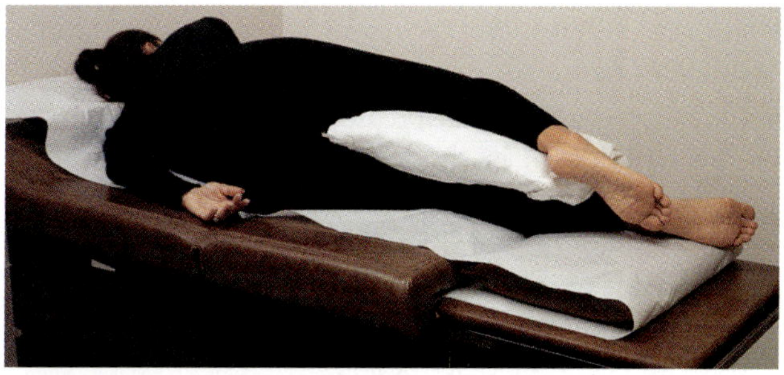

FIGURE 28-6 Sims' position.

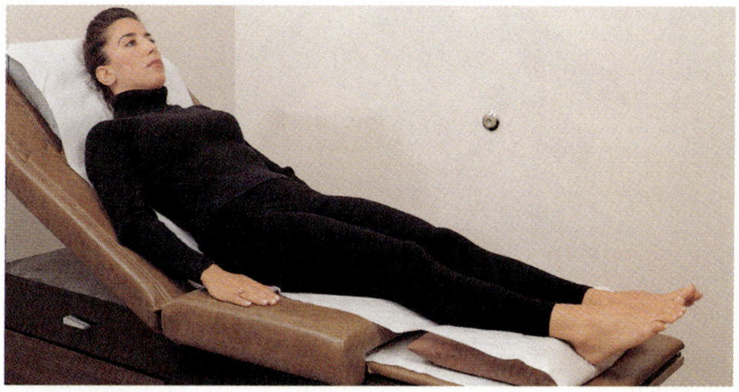

FIGURE 28-7 Semi-Fowler's position.

- The arms rest at the sides.
- One drape is usually enough.

Trendelenburg Position

The **Trendelenburg position** encourages circulation to the patient's heart and brain. It is used when the patient is in shock.

- Assist the patient to lie flat on the back with the head lower than the rest of the body.
- If possible, the lower half of the bed or table is tilted so the legs are slightly flexed (Figure 28-8). In an emergency, the entire bed frame may be supported on blocks, tilting the bed to a 45-degree angle. Some hospital beds, stretchers, and examination tables have a switch that enables the user to position the device in the Trendelenburg position quickly in emergencies.
- Beds that are electrically powered may be adjusted to this position.
- Shoulder braces may be needed to prevent the patient from slipping.
- One drape is usually sufficient.

Dorsal Lithotomy Position

The **dorsal lithotomy position** is frequently used for the pelvic examination of female patients. This is a difficult examination for most women, so make sure your draping makes the patient feel covered.

- Make sure the patient voids her bladder before the examination.
- The patient is positioned on her back.
- The knees are well separated and flexed.
- Usually this position is achieved by placing the feet in stirrups (Figure 28-9).
- One or two drapes may be used to cover the patient. The draping may be similar to draping for the knee-chest position.
- This position can be difficult and uncomfortable for the patient to maintain. Do not place the patient's legs in the stirrups until the physician is in the room and ready to begin the examination.

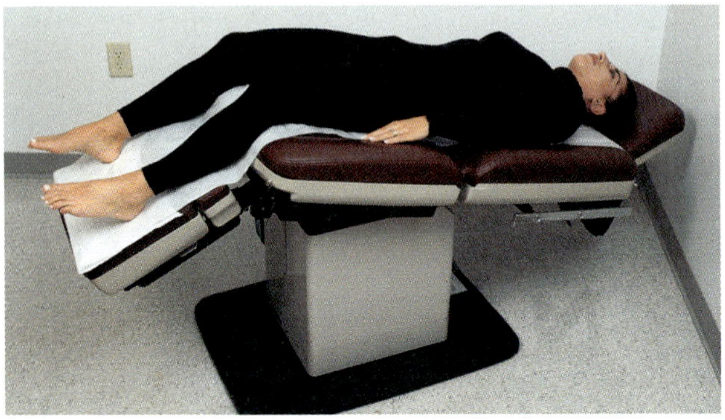

FIGURE 28-8 Trendelenburg position.

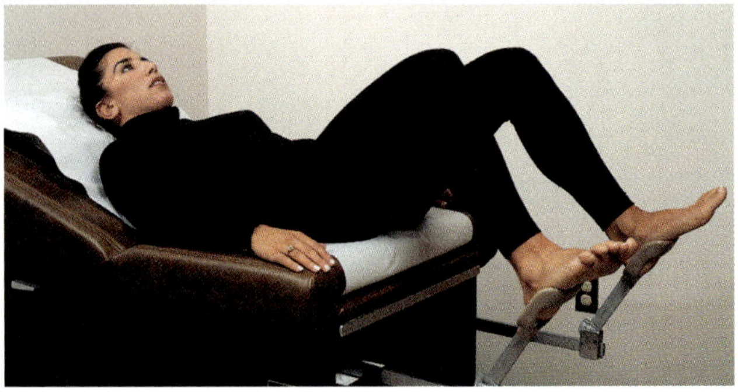

FIGURE 28-9 The patient's feet are placed in stirrups for the dorsal lithotomy position, with the knees flexed and separated.

PHYSICAL EXAMINATION

Some health care facilities have examining instruments and equipment collected on trays. At other facilities, you will gather the necessary equipment and assemble it (Figure 28-10).

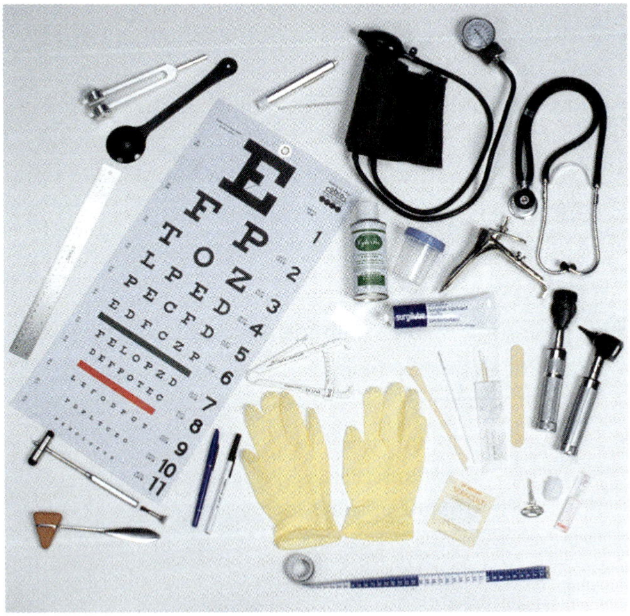

FIGURE 28-10 Equipment and supplies for the physical examination.

OSHA *Alert*

Apply the principles of standard precautions when assisting with a physical examination. Anticipate the equipment that will be needed and make sure it is available to you and to the physician or nurse who is doing the examination.

PROCEDURE 86

ASSISTING WITH A PHYSICAL EXAMINATION

1. Carry out beginning procedure actions.
2. Assemble equipment:
   - gloves
   - flashlight or penlight
   - **percussion hammer** (tests nerve reflex)
   - tongue depressors
   - thermometer
   - cotton balls
   - emesis basin (lined with paper towel)
   - specimen cup
   - vaginal speculum
   - cervical brush
   - cotton-tip applicator
   - cervical spatula
   - slide and fixative
   - lubricant
   - tape measure
   - nasal speculum
   - sterile needle
   - **otoscope** (used to examine ears)
   - **ophthalmoscope** (used to examine eyes)
   - blood pressure cuff (sphygmomanometer)
   - stethoscope
   - visual acuity chart
   - tuning fork
   - pen and paper
   - marking pen
   - guaiac material
   - goniometer
   - scale

Note: *A* ***speculum*** *is an instrument used to spread a body opening. If only a female pelvic examination is to be performed, the following equipment will be needed (Figure 28-11).*

   - gloves
   - linens for draping
   - microscope slides and cover slips
   - fixative spray
   - reagents

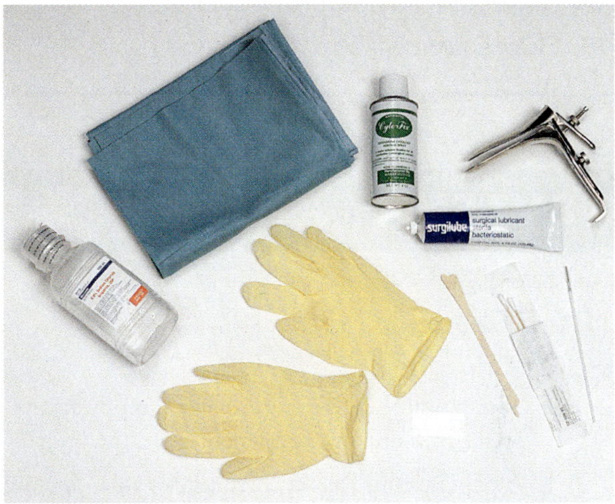

FIGURE 28-11 Equipment and supplies for the pelvic examination.

   - cotton-tipped applicators
   - vaginal speculum
   - spatulas
   - cytobrushes
   - lubricant
3. Ask the patient to void, if ambulatory. If the patient is in bed, follow the procedure for giving the bedpan or urinal.
4. Help the patient onto the examination table.

Note: *If the examination is done with the patient in bed, cover the patient with a bath blanket and fanfold the top bedding to the foot of the bed.*

5. Cover the patient with a drape.
6. Assist as the examination is performed.
   a. Provide privacy.
   b. Position the patient and equipment as necessary.
   c. Hand equipment as required to the examiner.
   d. Adjust lighting as necessary.
7. After the examination is complete, help the patient to:
   a. Sit up slowly.
   b. Get off the table and stand.
   c. Dress.
   d. Return to the unit or office.

continues

PROCEDURE 86

continued

8. Wash your hands and return to the examination room.
9. Put on gloves.
10. Clean equipment according to facility policy.
11. Care for specimens according to facility policy.
12. Remove gloves and dispose of properly.
13. Wash your hands.

REVIEW

A. True/False.

Mark the following true or false by circling T or F.

1. T F The physical examination helps the physician establish a nursing assessment.
2. T F A patient who feels covered is able to cooperate more fully.
3. T F Positions used for the physical examination can only be used for that purpose.
4. T F The nursing assistant performs the actual physical exam.
5. T F When a patient is placed in the Trendelenburg position, the feet must be at the same level as the knees.
6. T F When positioning a patient for a physical examination, you must maintain proper body mechanics.
7. T F Once you have the patient positioned for a physical examination, you should leave the room.
8. T F The nursing assistant assists in the physical assessment by draping and positioning the patient.
9. T F Lighting may have to be adjusted during the examination.
10. T F The semi-Fowler's position encourages blood flow to the head and heart.

B. Multiple Choice.

Select the one best answer for each of the following.

11. The basic examination position is
    - **a.** Sims'.
    - **b.** dorsal recumbent.
    - **c.** dorsal lithotomy.
    - **d.** Trendelenburg.
12. The patient is to have a pelvic examination. In what position should she be positioned?
    - **a.** Sims'
    - **b.** Lithotomy
    - **c.** Trendelenburg
    - **d.** Semi-Fowler's
13. Your female patient is to have a pelvic examination. Which instrument would you be sure to have ready?
    - **a.** Otoscope
    - **b.** Vaginal speculum
    - **c.** Nasal speculum
    - **d.** Ophthalmoscope
14. The patient has vaginal bleeding and the physician orders you to place her in a position that will increase blood flow to the head. Which position would you prepare for?
    - **a.** Sims'
    - **b.** Semi-Fowler's
    - **c.** Trendelenburg
    - **d.** Lithotomy
15. Stirrups are used in which position?
    - **a.** Dorsal lithotomy
    - **b.** Semi-Fowler's
    - **c.** Sims'
    - **d.** Trendelenburg

C. Matching.

Choose the correct word from Column II to match the word or phrases in Column I.

Column I	Column II
16. ____ instrument to examine the ear	**a.** apprehensive
17. ____ instrument to examine the eye	**b.** drape
18. ____ instrument to spread (dilate) a body opening	**c.** ophthalmoscope
19. ____ fearful	**d.** otoscope
20. ____ covering	**e.** speculum
	f. percussion hammer

D. Nursing Assistant Challenge.

Robert Ubek is to have a physical examination in the doctor's office. He is 88 years of age and appears very nervous. He tells you that he is afraid he has prostate cancer. You are to assist the doctor. Complete the following statements using words from the following list.

anticipate	off
dorsal recumbent	on
drape	reassure

21. One of your responsibilities will be to ______ the patient.

22. Because of Mr. Ubek's age, you will be especially careful in assisting him to get ______ and ______ the table.

23. You can help him feel more comfortable if you ______ him properly.

24. You can help the examination go more smoothly if you ______ the examiner's needs.

25. You will position Mr. Ubek in the ______ position to begin the examination.

EXPLORING THE WEB

Description	Location
The Complete Physical Exam	*http://www.mtmonthly.com*
Physical Exam Encyclopedia	*http://www.nlm.nih.gov/medlineplus/ency/article/002274.htm*
Physical Exam Terms and Phrases	*http://mtdesk.com*
Physical Examination by ADAM	*http://health.yahoo.com*
Screening Physical Examination	*http://www.meddean.luc.edu*
What to Expect from a Physical Exam	*http://webmd.lycos.com*

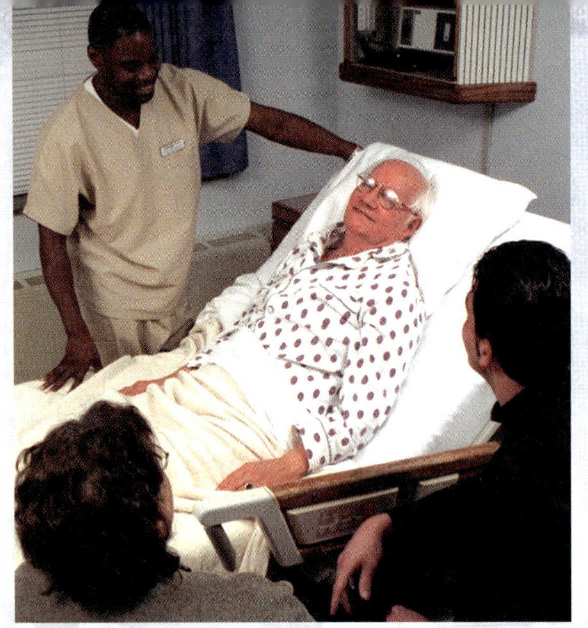

unit 29

The Surgical Patient

objectives

After completing this unit, you will be able to:

- Spell and define terms.
- Describe the concerns of patients who are about to have surgery.
- List the various types of anesthesia.
- Shave the area to be operated on.
- Prepare the patient's unit for the patient's return from the operating room.
- Give routine postoperative care when the patient returns to the room.
- Assist the patient with deep breathing and coughing.
- Apply elasticized stockings or bandages and pneumatic hosiery.
- Demonstrate the following procedures:
  - Procedure 87 Shaving the Operative Area
  - Procedure 88 Assisting the Patient to Deep Breathe and Cough
  - Procedure 89 Performing Postoperative Leg Exercises
  - Procedure 90 Applying Elasticized Stockings
  - Procedure 91 Applying Elastic Bandage
  - Procedure 92 Applying Pneumatic Compression Hosiery
  - Procedure 93 Assisting the Patient to Dangle

vocabulary

Learn the meaning and the correct spelling of the following words and phrases:

ambulation
anesthesia
anti-embolism hose
aspirate
atelectasis
bandages
binders
dangling
deep vein thrombosis (DVT)
depilatory
disruption
distention
drainage
dressings
embolus
general anesthetic
hypoallergenic tape
hypoxia
local anesthetic
Montgomery straps
nosocomial
NPO
operative
orifice
perioperative
postanesthesia care unit (PACU)
postoperative
preoperative
prosthesis
pulmonary embolism
recovery room
sequential compression therapy
singultus
spinal anesthesia
stable
surgical bed
TED hose
thrombophlebitis
umbilicus
vertigo

INTRODUCTION

Patients facing any surgical procedure tend to be fearful. Remember that these patients require great emotional as well as physical support (Figure 29-1). Such support should be given from the time the patient is admitted through the discharge.

Patients are concerned with:

- Disfigurement
- Pain
- Loss of control as they undergo anesthesia
- What serious conditions might be found
- Length and cost of recovery
- Possibility of death

Surgery is often associated with anxiety, pain, and discomfort. For this reason, medications are given before, during, and after surgery.

PAIN PERCEPTION

When a person feels pain sensations, the:

- pain receptors record the sensation.
- sensation is sent by the spinal nerves to the spinal cord and then to the brain.
- sensation is received and interpreted in the brain.

Before surgery, the patient is given medication to promote relaxation. During surgery, anesthetics are given to prevent pain (Figure 29-2). After surgery, medications are given to reduce discomfort.

ANESTHESIA

Anesthesia is given to prevent pain, to relax muscles, and to induce forgetfulness. The anesthetic agent (drug) and method of administration used are determined by the location and type of surgery to be performed, the length of time needed for surgery, and the patient's physical condition.

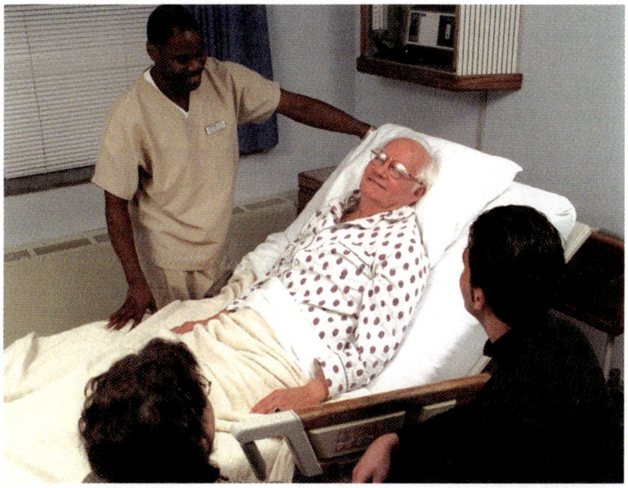

FIGURE 29-1 Patients and family members need support during the preoperative period.

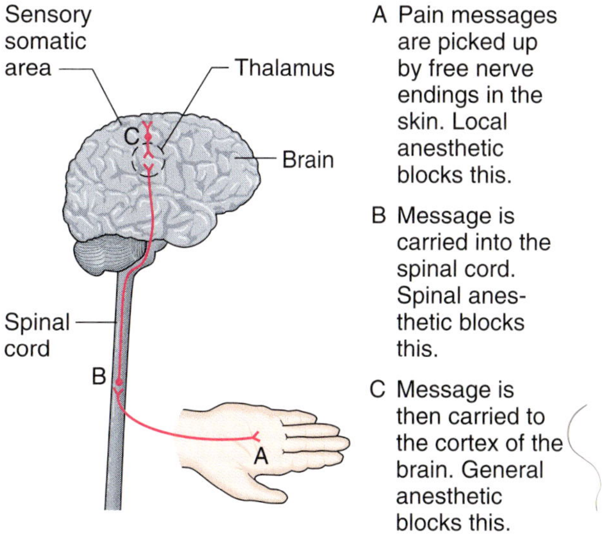

FIGURE 29-2 Anesthetics will block pain impulses at points A, B, or C.

There are two main types of anesthetics:

1. **General anesthetics**—These induce the patient to become unconscious.
2. **Local anesthetics**—These induce loss of feeling in a specific area.

General Anesthetics

General anesthetics block reception of pain in the brain. They are usually given in one of two ways:

1. Inhalation—Some gases that are used as anesthetics include nitrous oxide and cyclopropane.
   - Inhaled anesthetics are apt to make the patient secrete more mucus and to experience nausea.
   - Special attention must be given after surgery to keep the respiratory tract clear.
   - There is a real danger that the patient may **aspirate** (inhale) vomitus into the respiratory tract.
2. Intravenous—Drugs are introduced directly into the veins.
   - These drugs, such as sodium pentathol, act rapidly.
   - The patient quickly loses consciousness.
   - IV anesthetics are often used with other types of anesthesia for short operations.

Local Anesthetics

Local anesthetics act by:

1. Blocking pain receptors in the operative area.
   - Drugs such as procaine hydrochloride may be injected into the patient around the operative area.

- These drugs stop the sensation of pain only in that area.
- The patient remains awake but free from pain during the operation.

2. Blocking transmission of the pain sensation at the level of the spinal cord.
   - A drug injected into the spinal canal prevents feeling in any point below the level of the injection.
   - The patient remains awake.
   - This type of anesthesia is commonly used for abdominal surgery because it produces good relaxation of the muscles.
   - This technique is called **spinal anesthesia**.

After getting this type of anesthetic, the patient is unable to feel or move the legs for a period of time. If not prepared ahead of time, the patient may be frightened by this experience.

SURGICAL CARE

The care of the surgical patient (**perioperative**) can be divided into three parts:

- **Preoperative** (before surgery)
- **Operative** (in the operating room)
- **Postoperative** (after surgery)

PREOPERATIVE CARE

Preoperative care begins when surgery is planned by the physician with the patient. Your responsibilities begin when the patient is admitted to the hospital. Remember that you may answer general questions that the patient asks, but you must refer specific questions about the surgery, its possible outcome, and anesthesia to your team leader.

Although it is the responsibility of the physician and nurse to answer questions and give explanations, it is helpful if you are aware of the information that has been given. Refer any questions the patient has to the nurse.

Teaching

Time spent with the patient in the preoperative period is very helpful. Patients who are prepared are able to cooperate more successfully in their recovery. Ideally, this time is spent shortly after the patient's admission. Sometimes much of the information is given in the doctor's office or clinic.

During the preoperative period, the nurse will determine the patient's specific needs. The nurse also does preoperative teaching. The other staff members support this effort.

- Tests, medications, and preoperative procedures are explained.
- Questions regarding the postoperative period are answered.
- The patient is taught and given an opportunity to practice postoperative exercises, such as leg exercises and respiratory exercises.
- The patient and staff discuss the events of the preoperative period, and what the patient may experience while being taken to the operating room and being given anesthesia.
- The recovery period is outlined and the purpose of special procedures or equipment, such as tubes or intravenous fluid lines, that may be used after surgery is explained.
- Play therapy may be used to explain to children.
- Every effort is made to teach ways of decreasing discomfort and to assure the patient that means for pain relief will be available.
- Planning for the discharge period begins now.

Psychological Preparation

The nursing staff spends as much time as possible helping patients deal with their emotional stress.

All members of the health team need to be sensitive and responsive to the psychological needs of the patient. Because you will be in frequent contact with the patient, you may be the first person to recognize signs of fear or concern. Listen to what the patient says and observe the patient's body language carefully. Report your observations to the nurse so that appropriate nursing intervention may be carried out.

Build patient confidence by:

- Performing your work in an efficient, calm manner.
- Being available to listen.
- Explaining what you plan to do before carrying out any procedure.
- Encouraging the patient to participate in his own care as much as possible. This helps the patient feel he still has a measure of control over his life.
- Immediately transmitting requests for clergy visits.

Physical Preparation

The Evening Before Surgery. If the patient is in the hospital the evening before surgery, part of the surgical preparation may be done then. It usually includes:

- Bath or shower with surgical soap
- Enema
- Surgical prep (shaving of the operative site)
- Special tests
- Medication to ensure a good night's rest, when indicated
- Insertion of special tubes for draining body cavities
- Being placed on **NPO** (nothing by mouth) orders after midnight
- Removal of the water pitcher from the bedside table and having the NPO notice posted over the bed,

bedside stand, on the door, on the patient's chart, and on the Kardex.

Nosocomial infections are those acquired during the hospital stay. It is known that such infections:

- are more likely to occur the longer the patient is in the hospital.
- add days to the hospital stay.
- increase the cost of hospitalization.
- can be life-threatening.

To decrease costs and the potential for nosocomial infections, patients are often admitted on the morning of surgery and are sometimes discharged on the day of surgery or the day after. In this circumstance, much of the preoperative care must be done at home or immediately upon admission. This is called outpatient or "short-term" surgery.

The Surgical Prep Area. Skin preparation before surgery may or may not include hair removal. There is a trend away from removing the hair unless its thickness will interfere with the surgery. In fact, some studies have shown more infections among shaved patients compared with unshaved patients.

If shaving is ordered, it must be done according to the procedure provided. (See Procedure 87.) It must be performed skillfully in a well-lighted area. Also, the area to be washed and shaved will be larger than the surgical incision area (Figure 29-3A and Figure 29-3B). In some cases, a **depilatory** (hair-removing) cream will be ordered for use the night before surgery. If a depilatory is to be used, check the skin for sensitivity. Apply a small amount to the skin of the forearm and wait 10 minutes. If redness occurs, do not continue, but report to the nurse.

Skin preparation may be performed by:

- Special surgical prep team
- Operating room (OR) staff in the OR
- Nursing staff in the patient's unit just prior to surgery

SAFETY *Alert*

All personnel involved in perioperative care of the patient must be alert to make sure that the correct surgical procedure is done on the correct patient, and that the surgery is done on the correct site. This often involves marking the site of the surgery. Various forms and checklists are used to verify the patient and surgical site. Take your responsibilities for identifying the patient and operative site seriously. There is no room for error in this area of nursing practice.

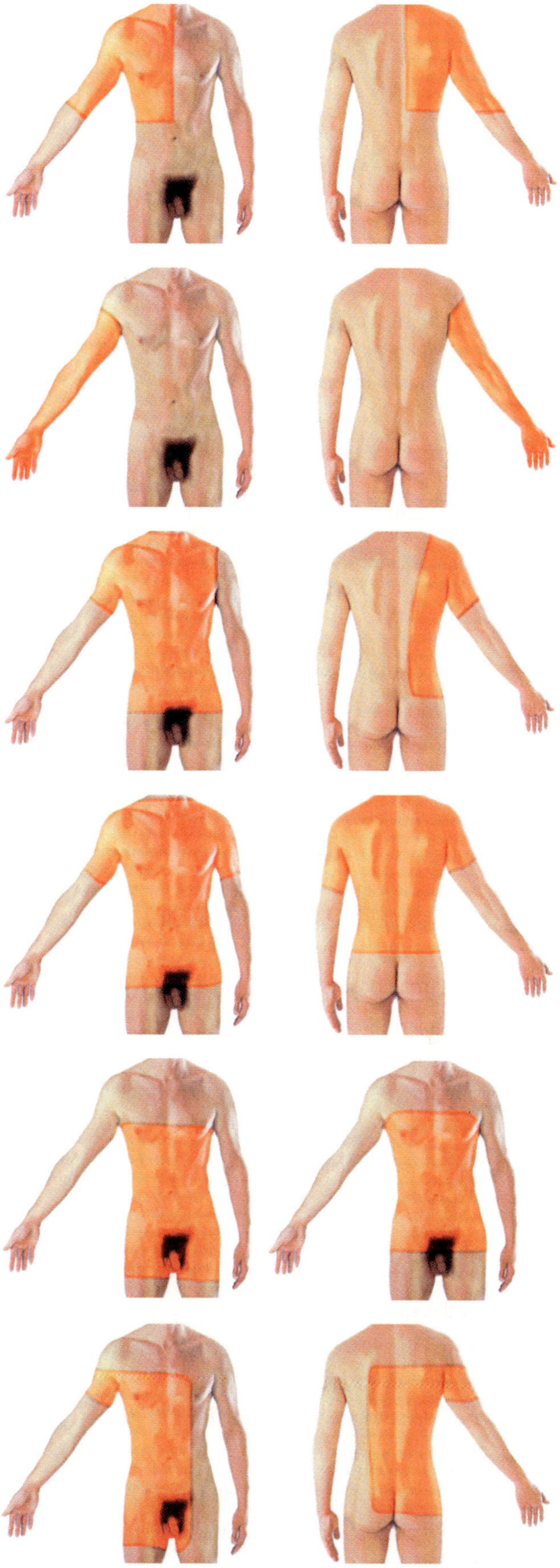

FIGURE 29-3A Surgical preparation sites for the upper extremities and torso.

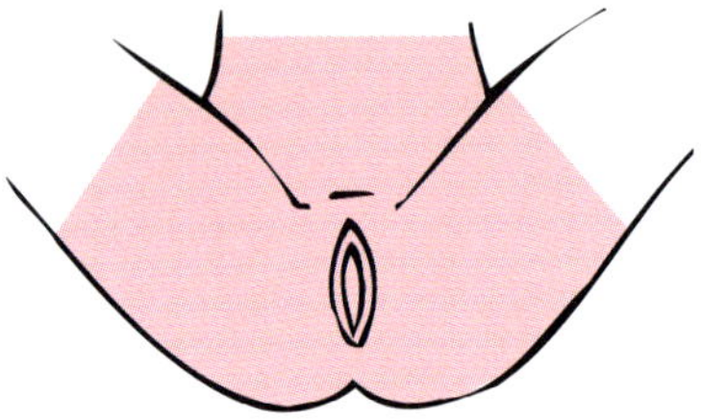

FIGURE 29-3B Surgical preparation sites for vaginal, rectal, and perineal surgery.

To prepare the surgical area by shaving:

- Make sure you know exactly what area is to be shaved. Most hospitals have routine prep areas.
- Do not shave the neck or face of a female patient. If in doubt, check with the nurse.
- Never shave the eyebrows.
- Be aware that the preparations for cranial surgery are usually performed after the patient has been medicated and taken to the operating suite. Doctors have special preferences in this regard.
- Remember that if a spinal anesthesia is to be given, the back may also be shaved.

Calm the patient's fears by explaining that the area prepared is much larger than the actual incision area. This is to prevent contamination of the surgical site, which may lead to possible complications after surgery.

PROCEDURE 87

SHAVING THE OPERATIVE AREA

1. Carry out beginning procedure actions.
2. Assemble equipment:
   - disposable gloves
   - bath blanket
   - individual prep pack, *or*
   - tray with razor and new razor blades, *or*
   - electric clipper—make sure the heads are disposable or, if reusable, that they have been sterilized
   - 2 small bowls
   - applicators
   - cleansing soap
   - lighting—for example, a spotlight or gooseneck lamp
   - 4 × 4 sponges
   - paper towels
   - towels or disposable Chux® (bed protector)
3. Determine the exact area to be prepped.
4. In the utility room:
   a. Fill the small bowls with warm water.
   b. Add cleansing soap to one.
   c. Adjust the razor and blade.
   d. Make sure the razor and blade are tight.
5. Cover the tray and take it to the bedside.
6. Drape the patient with a bath blanket. Place a towel or bed protector under the area to be shaved.
7. Put on disposable gloves.
8. If a safety razor and blade are used, soften hairs with soapy solution and wait 1 minute. This makes hair removal easier and helps avoid skin injury.
9. Holding the skin taut with one hand, lather the area to be shaved. If hair is very long, such as on the pubis and axilla, it may be clipped with scissors before shaving. Take care when clipping—do not nick the skin. If an electric clipper is used, attach the heads and check for security.
10. Shave the area with strokes in the same direction as the hair grows. Be careful not to cut the skin or to remove any warts or moles. Work carefully around such areas.
11. Using the applicators, clean the **umbilicus** (navel) and shave it if it is in the operative area.

SAFETY *Alert*

Hold the razor at a 45-degree angle. Maintain contact with the skin. Try to avoid lifting the razor and then putting it down again. Doing this increases the risk of nicks and cuts.

continues

PROCEDURE 87

continued

12. Check carefully for hairs after shaving is complete.
    - Unattached hairs are easily removed by gently pressing a piece of tape against the area.
    - Discard hair in a paper towel.
13. Cleanse the skin with warm, soapy water. Rinse and dry thoroughly.
14. Dispose of equipment according to facility policy.
15. Remove the towel from under the patient.
    - Make sure the side rails are up.
    - Make sure linen is dry.
    - Change, if necessary.
16. Remove and dispose of gloves according to facility policy.
17. Carry out procedure completion actions.

Immediate Preoperative Care. Approximately one hour before surgery, the patient will be given additional medication by the nurse. Your responsibilities regarding the patient must be completed before this time. You may be asked to do the following:

- Take and record vital signs (Figure 29-4) (see Section 6).
- Take care of valuables according to hospital policy. Remove dentures and any other **prosthesis** (artificial part), such as a hearing aid or glasses. See that they are safely marked with the patient's name and stored appropriately.
- Remove nail polish, makeup, hairpins, and jewelry. Long hair should be neatly braided or capped. Plain wedding bands may be taped in place.
- Dress the patient in a gown and cover the hair with a surgical cap.
- See that the patient voids and measure the urine. Drain the catheter, if present, and record.
- Make sure that the room is quiet and comfortable.

As soon as the nurse gives the preoperative medication:

- Be sure the side rails are in place for safety.

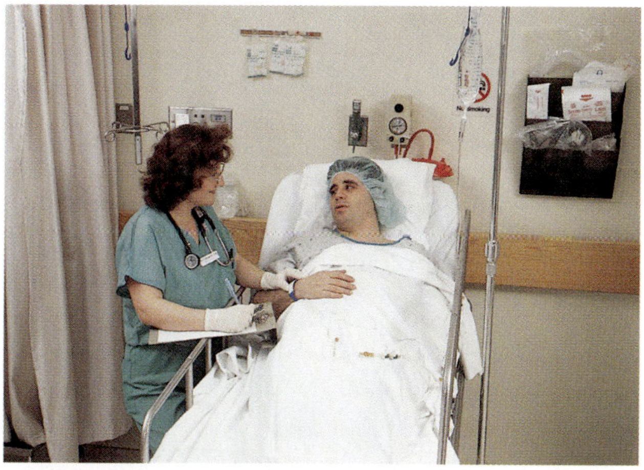

FIGURE 29-4 Taking vital signs is an important part of preoperative care.

- Remove all unnecessary equipment.
- Push the bedside table, overbed table, and chair out of the way to make room for the stretcher when it arrives from surgery.
- Complete the surgical checklist:
  1. Admission sheet
  2. Surgical consent
  3. Sterilization consent (if necessary)
  4. Consultation sheet (if necessary)
  5. History and physical
  6. Lab reports (pregnancy test also if necessary)
  7. Surgery prep done and charted, if required
  8. Latest TPR and blood pressure charted
  9. Preoperative medication given and charted (if required)
  10. Identification band on patient
  11. Fingernail polish and makeup removed
  12. Metallic objects removed (wedding ring may be taped)
  13. Dentures removed
  14. Other prostheses removed (such as artificial limb or eye, wigs and hairpieces)
  15. Glasses or contact lenses removed
  16. Bath blanket and head cap in place
  17. Bed in high position and side rails up after preop medication is given
  18. Patient has voided
  - Check off those duties to which you were assigned.
  - Note the time your patient leaves for surgery.
- Follow facility policy regarding visitors. Sometimes they are allowed to wait quietly with the patient. Sometimes they should be directed to the visitors' waiting room.
- Elevate the bed to stretcher height when the transporter arrives to take the patient to surgery.

The nurse and surgical attendant will check the patient's identification and surgical checklist before the patient is moved.

A staff member, and sometimes a family member, accompanies the patient to the doors of the operating room. You will probably be asked to assist in transferring the patient from the bed to the stretcher and, after surgery, from the stretcher to the bed. Review Procedures 24 and 25 in Unit 16.

DURING THE OPERATIVE PERIOD

While the patient is in the operating room, you will prepare the room for the patient's return.

- A special surgical bed will be prepared. This was described in Unit 23. The **surgical bed** is also called a postop bed or recovery bed.
- Everything should be removed from the top of the bedside stand except an emesis basin, tissue wipes, tongue depressors, and equipment to check vital signs.
- A pencil and small pad to record the signs should also be available.
- Check with your team leader for any special equipment, such as oxygen, IV poles, suction, or drainage bags, that might be necessary for your patient.
- Be watchful while carrying out your other assignments for the return of your patient from surgery.
- Follow facility policy regarding the location of visitors and family during surgery. They are sometimes permitted to wait in the patient's room. In most cases they are directed to a special waiting area.

POSTOPERATIVE CARE

During the immediate postoperative period, the patient recovers from anesthesia. For this period, the patient is placed in a special area called the **recovery room** (Figure 29-5). The recovery room is located next to the operating room and is sometimes called the **postanesthesia care unit** (**PACU**).

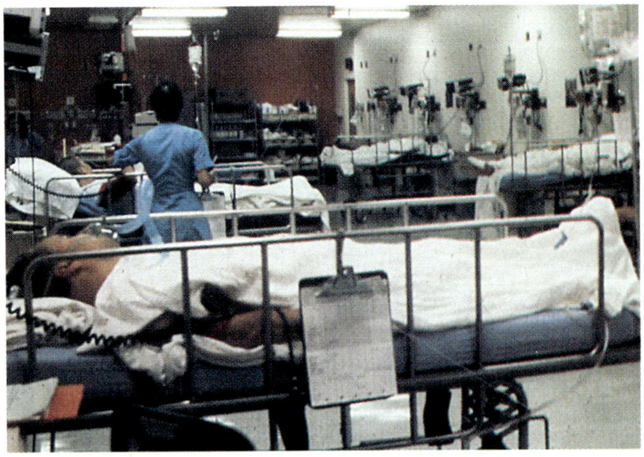

FIGURE 29-5 Postanesthesia Care Unit (PACU)—the unit where the patient wakes up from anesthesia after surgery. *(Courtesy of Memorial Medical Center of Long Beach, CA)*

SAFETY *Alert*

Remember that most patients receive many drugs when they are in surgery. Many of these drugs can alter the patient's mental status. The drugs are excreted from the body slowly. The patient may sleep soundly upon return to the unit. Keep the side rails up and follow all safety precautions until the patient is fully awake and the nurse instructs you that side rails are no longer necessary. Do not leave liquids at the bedside until the nurse instructs you that it is safe to do so. Check on the patient regularly.

When the patient's condition is stabilized, the patient is returned to the unit. Upon the patient's return from the recovery room, you should:

- Identify the patient.
- Assist in the transfer from stretcher to bed (see Unit 16).
- Never leave the unconscious patient alone at any time.
- Check with the nurse for any special instructions.
- Realize that the patient may be drowsy for several hours after return.
- Have an extra blanket available—many patients complain of feeling cold upon return (Figure 29-6).

The following are routine instructions to be followed unless otherwise ordered.

- Always wear gloves and follow standard precautions when contact with blood, body fluids, mucous membranes, or nonintact skin is likely.

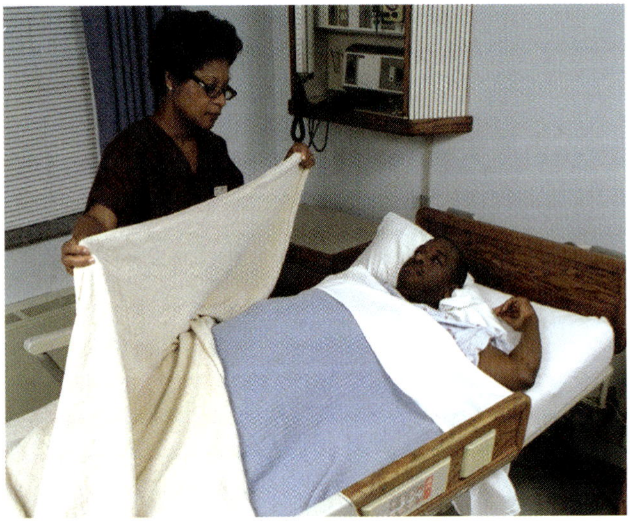

FIGURE 29-6 Patients may be cold after surgery. Cover them to prevent chilling.

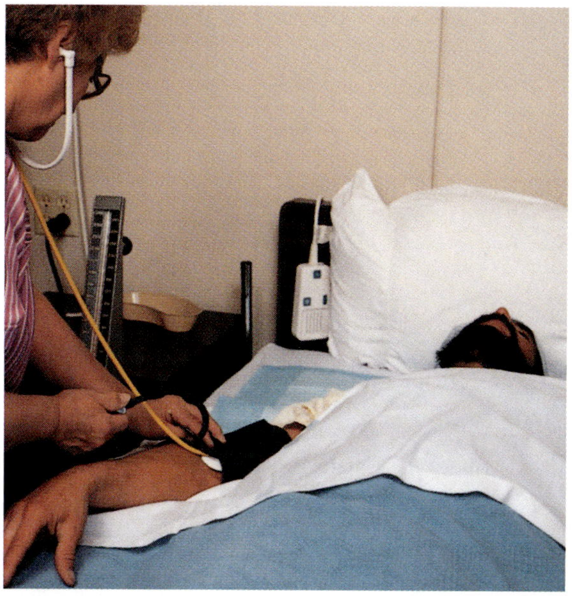

FIGURE 29-7 Check the vital signs regularly until they are stable.

- Take vital signs of the patient upon arrival on the unit (Figure 29-7) and every 15 minutes for four readings (see Section 6). The patient's temperature may not always be taken at this time.

  When taking postoperative vital signs, count pulse and respiration for one full minute. Most facilities have policies for postoperative vital signs at specified frequencies that decrease if the vital signs are **stable** (approximately the same), such as:
  - every 15 minutes for 1 hour
  - if stable, every 30 minutes for 1 hour
  - if stable, every hour for 2 hours
  - if stable, every 4 hours for 24 hours

  Always follow the protocol for vital signs used by your facility. The vital sign schedule may be altered by the RN if the patient's condition warrants. The physician may also order vital signs at a specifically designated frequency. Monitor the patient's level of consciousness (drowsy, unresponsive, alert) each time you check the vital signs.

  Many facilities consider pain to be the fifth vital sign, so you should ask the patient if he or she is having pain each time you check the vital signs. Inform the nurse if pain is present.

SAFETY *Alert*

Anesthesia reduces body temperature. Keep the patient warm. If the patient's temperature is below 97°F, inform the nurse promptly.

- Check dressings for amount and type of any drainage. The nurse may reinforce them as necessary.
- Check IV solution for flow rate. Restrain the infusion site whenever ordered by the physician and report to the nurse. Remember that the flow rate is ordered by the physician.
- Encourage the patient to breathe deeply, cough, and move in bed. Position should be changed every 2 hours.
- Turn the patient's head to one side and support if he is vomiting. Have an emesis basin ready, as well as tissues and wet cloth. If the patient is conscious, allow the patient to rinse the mouth with water after vomiting. Note the type and amount of vomitus and record on the output worksheet.
- Check the pulses distal to the operative site. Inform the nurse if the pulse is weak or cannot be felt.
- If the patient was given a spinal anesthetic:
  - Give extra care in turning frequently and maintaining proper alignment.
  - Remember that the patient will be unable to move independently until sensation and motor functions return. Make sure to calm the patient's fear about this.
  - Some physicians require that the patient remain flat on the back and without a pillow for 8 to 12 hours following spinal anesthesia, to avoid headaches.
  - Any complaints of a headache following spinal anesthesia should be reported promptly.
  - Provide extra blankets if the patient is cold.
- Be sure all drainage tubes have been connected (the nurse will usually attend to this). If you notice a tube clamped shut, check with the nurse.
- Measure and record the first postoperative voiding. Inform the nurse.
- Report any patient complaints of discomfort or pain to the nurse (Figure 29-8).

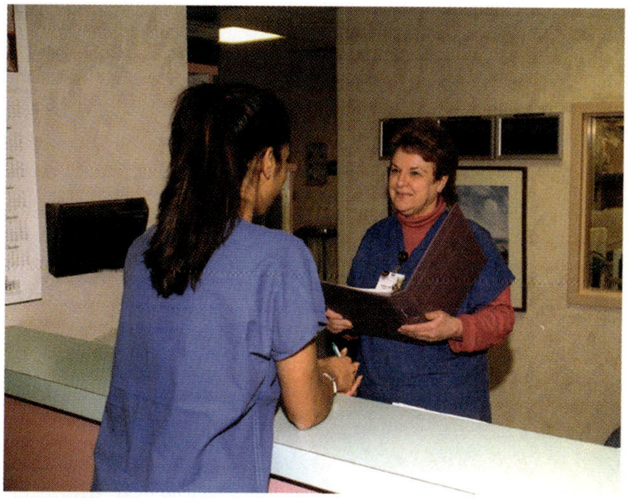

FIGURE 29-8 Report complaints of pain or discomfort to the nurse.

Tubes

Patients often return from surgery with a variety of tubes and drains in place.

- Some tubes may deliver materials into the patient. Examples are oxygen tubes or intravenous tubes.
- Other tubes may have been placed in the patient to provide **drainage** from wounds or body cavities. Examples are drains in the incision or urinary catheters.

The following are some special precautions to be taken:

- Always wear gloves if contact with drainage from the tube is likely.
- Learn the type, purpose, and location of each tube.
- Check drainage for character and amount.
- Check for obstructions to the tube system.
- Check flow rate of infusions from intravenous lines.
- Keep **orifices** (body openings) clear of secretions and discharge.
- Never disconnect tubes or raise drainage bottles above the level of the drainage site.
- Never lower infusion bottles below the level of the infusion site.
- Never put stress on the tubes when moving the patient or giving care.
- Restrain infusion sites as necessary to prevent dislocation.

Note: A physician's order is needed.

- Monitor levels of infusions and report to the nurse before they run out.
- Report any signs of leakage or disconnected tubes immediately.
- Report pain, discoloration, or swelling at sites or drainage and infusion.

Dressings and Bandages

Caring for surgical wounds, injuries, and ulcers is very important. **Dressings** are gauze, film, or other synthetic substances that cover a wound, ulcer, or injury. Some dressings have an adhesive backing. Some are affixed with tape. Many different types of tape are available in the health care facility. Some patients need special **hypoallergenic tape**, which reduces the incidence of a skin reaction in patients who are allergic to the adhesive backing. **Bandages** are sometimes used to hold dressings in place. These are fabric, gauze, net, or elasticized materials used to cover the dressing and keep it securely in place. Bandages are available in different sizes and shapes. Gauze bandages are commonly used to cover dressings. Elastic bandages are used to reduce edema and support injured body parts. When wrapping bandages, avoid wrapping them so tightly that they restrict circulation.

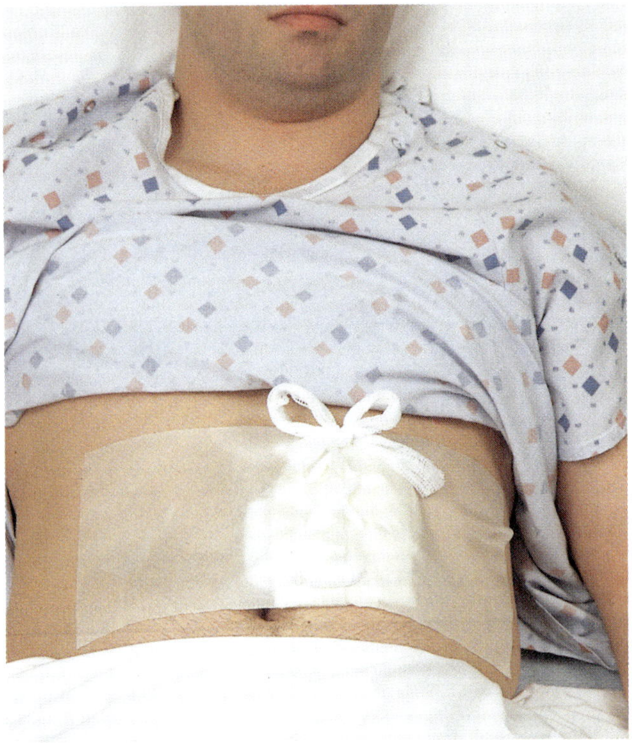

FIGURE 29-9 Montgomery straps hold dressings securely in place so they can be observed, changed, and reinforced without tape. This is much less traumatic for the patient.

Occasionally, **Montgomery straps** (Figure 29-9) are used to hold dressings in place. These are long strips of adhesive attached to the skin on either side of the wound. They are less traumatic to the skin because the adhesive is not removed with each dressing change unless the straps are soiled. After the dressing is in place, the straps are tied to hold the dressing securely. **Binders** (Figure 29-10) may also be used to hold dressings in place.

Drainage

When a body cavity is the operative site, it may be necessary to drain fluid such as blood, pus, serous drainage caused by tissue trauma, or gastric contents from it before or after surgery. Always wear gloves if contact with drainage is likely. The drainage outlet may be a:

- Catheter

INFECTION CONTROL Alert

Body sites with tubes, drains, and surgical dressings are managed using sterile technique. Never open a tube or drain or remove a dressing. The nurse will use sterile technique to manage these areas.

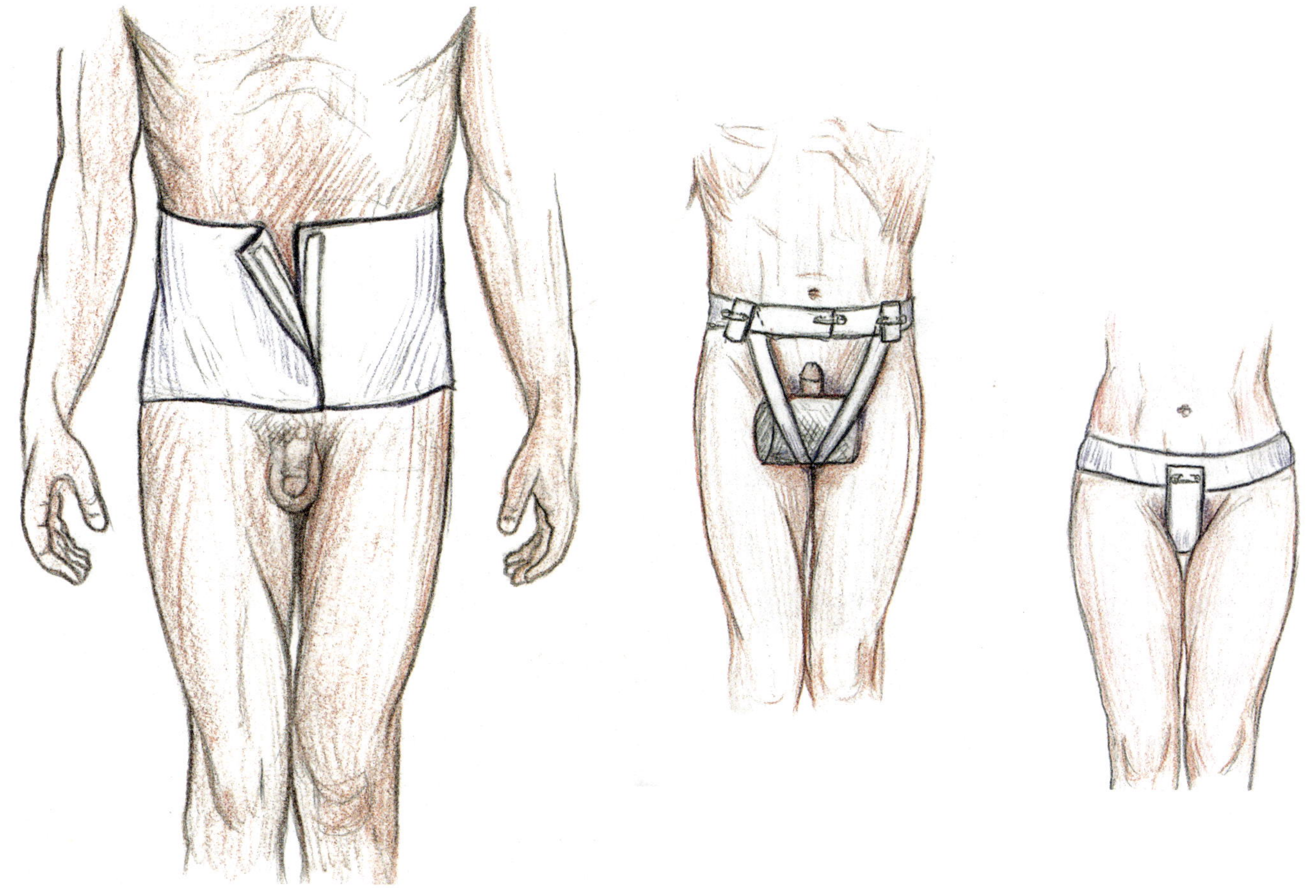

FIGURE 29-10 Various surgical binders support the body part and hold dressings in place.

- T-tube
- Jackson-Pratt (J–P)® or Hemovac® drain
- Penrose drain
- Cigarette drain

When such a drain is in place, the drainage accumulates on the dressing (Figure 29-11). You should:

- note the amount and character of the drainage.
- inform the nurse when the dressing needs to be changed or reinforced.

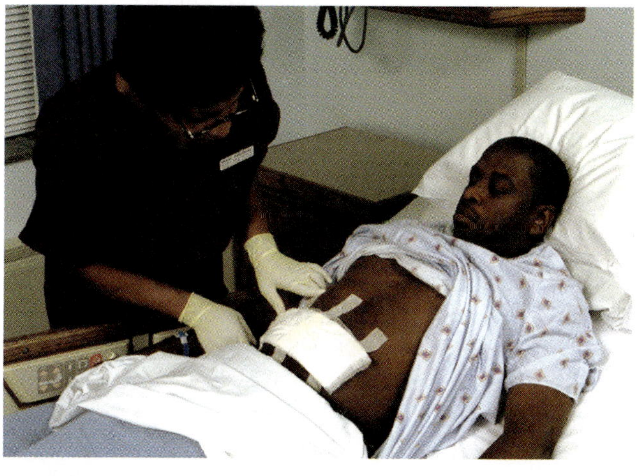

FIGURE 29-11 Check the dressings regularly for drainage or bleeding.

At times, the withdrawal of fluids is controlled by attaching the drainage tube to a connecting tube and then a suction apparatus. The drainage accumulates in a container. The container is emptied and the contents measured at the end of each shift. The Jackson-Pratt or Hemovac drains are closed drainage systems. The drains are placed directly in the wound, and drainage goes directly into an expandable container. A record of the amount and character of the drainage is entered in both the output chart and the nurses' notes.

It is your responsibility to:

- Report either heavy or light drainage.
- Report a change in the character or amount of the drainage.
- Make sure that the flow of drainage is not blocked by kinking of the tube (Figure 29-12).

Never assume responsibility for chest drainage or attempt to empty chest bottles. Chest bottles and irrigations require the nurse's or physician's attention.

Careful preoperative preparation and postoperative care can help limit the extent of postoperative discomfort and complication.

The patient must be carefully observed, especially during the first 24 hours, for possible complications. Possible

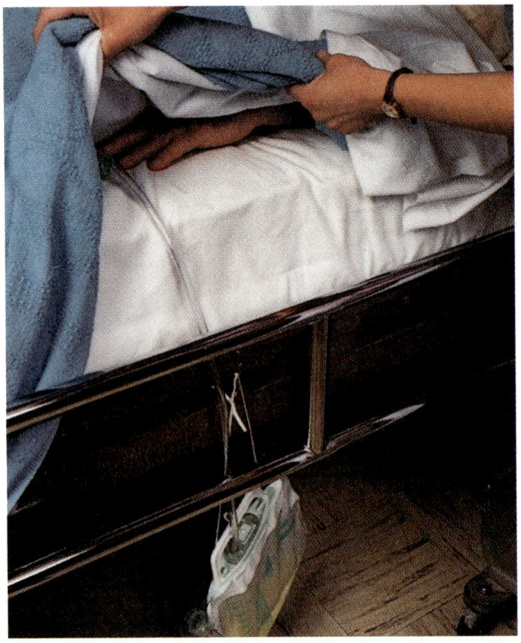

FIGURE 29-12 Monitor the drainage tubes to make sure they are not twisted, kinked, or obstructed.

postoperative discomfort and complications and appropriate nursing assistant actions are summarized in Table 29-1. When the patient has responded sufficiently and vital signs are stable, the patient may be refreshed by:

- washing the hands and face.
- changing the linen.
- being given a light backrub.

The patient is now ready to participate more actively in recovery. Exercises taught in the preoperative period are practiced, including:

- Deep breathing and coughing
- Leg exercises.

Deep Breathing and Coughing

SAFETY *Alert*

Although we routinely encourage postoperative patients to cough and deep breathe, there are a few exceptions you must be aware of. Avoid this procedure with patients who have had eye, nose, or neurologic surgery. Coughing and deep breathing will increase pressure, causing complications in these patients. Check with the nurse if you are unsure of what action to take.

TABLE 29-1 POSTOPERATIVE COMPLICATIONS AND NURSING ASSISTANT ACTIONS

Possible Discomfort	Report	What You Can Do*
Thirst	Patient complaints of dryness of lips, mouth, and skin	Carefully check I&O. Give ice chips or increase fluid intake by mouth with permission. Monitor IV if ordered. Give mouth care. Check BP and pulse. Watch for signs of shock and hemorrhage.
Singultus (hiccups)—intermittent spasms of the diaphragm	Incidence of hiccups	Allow the patient to rest; hiccups can be tiring. Support the incisional area. Assist the patient to breathe into a paper bag.
Pain	Location, intensity, type	Change position. Apply warmth if instructed. Monitor carefully for and report effects of medication given by nurse.
Distention (accumulation of gas in bowel)	Distention of abdomen, complaints of pain	Increase mobility. Insert a rectal tube if instructed and permitted.
Nausea, vomiting	Nausea, character of vomitus	Keep an emesis basin at the bedside. Monitor IV fluids, which are substituted for oral fluids. Give mouth care. Limit fluids by mouth. Encourage the patient to breathe deeply.

continues

TABLE 29-1 *continued*

Possible Discomfort	Report	What You Can Do*
Urinary retention	Amount and time of first voiding. Distention, restlessness, imbalance between I&O	Monitor I&O carefully. Check for distention.
Hemorrhage (excessive blood loss)	Fall in blood pressure; cold, moist skin; weak, rapid pulse; restlessness; pallor/cyanosis; condition of dressing; thirst	Report immediately to nurse. Keep the patient quiet. Check vital signs.
Shock	Fall in blood pressure; weak, rapid pulse; cold, moist skin; pallor	Report immediately to nurse. Keep the patient quiet. Monitor ordered oxygen. Be prepared to follow additional instructions.
Hypoxia (lack of oxygen)	Restlessness, dyspnea, crowing sounds to respirations, pounding pulse, perspiring	Report immediately to nurse. Monitor oxygen, if ordered.
Atelectasis (failure of lungs to expand)	Dyspnea; cyanosis/pallor	Report immediately to nurse.
Wound infection	Increased pain in incisional area; fever; chills, anorexia, increased drainage on dressing	Be observant. Report findings promptly to nurse. Check dressing.
Wound **disruption** (separation of wound edges)	Pinkish drainage. Complaints by the patient that he "feels open," "broken," "given away"	Report immediately to nurse. Keep the patient quiet. Support incisional area.
Pulmonary emboli	Anxiety, difficulty breathing; feelings of "heaviness in chest," cyanosis, chest pain	Keep the patient quiet. Report immediately to nurse. Elevate head of bed.

*In all cases, be prepared to follow the nurse's additional instructions.

Deep breathing and coughing clear the air passages. This helps to prevent postoperative respiratory complications such as pneumonia and atelectasis, which is the collapse of the alveolar air sacs. This may be an uncomfortable task when the patient has a new incision and feels fatigued. (See Procedure 88.) You can best assist the patient by:

- Explaining the value of the exercise and carrying out the following procedure.
- Checking with the nurse to see if medication for pain is to be administered before the exercise. If so, wait for 45 minutes after the medication has been given before carrying out the exercise.
- Learning from the nurse how many deep breaths and coughs should be attempted. The usual number is 5 to 10 breaths and 2 to 3 coughs.
- Using a pillow or binder to support the incision during the procedure.

OSHA *Alert*

Apply the principles of standard precautions when assisting with coughing and deep breathing procedures. If the patient is expelling loose secretions, select and wear appropriate protective equipment, including gloves, gown, mask, and face shield. Show the patient how to contain secretions in a tissue. Assist him or her with handwashing after the activity.

PROCEDURE 88

ASSISTING THE PATIENT TO DEEP BREATHE AND COUGH

1. Carry out beginning procedure actions.
2. Assemble equipment:
   - disposable gloves
   - a pillowcase-covered pillow or binder, if ordered
   - tissues
   - emesis basin
3. Elevate the head of the bed and assist the patient to assume a comfortable semi-Fowler's position.
4. Have the patient place his hands on either side of his rib cage or over the operative site (Figure 29-13). A pillow over the operative site can be used to support an incision during respiratory exercises.
5. Ask the patient to take as deep a breath as possible and hold it for 3 to 5 seconds; then exhale slowly through pursed lips.
6. Repeat this exercise about five times unless the patient seems too tired. If so, stop the procedure and report to nurse.
7. Place the pillow across the incision line as a brace. Have the patient hold the pillow on either side or have the patient interlace fingers across the incision to act as a brace.
8. Pass tissues to the patient and instruct the patient to take a deep breath and cough forcefully twice with the mouth open, collecting any secretions that are brought up in tissues (Figure 29-14).
9. Put on disposable gloves to handle the tissues.
10. Dispose of tissues in an emesis basin.
11. Assist the patient to assume a new, comfortable position.
12. Clean the emesis basin.
13. Remove and dispose of gloves according to facility policy.
14. Carry out procedure completion actions.
15. Report to nurse on the number of times the patient performed each exercise, how the patient tolerated the exercise, and the type and amount of any sputum coughed up.
    - Be sure the patient does not become overly fatigued.
    - Encourage the patient to cough and clear the respiratory passages.
    - Report to your team leader if the patient seems overly fatigued during the procedure.
    - Carefully observe and report any unusual responses such as pain, dizziness, or throat and airway irritation.

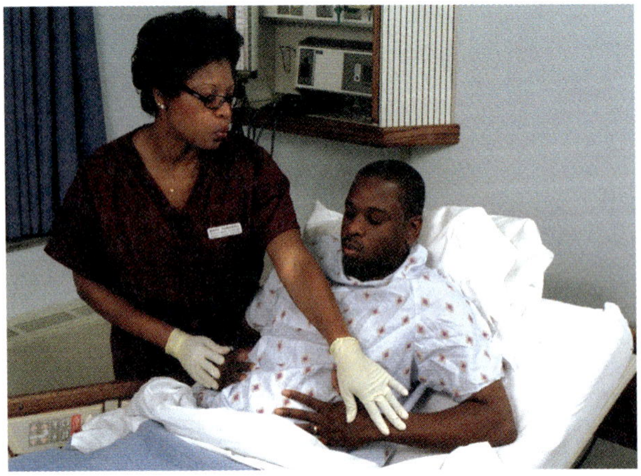

FIGURE 29-13 Encourage the patient to perform deep breathing exercises.

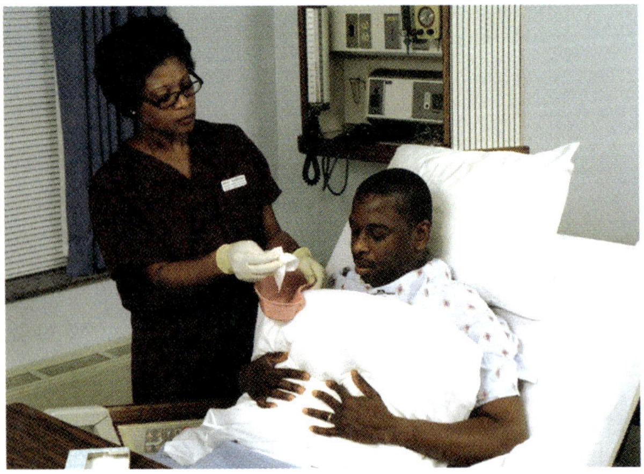

FIGURE 29-14 A pillow helps support the abdomen and splint the incision during coughing and deep breathing.

Leg Exercises

Leg exercises following surgery encourage steady circulation. This helps to prevent another serious complication of the postoperative period—the development of blood clots. (See Procedure 89.)

A blood clot or **deep vein thrombosis (DVT)** could develop in the venous system and block the essential blood flow. A small piece of thrombus broken off (**embolus**) could travel throughout the vascular system and block a vessel in the lungs.

A specific order must be written for leg exercises when there has been surgery on the legs themselves. Otherwise, leg exercises are routinely performed by the patient. If the patient is very weak, you may need to assist.

- Encourage leg exercises and be sure they have been performed.
- Each exercise should be performed 3 to 5 times at least every 1 or 2 hours, and at other times as well.
- Carry out leg exercises as you assist with position changes.
- Apply or reapply support hose (TED) after exercises if ordered.

PROCEDURE 89

PERFORMING POSTOPERATIVE LEG EXERCISES

1. Carry out beginning procedure actions.
2. Explain how the exercise is to be performed. Have the patient:
   a. Brace the incisional area with laced hands.
   b. Rotate each ankle by drawing imaginary circles with the toes.
   c. Dorsiflex (bring toes toward knee) and plantar flex (point toes and foot down) each ankle (Figure 29-15).
   d. Flex and extend each knee.
   e. Flex and extend each hip.
   f. Repeat each exercise 3 to 5 times. Assist as needed.
3. Lower the side rail.
4. Cover the patient with a bath blanket and draw the top bedding to the foot of the bed.
5. Supervise exercises or assist. Apply or reapply support hose (TED hose) as ordered after exercises.
6. Draw bedding up and remove the bath blanket.
7. Fold the bath blanket and place in the bedside stand for reuse.
8. Carry out procedure completion actions. Report to nurse on the number of exercises done and how they were tolerated by the patient.

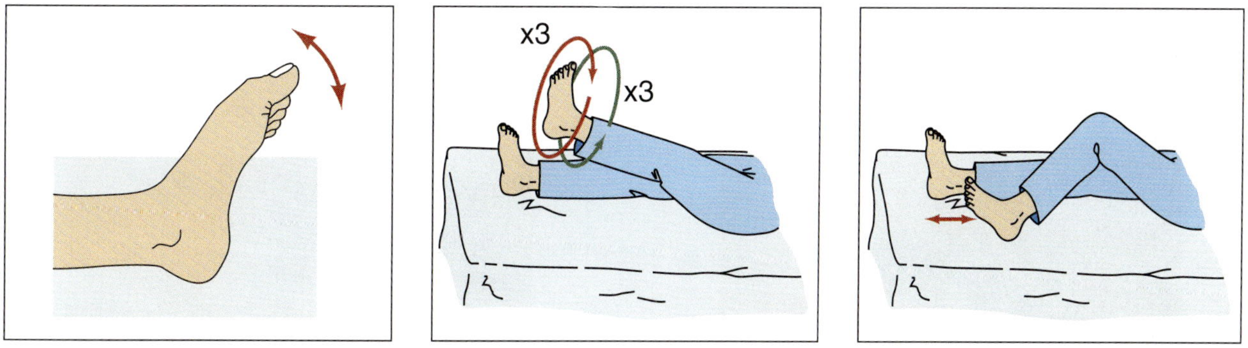

A. Curl the toes down and up. Repeat 5 times.

B. Make circles with the feet clockwise 3 times and counterclockwise 3 times. Repeat 5 times.

C. Slide one leg up and down in bed. Do the same with the other leg. Repeat 5 times.

FIGURE 29-15 Help the patient perform leg exercises to encourage circulation.

Elasticized Stockings

Elasticized stockings, called **TED hose** or **anti-embolism hose**, or Ace bandages that extend from the ankle or foot to calf or mid-thigh, are often applied during the preoperative and postoperative periods to support the veins of the legs. This reduces the incidence of **thrombophlebitis**, which is inflammation of the veins that can lead to blood clots. The stockings must be applied smoothly and evenly before the patient gets out of bed. They should be removed and reapplied at least every eight hours—more often if necessary or as ordered.

Several different types of anti-embolism hose are used. Some have closed toes, but most have an opening near the toe end. The hole is positioned on the top or the bottom of the foot, just proximal to the toes. Check the heel placement on the stocking. By using the heel as a landmark, you will see where to position the hole in the stocking. (Refer to Procedure 90.)

Make sure the legs are dry before attempting to apply the hose. Elastic hosiery fit tightly. An apparatus is used in some facilities to make them easier to apply. If this is not available, the nurse may permit you to dust the legs lightly with baby powder, making the hose easier to apply. Avoid using powders if the patient has respiratory difficulty, a rash, or dressings on the legs.

PROCEDURE 90

APPLYING ELASTICIZED STOCKINGS

1. Carry out beginning procedure actions.
2. Assemble equipment:
   - elasticized stockings of proper length and size
3. Always apply stockings with the patient lying down. Expose one leg at a time.
4. Grasp the stocking with both hands at the top and roll it toward the toe end (Figure 29-16A).
5. Adjust over the patient's toes, positioning the opening at the base of the toes (unless the toes are to be covered) (Figure 29-16B). Remember that the raised seams should be on the outside.
6. Apply the stocking to the leg by rolling it upward toward the body (Figure 29-16C).
7. Check to be sure the stocking is applied evenly and smoothly and that there are no wrinkles (Figure 29-16D).
8. Repeat the procedure on the opposite leg.
9. Carry out procedure completion actions.

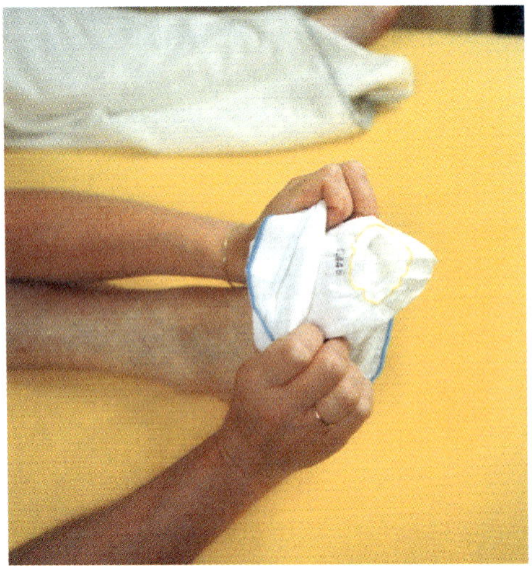

FIGURE 29-16A Gather the stocking and slip it over the patient's toes.

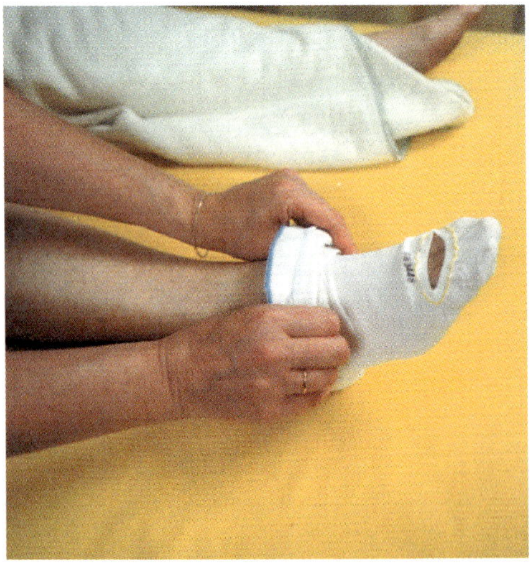

FIGURE 29-16B Position the opening on the top of the foot, at the base of the toes.

continues

PROCEDURE 90

continued

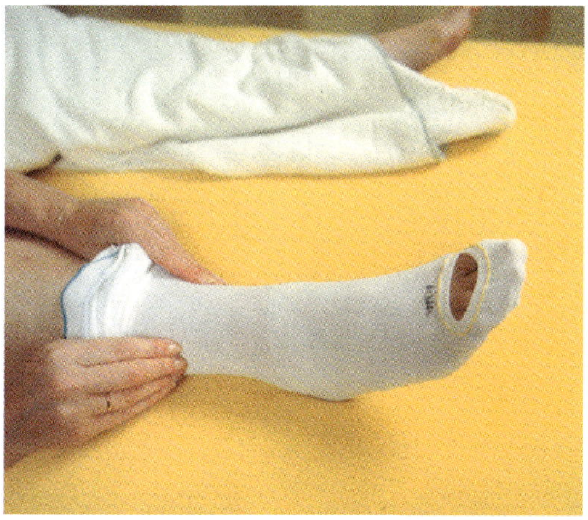

FIGURE 29-16C Draw the stocking smoothly up to the knee.

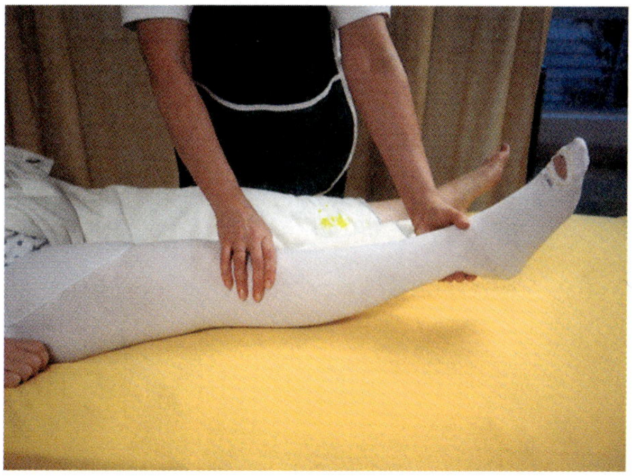

FIGURE 29-16D Check to make sure the stocking is free of wrinkles.

Elastic Bandage

An elasticized bandage (Ace bandage) may be used to keep dressings in place, especially on an extremity or on the head. You may need to remove and reapply the bandage once or twice on your shift. Elastic bandages are also used on nonsurgical patients, to promote venous blood flow in the legs, and for injuries of the musculoskeletal system, to reduce swelling. Elastic bandages come in 2-inch to 6-inch widths and in 4-foot and 6-foot lengths (Figure 29-17). Check with the nurse for the appropriate size bandage. (Refer to Procedure 91.)

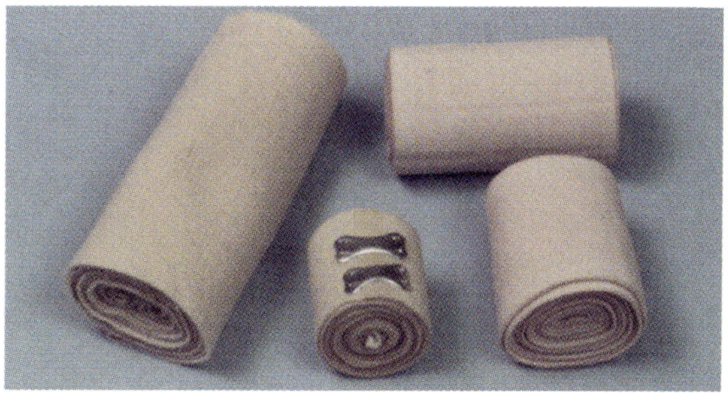

FIGURE 29-17 Elastic bandages are available in a variety of widths.

PROCEDURE 91

APPLYING ELASTIC BANDAGE

1. Carry out beginning procedure actions.
2. Assemble equipment:
   - appropriate size bandage (check for cleanliness)
   - tape, pins, or self-closures that come with bandage
3. Check the area to be bandaged.
   a. If there are lesions or signs of skin breakdown, report to the nurse before bandaging.
   b. If there are dressings underneath the bandage, the nurse may want to check them before you reapply the bandage.
   c. If an arm or leg is to be bandaged, elevate it for 15 to 30 minutes before application to promote venous blood flow.
   d. Apply the bandage so that two skin surfaces do not rub together (toes, fingers, under breasts and arms). Place gauze or cotton to prevent friction (Figure 29-18A).

continues

PROCEDURE 91

continued

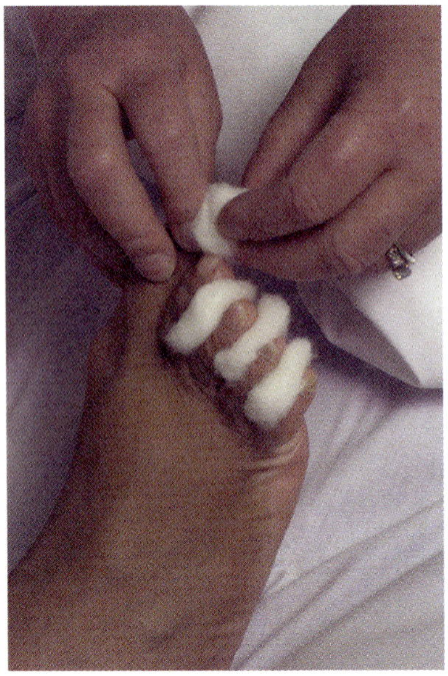

FIGURE 29-18A Pad the toes with cotton to keep them from rubbing together.

4. Hold the bandage with the roll facing upward in one hand and the free end of the bandage in your other hand (Figure 29-18B).
   a. Hold the roll close to the part being bandaged so that pressure is even.
   b. When bandaging an extremity, always wrap from the distal (far) area to the proximal (near) area (Figure 29-18C).
   c. Unroll the bandage as you wrap the body part. Never unroll the entire bandage at once.
5. Use appropriate bandaging technique (Figure 29-18D). Overlap each layer of bandage by one-half the width of the strip.
6. When finished rolling, secure the bandage with pins, tape, or self-closures. Avoid using the clips that may come with the bandage, if possible. They tend to come loose and could injure the patient's skin. The bandage should be smooth and wrinkle-free.
7. Check distal circulation just after the bandage has been applied and once or twice every 8 hours thereafter (check the skin under the bandage for color and temperature; note patient complaints of burning, tingling, or other discomfort).
8. Remove and reapply the bandage every shift, or more often if needed. The patient should have two bandages so that they can be laundered daily. Ask the nurse whether the bandage is to be worn continuously or only at specified times.
9. Carry out procedure completion actions.

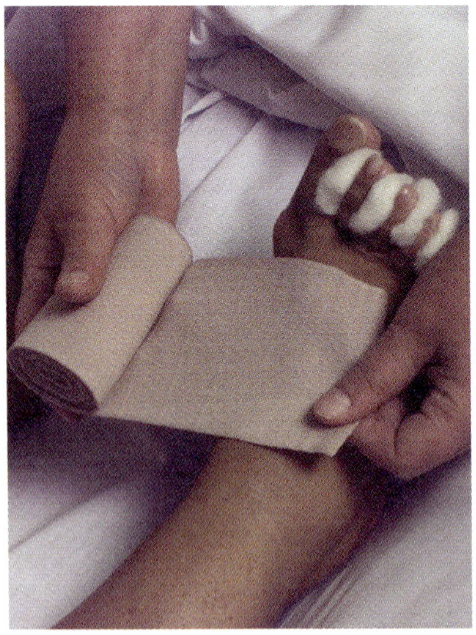

FIGURE 29-18B Hold the bandage with the roll facing upward in one hand and the free end of the bandage in your other hand.

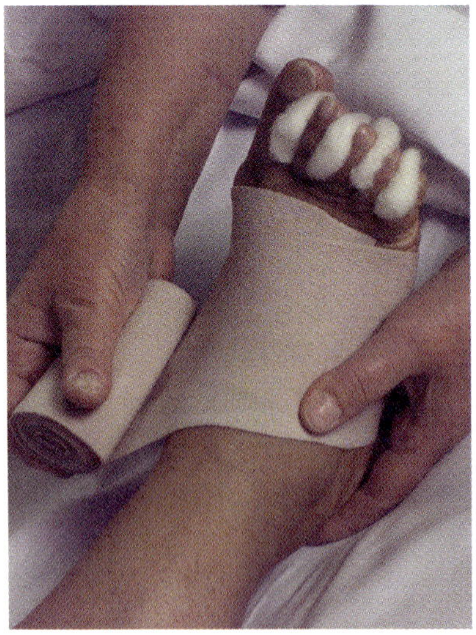

FIGURE 29-18C Always wrap from distal to proximal.

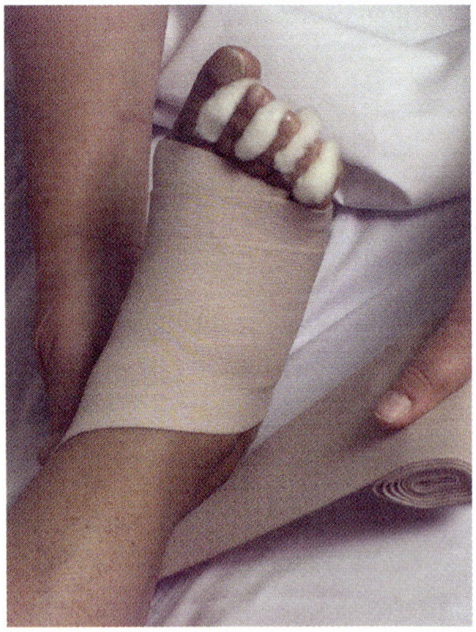

FIGURE 29-18D Use the correct bandaging technique. Overlap each layer of bandage by one-half the width of the strip. The finished bandage should be smooth and wrinkle-free.

Sequential Compression Therapy

Deep vein thrombosis and **pulmonary embolism** (blood clot in the lungs) are serious postoperative complications. Approximately 10% of all patients with DVT die from pulmonary embolism. Most have no symptoms until they develop the pulmonary embolus. The femoral vein, the large blood vessel in the groin, is particularly susceptible to clot formation. Because of the high risk and serious consequences associated with blood clots, the physician may order **sequential compression therapy** to reduce the risk. Sequential compression therapy massages the legs using a milking, wavelike motion.

Pneumatic hosiery (Figure 29-19) are also called *sequential compression hosiery*. This device prevents blood clots by massaging the legs mechanically. Pneumatic hosiery inflate and deflate rhythmically to produce the milking, wavelike massaging motion. The device should not be used on patients with lower leg ulcers, blood clots, massive edema, deformities, infected or broken skin, or arterial disease. Shiny, hairless skin is an indication of arterial problems. If you observe any hard nodules, red areas, or warm areas on the patient's lower legs, inform the nurse before applying the hosiery.

Measuring and Connecting the Hosiery. Before beginning this procedure, you must determine the proper size hosiery for the patient. Do this by measuring the circumference of the patient's upper thigh with a tape measure when she is in bed. Hold the measure snugly against the leg and note the circumference. Compare the measurement with the sizing chart, and select the proper size hosiery.

Familiarize yourself with the hosiery and compression controller if you have not used them before. Open the package and lay the hose on a flat surface. Open them completely, with the cotton lining facing up. Inside you will notice markings for the ankle and knee. When you apply the garment to the patient's leg, line it up exactly with these landmarks. Next, familiarize yourself with the compression controller. The device may have a cooling adjustment. This is used to cool the patient. It is turned off during routine use. Follow your facility policy and the nurse's instructions for activating this feature. The controller also has arrows to adjust the pressure inside the hose. It should be set at 35 mm Hg to 55 mm Hg. The unit may automatically set at 45 mm Hg, the midway point. The nurse will set the unit or instruct you on the setting to use.

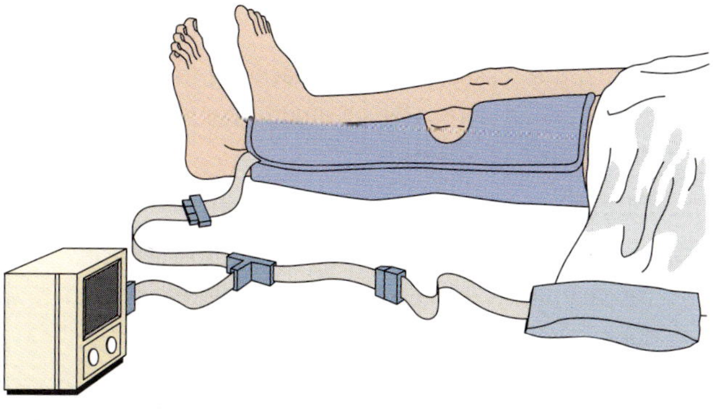

FIGURE 29-19 Pneumatic compression hosiery is used to prevent blood clots.

Both hosiery must be connected to the controller for the unit to operate. Position the arrows on the hose opposite the arrows on the tubing. Push the ends together firmly until you hear a clicking sound. If the patient will be using only one sleeve, such as when she has a cast on one leg, leave the unused sleeve in the sealed plastic bag. Cut a small hole in the bag and connect the tubing.

Applying Pneumatic Hosiery. Before applying the hosiery, palpate the pedal (Figure 29-20A) and posterior tibial pulses (Figure 29-20B). In most facilities, staff mark the location of these pulses with a marker, making a small

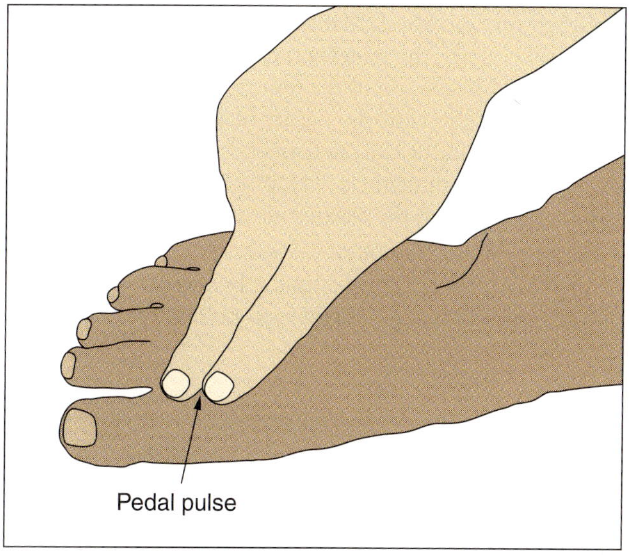

FIGURE 29-20A The pedal (dorsalis pedis) pulse.

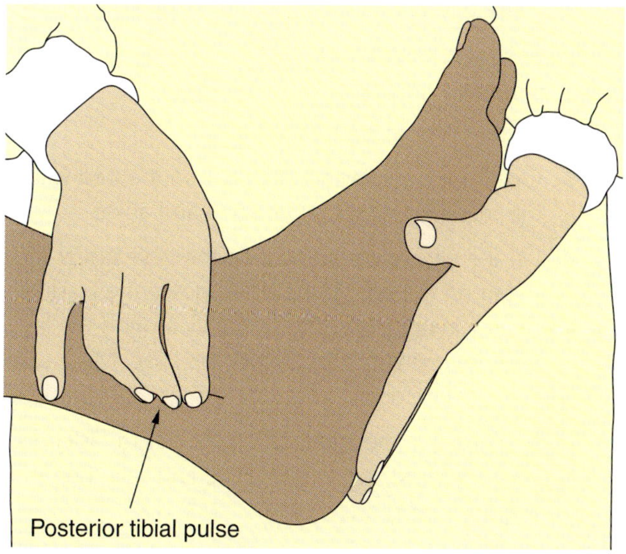

FIGURE 29-20B The posterior tibial pulse.

"X" on the patient's skin. Compare the movement, sensation, and color in both feet. If abnormalities are noted, consult the nurse before continuing. The nurse will assess the patient's legs and check for contraindications. Follow the nurse's instructions.

Pneumatic hosiery may be applied over anti-embolism hose, but both the sleeves and the anti-embolism hose must be smooth and wrinkle-free to reduce the risk of skin breakdown. The device is used 24 hours a day, when the patient is lying down, until the patient is completely ambulatory. It may be removed for bathing and ambulation, then reapplied immediately. The nurse may instruct the patient to perform certain leg exercises while the device is being used. (Refer to Procedure 92.)

Caring for the Patient with Pneumatic Hosiery. The compression controller has a visual display that notes which chamber is inflated. When the chambers decompress, the unit will say "vent." Make sure the audible alarm is turned on, and check that the key has been removed. If the alarm sounds, the panel will display a message code. A card in a slot in the top of the unit will display the numerical message code with the nature of the problem. Follow the directions on the card to correct the problem, or notify the nurse, according to facility policy. The hose deflates automatically when the alarm sounds.

Turn the power off and remove the hose every 4 hours. Disconnect the sleeves from the tubing by releasing the latches on each side of the connectors, then pulling the connectors apart. Observe the skin under the device, and provide skin care as ordered. Avoid massaging the legs. Massage may dislodge a blood clot, which will quickly migrate to the lungs. Inform the nurse when you will be removing the device so that he or she can assess the patient's legs.

Use of the hose will be discontinued when the patient is fully ambulatory. The unit is not disposable. Clean and store the device according to facility policy after use, or return it to central supply.

Documentation. Follow your facility policy for documenting use of the pneumatic compression device. You may be asked to document the procedure, pulse checks in the feet, skin color, the patient's response, and the settings, including use of the alarm and cooling settings.

Initial Ambulation

Some time after surgery, a patient is permitted to sit up with the legs over the edge of the bed. This position is called **dangling**.

- Watch carefully for signs of fatigue or dizziness (**vertigo**).
- Assist the patient to assume the position slowly.

The first **ambulation** (walk) is usually short. The patient usually dangles for a short time before ambulating. Dangling is an important part of postoperative care because it stimulates circulation and helps prevent the formation of blood clots (thrombi). (Refer to Procedure 93.)

PROCEDURE 92

APPLYING PNEUMATIC COMPRESSION HOSIERY

1. Carry out beginning procedure actions.
2. Assemble equipment:
   - hosiery of proper size
   - compression controller
3. Open the hose, laying them flat on the bed with the markings opposite the knee and ankle.
4. Lift the patient's leg, and slide the hose under it. Begin on the side of the leg opposite the plastic tubing. Wrap the sleeve smoothly around the leg with the opening in front, over the knee. Make sure there are no dents, folds, or creases in the garment.
5. Beginning at the ankle, fasten the Velcro fasteners securely. Next, secure the ankle and calf, then the thigh.
6. Check the fit by inserting two fingers between the sleeve and the patient's leg. The fit should feel snug and secure, but not tight.
7. Wrap the other leg in the same manner, beginning on the side opposite the plastic tubing. After wrapping the leg, check the fit.
8. Attach the plastic tubing on each leg to the compression controller by lining up the arrows on the tubing.
9. Plug the controller in and turn on the power.
10. Remain with the patient for one complete cycle (usually 60 to 90 seconds) to ensure that she tolerates the procedure.
11. Carry out procedure completion actions.

PROCEDURE 93

ASSISTING THE PATIENT TO DANGLE

1. Carry out beginning procedure actions.
2. Assemble equipment:
   - bath blanket
   - pillow
3. Check the pulse (see Unit 19).
4. Lower the side rail nearest to you. Lock the bed at the lowest position.
5. Drape the patient with a bath blanket and fanfold the top bedcovers to the foot of the bed.
6. Gradually elevate the head of the bed.
7. Help the patient to put on a bathrobe.
8. Place one arm around the patient's shoulders and the other arm under the knees.
9. Gently and slowly turn the patient toward you. Allow the patient's legs to hang over the side of the bed.
10. Roll a pillow and tuck it firmly against the patient's back for support.
11. After putting slippers on the patient, ask the patient to swing the legs.
12. Have the patient dangle as long as ordered.
    - If the patient becomes dizzy or faint, help him lie down.
    - Report to the supervising nurse immediately.
13. Check the patient's pulse.
14. Rearrange the pillow at the head of the bed. Remove the patient's bathrobe and slippers.
15. Place one arm around the patient's shoulders and the other arm under the knees. Gently and slowly swing the patient's legs onto the bed.
16. Check the patient's pulse. Lower the head of the bed and raise the side rails.
17. Carry out procedure completion actions. Remember to wash your hands, report completion of your task, and document the time dangled (duration), pulse, and the patient's reaction.

SAFETY *Alert*

Remain next to the patient during the first dangling and ambulation. For patient safety, do not turn your back or leave the bedside. These precautions will probably not be necessary as the patient recovers and gains strength. Use common sense and follow the care plan and the nurse's instructions.

The patient may need assistance the first few times he stands up to ambulate. The anesthesia and medications administered before, during, and after surgery may affect the patient's balance, endurance, and strength. There may be drainage tubes or an intravenous feeding that must be moved with the patient (Figure 29-21).

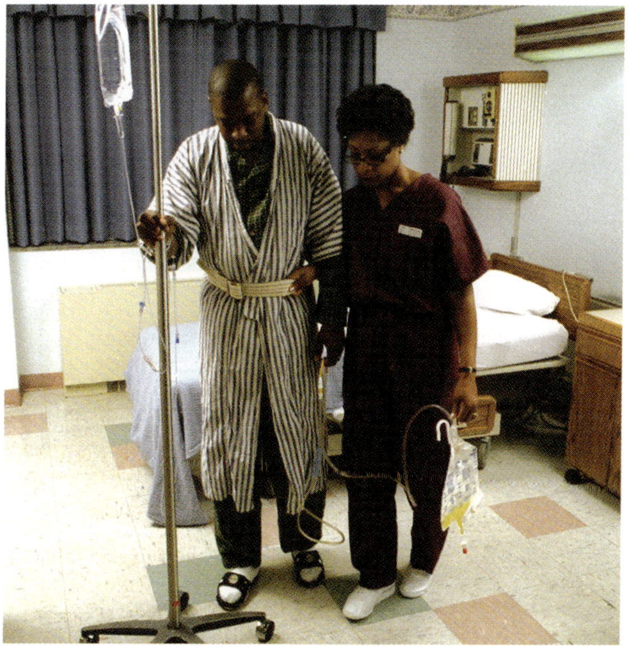

FIGURE 29-21 Drainage tubes and intravenous lines may be in place after surgery. Carefully move these with the patient.

guidelines *for*

Assisting the Patient in Initial Ambulation

- Check with the nurse to see if a transfer belt can be used.
- Assist the patient to sit on the edge of the bed with the bed in low position.
- Assist the patient to put on footwear appropriate to the floor surface. Never allow a patient to ambulate with bare feet or socks.
- Take the patient's pulse before and after standing. If there is more than 10 points difference, return the patient to bed and inform the nurse.
- If the patient becomes dizzy or faint, return the patient to bed and inform the nurse.
- Walk with the patient as instructed in Unit 17.

REVIEW

A. True/False.

Mark the following true or false by circling T or F.

1. T F Patients receiving local anesthetics lose consciousness during the surgery.

2. T F When spinal anesthetics are used, patients may lose feeling and movement in their legs.

3. T F Preoperative teaching has little effect on the patient's postoperative recovery.

4. T F You help build patient confidence when you explain what you plan to do when carrying out procedures.

5. T F Skin preparation involves shaving an area larger than the size of the incision.

6. T F The nursing assistant has no responsibilities related to the patient while the patient is in surgery.

7. T F Patients should be dangled without incident before initial ambulation.

8. T F Patients who are unconscious following surgery should not be left alone.

9. T F Nosocomial infections do not affect the cost or length of hospital stay.

10. T F Patients who are faced with surgery are often filled with apprehension and fears.

B. Matching.

Choose the correct word or phrase from Column II to match each item in Column I.

Column I	Column II
11. ____ inflammation of a vein leading to clot formation	**a.** ambulation
12. ____ period before surgery	**b.** orifice
13. ____ medicine given to prevent pain	**c.** nosocomial
14. ____ hospital-acquired	**d.** PACU
15. ____ opening	**e.** umbilicus
16. ____ walking	**f.** vertigo
17. ____ dizziness	**g.** anesthesia
18. ____ lung collapse	**h.** preoperative
19. ____ blood clot	**i.** aspiration
20. ____ area where immediate postoperative care is given	**j.** embolism
	k. atelectasis
	l. thrombophlebitis

C. Multiple Choice

Select the one best answer for each of the following.

21. When assisting a patient with coughing and deep breathing exercises, teach him or her to

a. inhale through the nose.
b. inhale through the mouth.
c. exhale through the nose.
d. keep the hands behind the neck to expand the lungs fully.

22. The main purpose of coughing and deep breathing exercises is to prevent
- **a.** pneumonia.
- **b.** dizziness.
- **c.** pain.
- **d.** anxiety.

23. The main purpose of pneumatic compression hosiery is to prevent
- **a.** edema.
- **b.** pneumonia.
- **c.** blood clots.
- **d.** pain.

24. Pneumatic compression hosiery are contraindicated
- **a.** in patients who have had abdominal surgery.
- **b.** if the patient is using oxygen.
- **c.** if a rash or open areas are present.
- **d.** for patients with a cast on one leg.

25. Check the postoperative patient's vital signs every
- **a.** 5 minutes for the first hour, then every 15 minutes for 4 hours.
- **b.** 15 minutes for an hour, then every 30 minutes for an hour.
- **c.** 30 minutes for 4 hours, then every 8 hours for 72 hours.
- **d.** 60 minutes for 4 hours, then every 4 hours for 16 hours.

D. Nursing Assistant Challenge.

Mr. Dovetski is a 47-year-old patient on the surgical unit. He has had abdominal surgery. When he is returned to his room from surgery, you note that he has a Foley catheter, an intravenous feeding running, dressings on the abdominal incision, and elastic stockings. Think about what procedures you will include in your care of Mr. Dovetski.

26. How often will you take his vital signs? Which procedures are included in vital signs? What are the "normal" ranges for each vital sign for a person of this age? If there are changes in the vital signs, these changes may be indications of what complications?

27. What observations will you make regarding the Foley catheter? Why do you think he has the catheter in place?

28. What observations will you make regarding the intravenous feeding? Why do you think the physician ordered an IV?

29. You know you will need to have Mr. Dovetski perform deep breathing exercises and deep coughing. Why is this important? How can you help him do the exercises with the least discomfort?

30. Why do you think he has elastic stockings on? How often should you take the stockings off and reapply them? What do you need to remember when putting the stockings back on?

31. How will you report any complaints of pain?

32. How will you check for bleeding from the incision?

EXPLORING THE WEB

Description	Location
Articles on preoperative and postoperative infection control	*http://www.infectioncontroltoday.com*
Nutrition and the surgical patient	*http://www.facs.org*
Perioperative client needs	*http://www.delmarhealthcare.com/pdf/0766824527.pdf*
Perioperative nursing slides	*http://www.indstate.edu*
Postoperative care of children	*http://www.musckids.com*
Preoperative and postoperative care procedures	*http://www.delmarhealthcare.com/olcs/acello/11checklists.pdf*
Procedure for transferring a patient to the OR	*http://www.cc.nih.gov/nursingnew*
Association of PeriOperative Registered Nurses	*http://www.aorn.org*
Guidelines for Preventing Surgical Site Infection	*http://www.nailm.com*
Nursing Specialties Perioperative Nursing	*http://allnurses.com/Nursing_Specialties*
PowerPoint Slides: Perioperative Care	*http://nursing.uaa.alaska.edu*

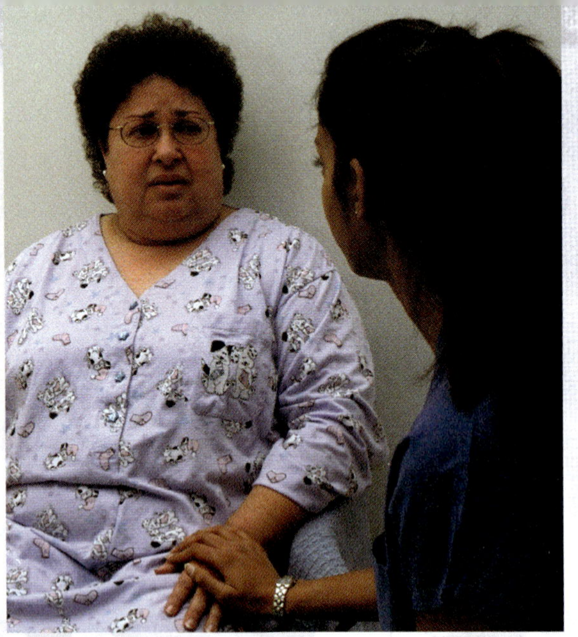

unit **30**

Caring for the Emotionally Stressed Patient

objectives

After completing this unit, you will be able to:

- Spell and define terms.
- Define mental health.
- Explain the interrelatedness of physical and mental health.
- Understand mental health as a process of adaptations.
- Identify commonly used defense mechanisms.
- Describe ways to help patients cope with stressful situations.
- Identify the signs and symptoms of maladaptive behaviors that should be documented and reported.
- List nursing assistant measures in providing care for patients with adaptive and maladaptive reactions.
- Identify professional boundaries in relationships with patients and families.

vocabulary

Learn the meaning and the correct spelling of the following words and phrases:

adaptation	denial	mental illness	reality orientation
agitation	depression	paranoia	repression
alcoholism	disorientation	professional boundaries	stressors
coping	enabling	projection	suicide
defense mechanisms	hypochondriasis	reaction formation	suppression
delusions	maladaptive behavior		

INTRODUCTION

There are varying degrees and differing aspects of health. A person who is in poor physical health may be mentally healthy. Because of good mental health, the person may be self-reliant and able to make decisions and to live an effective, productive life (Figure 30-1).

In contrast, a person with good physical health may not be able to cope with and adapt to changes. This inability limits the person's chances to participate successfully in society.

MENTAL HEALTH

Mental health means exhibiting behaviors that reflect a person's **adaptation** or adjustment to the multiple stresses of life, such as:

- Illness
- Hospitalization
- Loss of a loved one
- Loss of a job
- Loss of status

Stresses or **stressors** are situations, feelings, or conditions that cause a person to be anxious about his or her physical or emotional well-being. Good mental health leads to positive adaptations. Poor mental health is demonstrated by maladaptive behaviors (behaviors that harm the person or her adjustment).

Physical and mental health are interrelated. Physical illness is often preceded by stressful life situations. Ill health causes emotional stress. It is easy to understand that each of these factors contributes to the total health pattern of each person.

Ways of **coping** with (handling) stressful situations (Figure 30-2) are learned early in life. As people grow, they find the behaviors that work best for them. They learn to use those behaviors to reduce stress and protect self-esteem. These coping patterns become part of the individual's habitual responses, becoming more and more obvious as the person ages.

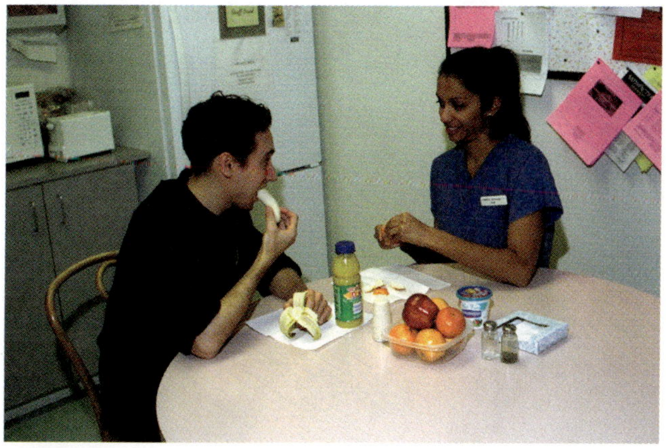

FIGURE 30-1 A mentally healthy person leads a productive life.

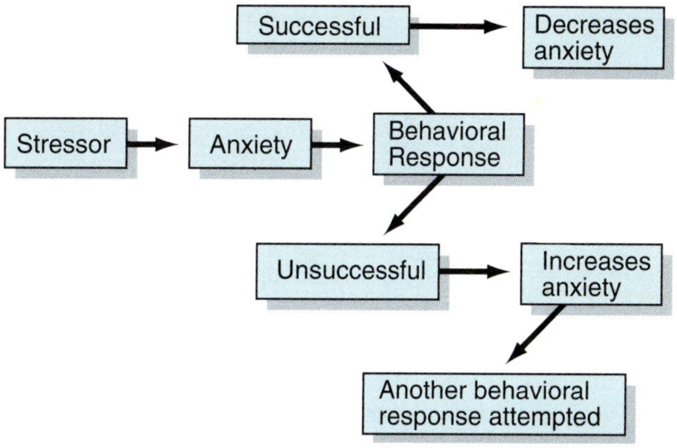

FIGURE 30-2 Each individual has different ways of coping with stress.

DEFENSE MECHANISMS

When any person feels unable to cope with stress and the situation threatens self-esteem, the person tends to act in protective ways. These ways are called **defense mechanisms**. A diagnosis of cancer, for instance, may be so overwhelming that a person must temporarily defend himself against acknowledging the truth. Everyone uses these defense-oriented behaviors from time to time to protect themselves. You use them. Patients use them. Your coworkers use them.

You must recognize and understand the need to use defense mechanisms. Do not be critical of their occasional use. Most people do not use one mechanism all the time. They usually rely on a combination of defenses. They may not even be aware that they are behaving in a defensive way.

Defensive behavior becomes harmful only when it is the major means of coping with stress. In such cases, the person continuously avoids recognizing and responding to reality with problem-solving methods. The person's stress is temporarily reduced, but the stressor (feeling or situation) is not resolved. Such a person needs counseling from a trained mental health provider.

Some of the commonly used defense mechanisms include:

- **Repression**—The involuntary exclusion from awareness of a painful or conflict-creating thought, memory, feeling, or impulse. For example, a woman has a lump in her breast, but refuses to go to a physician for examination and diagnosis. She has recently lost her husband, her house, and her job. She feels that she cannot "acknowledge" any other illness or crisis, so she unconsciously represses the knowledge of the lump in her breast. She is not going to take the chance that the lump may be cancer. She cannot face the possibility of a terminal disease.
- **Suppression**—This mechanism differs from repression because the person is aware of the unacceptable feelings and thoughts but deliberately refuses to acknowledge them. For example, a man becomes immobilized with the fear of rejection by his wife if he tells her he has a diagnosis of AIDS. Therefore, he consciously suppresses

the knowledge of the AIDS diagnosis because he cannot handle the anxiety associated with telling his wife.

- **Projection**—A person's own unacceptable feelings and thoughts are attributed to others. The person blames others for his own shortcomings. For example, a person blames his wife or family for his alcoholism and loss of jobs. He projects his failings onto his wife and children.
- **Denial**—Blocking out painful or anxiety-producing events or feelings. This is one of the most common defenses against the stress of diagnosis and illness. For example, a patient with very high blood pressure refuses to stop smoking. She continues to eat a diet high in fats. She cannot deal with her fear of disability and unemployment, so she refuses to accept the seriousness of her condition.
- **Reaction formation**—A person using this defense mechanism represses the reality of a situation and then behaves in a manner that is the exact opposite of the real feelings. For example, a woman dislikes one nursing assistant but is fearful that if she expresses that feeling, the assistant will be less caring. This patient may be overly friendly and cooperative with that assistant.

Other adaptive behaviors are as follows:

- Displacement—Substituting an object or person for another and behaving as if it were the original object or person. *Example:* Being angry with the nursing assistant because another patient is annoying.
- Identification—Behaving like another person whom one holds as an ideal. *Example:* Speaking to coworkers with the same tone the supervisor uses with you.
- Compensation—Excelling in one area to make up for feelings of failure in another. *Example:* The nursing assistant who overachieves in the skill area because her ability to read written directions is poor.
- Conversion—Offering a socially acceptable reason to avoid an unpleasant situation. *Example:* The nursing assistant who calls saying she cannot report for duty because she has the flu, when she is just tired from staying up too late.
- Fantasy—The use of imagination to solve problems. *Example:* The supervisor criticizes the nursing assistant, who then daydreams of a time when she is the head of nursing and can fire the supervisor.
- Undoing—A method of reversing something wrong that was done. *Example:* The person who used his hands to hurt another may wash his hands repeatedly to try to undo the deed.

ASSISTING PATIENTS TO COPE

Here are some ways to help patients become better able to cope and adapt:

- Be a good listener.
- Try to determine the source of stress so it can be removed and the stress reduced.

DIFFICULT *Situations*

Patients with coping and behavior problems usually have a behavior management care plan that lists steps to follow when certain problems are exhibited. Become familiar with the care plan. Implement the approaches in the order listed. Modify your behavior in response to the patient's behavior by monitoring how the patient responds to you, then adjusting your approach to achieve results. Vary routines and equipment, if necessary. Put yourself in the patient's shoes and try to understand what is happening.

- Be sensitive to nonverbal messages (body language) that may give clues to the source of stress.
- Treat the person with respect, recognizing him as a unique individual.
- Understand the behavior in the same way the patient is viewing it, without labeling the behavior and passing judgment.
- Let the patient know that you are reliable and that you respect her privacy and feelings.
- Never argue, enter into a power struggle, or debate with a patient, even when you know the patient is wrong.
- Be supportive of the person's own attempts to overcome the stress (Figure 30-3).

Remember that illness, age, and separation from family and home are major stress factors.

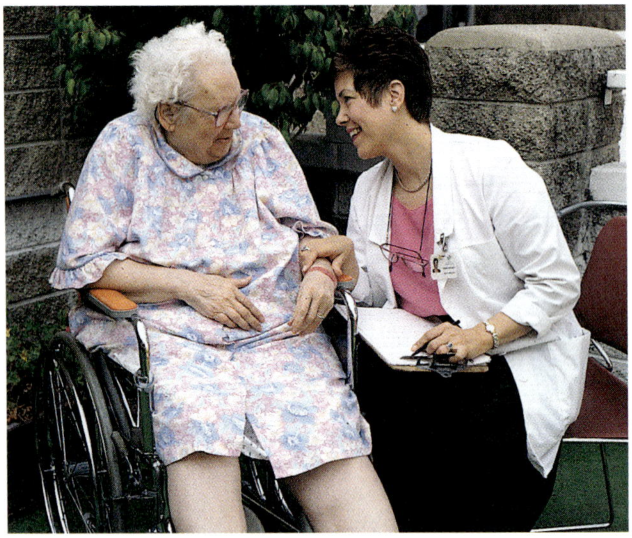

FIGURE 30-3 Staff can help patients find acceptable ways of coping with stress.

THE DEMANDING PATIENT

In every nursing care situation, you will meet patients who are very demanding. This can be a difficult experience for everyone if it is not handled correctly.

Being demanding is another way in which patients show their frustration. It is a coping behavior. Patients who are very demanding are usually frustrated by their loss of control. To be successful in caring for these patients, the nursing assistant must:

- Try to learn and understand the factors that are causing the demanding behavior.
- Show that you care about the patient's situation, but keep control of your emotions.
- Maintain open communications by listening to the patient's words and by being sensitive to the patient's body language.
- Provide opportunities that allow the patient to regain some control by making choices.
- Be consistent in the manner of care. This builds the patient's sense of security (Figure 30-4).
- Do not take the patient's demands personally.
- Report observations to the supervisor with suggestions for changes in the care plan.

ALCOHOLISM

Some people use alcohol as a means of coping with stress. The National Institute for Alcohol Abuse reports that two-thirds of the senior population uses alcohol. Fifteen percent of them become alcoholics. **Alcoholism** is regarded as a disease. Factors that contribute to the excessive use of alcohol include:

- Retirement
- Lowered income

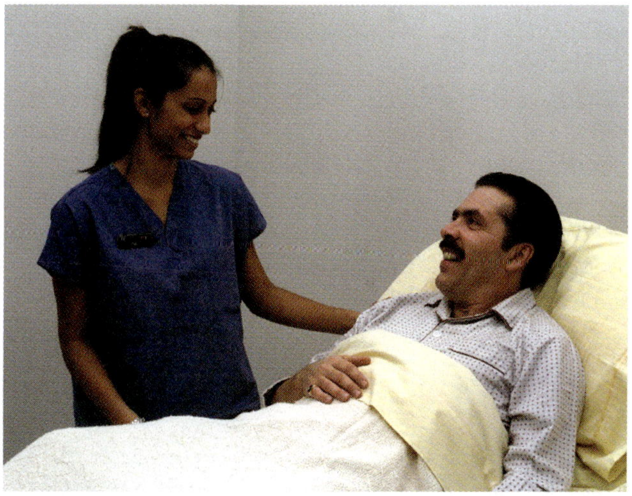

FIGURE 30-4 Being attentive and consistent builds the patient's security.

- Grief
- Loss of spouse and/or friends
- Loneliness
- Stress in the family
- Decline in health
- Pain

Alcohol toxicity may be associated with an acute onset of:

- Altered levels of awareness
- Mild confusion
- Progressive stupor
- Acute delirium
- Disorientation similar to that seen in irreversible brain syndrome

Alcohol slows down brain activity. It impairs mental alertness, judgment, physical coordination, and reaction time—increasing the risk of falls and accidents.

Alcohol can affect the body in unusual ways. It can make it difficult to diagnose diseases and conditions of the cardiovascular system. It can mask pain that might otherwise serve as a warning sign of heart attack. Alcohol can also produce:

- Symptoms similar to dementia
- Forgetfulness
- Reduced attention
- Restlessness
- Impatience
- Agitation
- Confusion

Alcohol is a drug. It mixes unfavorably with many other drugs (Table 30-1). The use of alcohol can cause some drugs to metabolize more rapidly, producing exaggerated responses. Such drugs include:

- Anticonvulsants
- Anticoagulants
- Antidiabetic drugs
- Diuretics

The alcoholic in withdrawal feels depressed and defensive. He needs to identify the stressors that bring on his need for alcohol and to find new ways of coping. This process takes professional skill, but you can:

- not allow the alcoholic to manipulate you.
- listen with empathy (Figure 30-5).
- reflect the person's ideas and thoughts.
- be sure alcohol is not available.
- be consistent in the limits that have been set.

Care of the intoxicated patient includes:

- caution during feeding to prevent choking or strangling.
- supervision of activities to prevent injury and falls.
- safety checks during bathing to prevent burns.
- close supervision if there is confusion or delirium.

TABLE 30-1 COMMON ALCOHOL-DRUG INTERACTIONS

Drug Taken by Patient	Effects to Report
Narcotics	Increased central nervous system (CNS) depression with acute intoxication
Salicylates	Gastrointestinal bleeding
Sedatives and psychotropic drugs	Increased CNS depression with acute intoxication
Barbiturates	Decreased sedative effect after chronic alcohol abuse
Chloral hydrate	Prolonged hypnotic effects
Chlordiazepoxide (Librium, Librax)	Increased CNS depression
Chlorpromazine (Thorazine)	Increased CNS depression
Diazepam (Valium)	Increased CNS depression
Oxazepam (Serax)	Increased CNS depression
Antihistamines	Increased CNS depression
Antabuse	Flushing, vomiting, excessive sweating, hyperventilation, confusion, and drowsiness

Problem drinkers and alcoholics have a good chance for recovery. Getting help should start with the family physician, a member of the clergy, the local mental health association, or the local chapter of Alcoholics Anonymous.

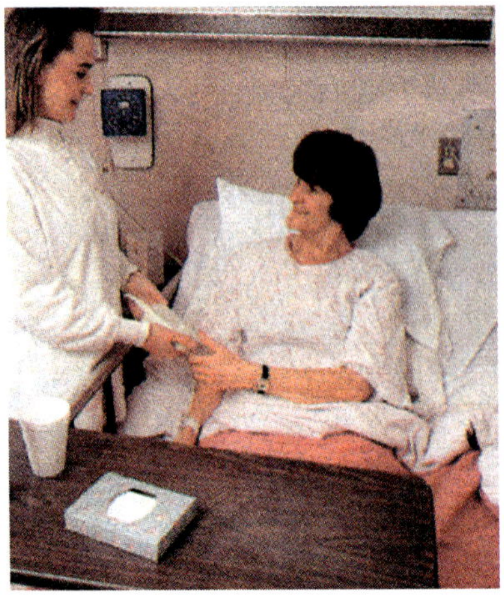

FIGURE 30-5
Listen with empathy.

MALADAPTIVE BEHAVIORS

Mental illness or **maladaptive behavior** occurs when behaviors and responses disrupt the person's ability to function smoothly within the family, environment, or community.

You must be careful about labeling anyone as mentally ill. Even when an official diagnosis of mental illness has been made, take care not to stereotype the patient.

Remember that stereotypes are often associated with *myths* (false beliefs). It is far better to view the person as an individual who is demonstrating poor behavioral responses.

As a nursing assistant, you need to be aware that sometimes signs and symptoms such as fatigue, loss of appetite, insomnia, and pain may reflect either physical or emotional stress. Note and report any unusual behavior or symptoms. Be careful, however, to be objective. Do not make judgments about your findings.

Remember also that confusion, disorientation, and aggressive behavior may only be temporary responses to a fever, drug interaction, or a full bladder. Continuation of such behavior may be the result of organic brain changes. Blaming and judging a patient is inappropriate and unhelpful.

Assessing the Patient's Behavior

An initial assessment of the patient's mental and emotional state will be made by the licensed care provider. Because you make frequent contact with the patient, you can make a valuable contribution to the nursing assessment process by making careful and sensitive objective observations.

Report observations regarding:

- Physical responses related to eating, personal hygiene, sleeping, participation in activities, or any strange or unusual behaviors
- Emotional responses related to interactions between the patient and yourself or between the patient and other patients, emotional outbursts, or inappropriate responses
- Patient behavior as it relates to judgment and affects memory, comprehension, and orientation

When working in long-term care, you will find many people whose coping ability has failed and so are demonstrating maladaptive behaviors. The many losses these people have suffered add to their inability to cope. Physical problems make dealing with reality more difficult.

Common maladaptive responses result in:

- Depression
- Disorientation or delirium
- Agitation
- Paranoia

Tips: Reward patients for positive behavior. Behavior that is rewarded is usually repeated. The goal is to show the patient a healthy way of directing energy. Verbal praise, positive feedback, and other signs of approval are rewards. Nonverbal rewards such as a hug, smile, or pat on the back may also be used, when appropriate. Snacks and privileges are sometimes used as rewards.

Depression

Depression is the most common functional disorder in older people (Figure 30-6), but younger people also may experience depression. Depression may be shown in a variety of ways:

- Preoccupation with constipation
- Flatulence
- Bad taste in the mouth
- Burning tongue
- Vague oral discomforts associated with dentures
- Burning on urination
- Pain in lower abdomen
- Crying spells
- Trouble sleeping (insomnia)
- Excessive sleep
- Loss of appetite or increased appetite
- Significant weight loss or weight gain
- Fatigue
- Headaches
- Backaches
- Stiff joints
- Apathy
- Impaired concentration
- Lethargy
- Agitation
- Poor personal hygiene
- Feeling of dejection
- Less interest in sex
- Depressed mood most of the day, nearly every day (irritability in children)

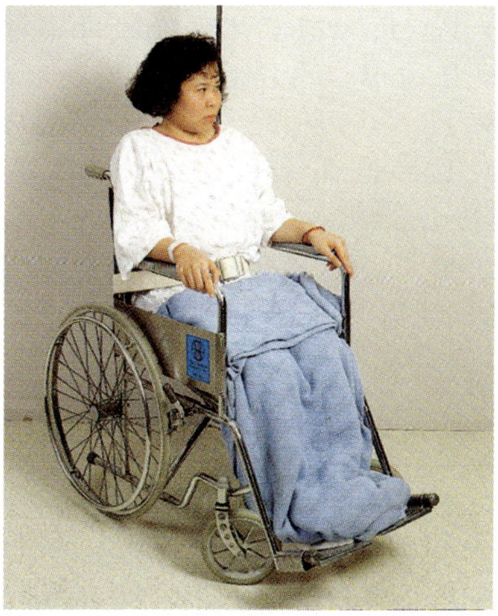

FIGURE 30-6 Withdrawal is common when a person is depressed.

- Markedly diminished interest or pleasure in almost all activities, most of the day and nearly every day
- Psychomotor agitation or retardation
- Feelings of worthlessness or guilt
- Recurrent thoughts of death or suicide

Depression is often masked by symptoms that make it seem as though the patient is physically ill. Your observations are doubly important because a patient who is depressed may actually have minor or major illnesses. These infirmities may in turn cause depression. Remember, physical and mental health are interrelated.

Some drugs that are used to treat actual physical illness in the elderly may cause depression. They are:

- Digitalis
- Reserpine
- Inderal
- Diuretics
- Most of the antihypertensive drugs

If your patient is receiving any of these drugs, be alert for signs of depression. If the depression is drug-induced, it will be relieved when the drug is withdrawn.

Severely depressed patients may be treated with:

- Antidepressants
- Electroshock therapy (in severe cases)
- Talk therapy

A mental health clinical nurse specialist, psychologist, or psychiatrist will direct and support the staff efforts.

When depression is severe, suicidal thoughts and attempts are a real possibility. You must be sensitive to the possibility of such a situation and report and document your observations. The suicidal patient must be carefully protected. Watch for and report:

- Change in response such as deepening depression or sudden elevation of mood
- Evidence of withdrawal or secretiveness
- Sudden loss of a support system (such as the death of a family member)
- Repeated, prolonged, or sporadic refusal of food (oral or through nasal tubes), care, medications, or fluids
- Hoarding of medication (stockpiling of pills)
- Sudden decision to donate body parts to a medical school
- Changes in behavior, especially episodes of depression, screaming, hitting, throwing things, or a sudden failure to get along with family, friends, or peers
- Sudden interest or disinterest in religion
- Purchase of a gun
- Purchase of razor blades and hiding them
- Statements such as: "I just want out," "I want to end it all," "I'll never get well," "I'm going to kill myself," or "You would be better off without me."

guidelines *for*

Assisting the Patient Who Is Depressed

- Reinforce the person's self-concept by emphasizing her continued value to society and helping the patient to use the support systems that are available (Figure 30-7).
- Do not act in a pitying way. This only validates the person's depressed feelings.
- Make sure physical supports, such as eyeglasses and hearing aids, are in place. These help the person to focus on reality.
- Report all complaints so that actual physical problems may be identified and corrected rather than being attributed to the depression.
- Provide the person with activities within her limitations to help her think beyond herself. For example, engage the person in some meaningful activity such as reading, making puzzles, or conversing with others (Figure 30-8).
- Avoid tiring activities.
- Use simple language and speak slowly when giving instructions.
- Monitor elimination carefully; constipation is common.
- Provide fluids frequently, because the depressed patient may be too preoccupied to drink.
- Be alert to the potential for **suicide** (the taking of one's own life).

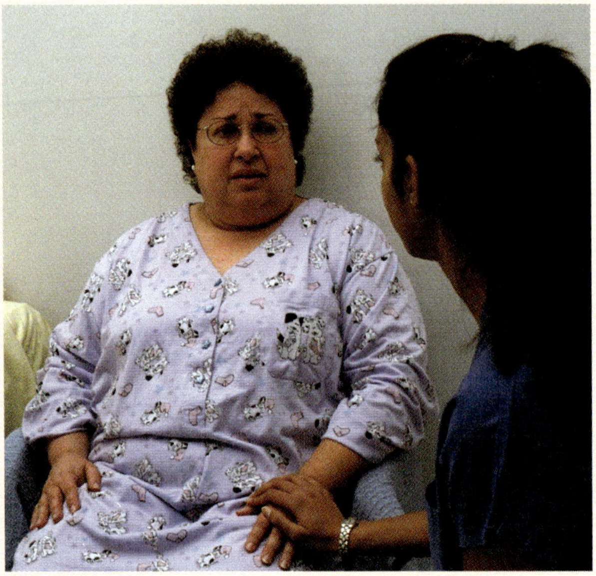

FIGURE 30-7 Try to reinforce the depressed person's sense of self-worth.

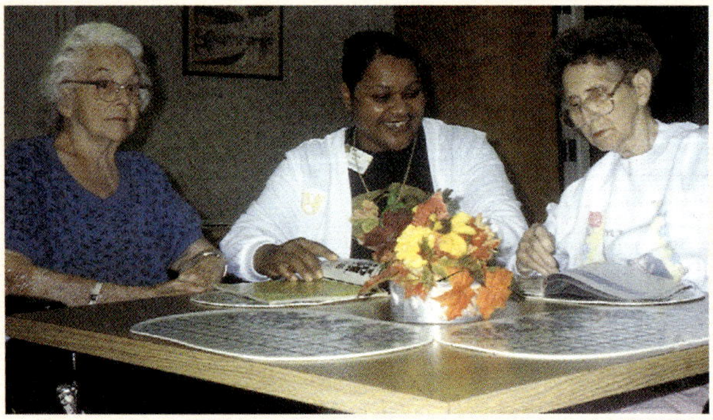

FIGURE 30-8 Socializing with others may help a person who is depressed.

- Increased use of alcohol and drugs
- Behavioral manifestations of anger, hostility, belligerence, loss of interest, or inability to concentrate
- Inability to do simple tasks, confusion, slurred speech, or retarded motor skills
- Deep preoccupation with something that cannot be explained

Nursing Care of a Patient with the Potential for Suicide. Never assume that a suicide attempt is a means of getting the attention of the staff or family. At least 15% of people who try to commit suicide do it again. Keep in mind the at-risk individuals. These include:

- White males over the age of 65 who live alone
- The very old (75 years and above)
- Persons with a recent diagnosis of a terminal illness
- Persons with unrelieved chronic pain
- Those suffering the sudden loss of a spouse
- The elderly with recent multiple losses

Be aware that the suicide rate is higher in acute medical units than it is on psychiatric units. Most of the suicides occur while the patient is under the supervision of a health provider, who frequently either misses or ignores the clues of suicide. Suicide attempts may occur either when the patient is successfully recovering or is getting worse. It is the responsibility of all staff members to observe their patients carefully and immediately report any signs of depression and/or suicide. You should:

- Be observant for clues to suicide attempts, and report them to the appropriate person.

- Be consistent in approaches and care.
- Encourage the patient to review his life, emphasizing the positive aspects.
- Give the patient hope while being realistic (Figure 30-9).
- Work to restore the person's self-esteem, self-worth, and self-respect, to preserve positive self-concept.
- Help the patient find a support network within the family, religious groups, and self-help groups.
- Make the person feel accepted as a unique, valued person.
- Never ignore the person's statements or threats about suicide.

Disorientation (Disordered Consciousness)

Disorientation is a condition in which a person shows a lack of reality awareness with regard to time, person, or place (Figure 30-10). In some cases, the disorientation is mild, sometimes severe; sometimes temporary but at times prolonged. It is important to report patient behavior, actions, and responses. The disoriented person has impaired:

- Judgment
- Memory
- Comprehension
- Orientation

Physical ailments and stresses that can bring about a disoriented state include:

- Recovery from surgery
- Pneumonia
- Myocardial infarction
- Renal infection
- Head trauma
- Organic brain disease
- Fevers

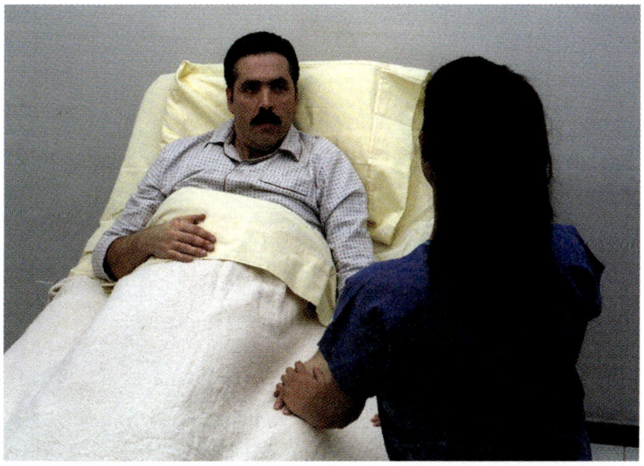

FIGURE 30-9 Be hopeful but realistic with a depressed person who is at risk of suicide.

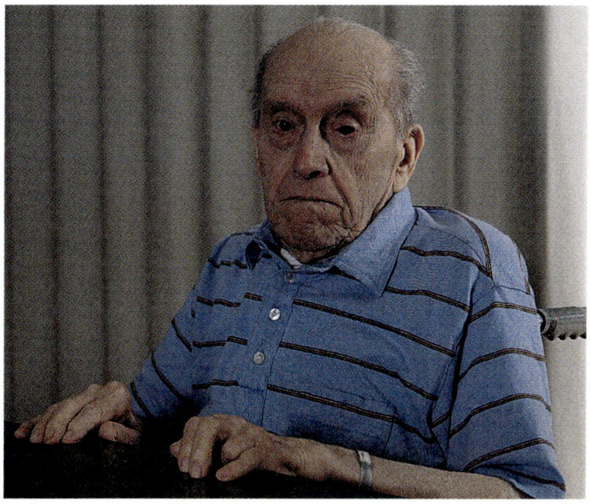

FIGURE 30-10 The person who is disoriented lacks awareness of reality.

- Dehydration
- Malnutrition
- Drug interaction

The signs and symptoms that identify the disoriented person are:

- Inability to think clearly
- Bewilderment
- Faulty memory
- Inability to follow directions
- Misinterpretation of stimuli
- Confusion about time
- Confusion about place
- Confusion about who he or she is

Nursing Assistant Responsibilities. The nursing assistant must realize that disoriented people cannot be responsible for their actions or for protecting themselves adequately. The patient's sensory misinterpretations (delusions or hallucinations) may put others at risk. The disorientation does not allow the patient to take action for self-protection. *Protection of the patient is the most important nursing responsibility.* In addition, you should:

- Be calm and gentle when approaching the patient. Disoriented patients are startled by even minor stimuli.
- Give instructions slowly, clearly, and in simple words.
- Give only one instruction at a time.
- Provide activities of short length that do not require much concentration.
- Build the patient's self-esteem with the reward of positive comments.
- Assist patients to participate in reality orientation activities (Figure 30-11). **Reality orientation** is making the disoriented patient aware of person, place, and time by visual reminders, activities, and verbal cues. See the guidelines for reality orientation activities.
- Maintain a constant, limited routine.

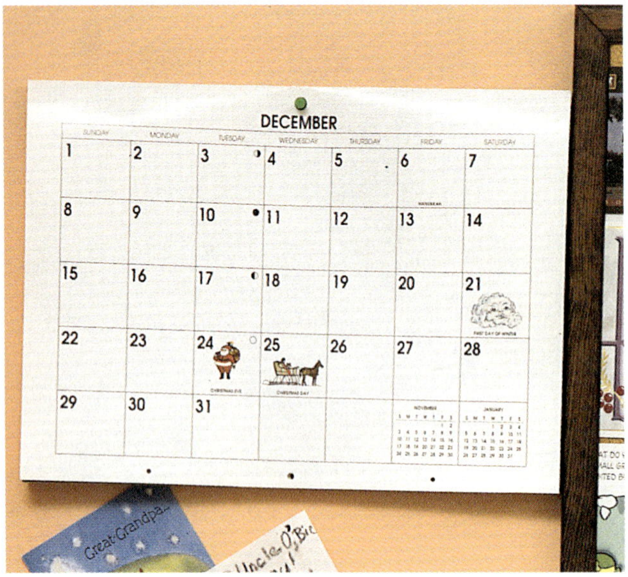

FIGURE 30-11 Calendars and clocks may help maintain orientation.

guidelines *for* Reality Orientation

- Address the patient by name with each contact.
- Identify yourself to the patient each time there is contact.
- Avoid reinforcing illusions, delusions, or hallucinations.
- Keep glasses, dentures, and hearing aids in place.
- Speak often with the patient.
- Be patient and repeat instructions.
- Keep clock and calendar in view.
- Encourage the presence of and refer to familiar objects.
- Post an activity board and draw attention to it.
- Call attention to color-coding of facility areas.
- Introduce day, date, time, season, and weather into conversation.

- Use restraints only when absolutely necessary and with a physician's order, making sure all safety practices are followed. Medications that chemically restrain patient responses and the presence of a friend or family member may make physical restraints unnecessary.
- Reduce disorientation by keeping rooms well lighted, cool, and quiet. Also, provide reality orientation according to the nursing care plan.
- Make sure patients wear glasses and hearing aids, if used.

To maintain a safe environment for disoriented patients:

- Keep all sharps, such as knives, out of reach.
- Remove and store valuable or breakable items. If patient is at home, make sure the family knows where you put these items.
- Use sturdy chairs and couches.
- Put rails on windows that are close to the floor.
- Provide adequate lighting.
- Protect stairways with gates.
- Do not permit poisonous plants.
- Control matches and smoking materials.
- Supervise use of stoves and appliances.
- Keep all medications out of reach.

Agitation

Agitation is defined as inappropriate verbal, vocal, or motor activity due to causes other than disorientation or real need. It includes behavior such as:

- Aimless wandering
- Pacing
- Cursing
- Screaming
- Repeatedly asking the same question
- Spitting
- Biting
- Fighting or arguing constantly
- Demanding attention
- Restlessness
- Constant activity

Agitation is a significant problem for the elderly, their families, and the nursing staff. It is probably one of the foremost management problems in acute care hospitals, in home care, and in long-term care facilities.

The major factors contributing to agitation are:

- Noise
- Frustration at loss of control
- Feelings that the patient's space has been invaded
- Loneliness and need for attention
- Unresolved personal difficulties in the patient's past
- Drug interactions
- Organic brain disease
- Boredom
- Behavior of others around the patient
- Depression
- Constipation
- Restraints
- Too much sensory stimulation

Study this list carefully, because your awareness can lead to early intervention. Early intervention can often prevent serious problems.

guidelines *for*

Managing the Patient Who Is Agitated

- Do not argue with or confront the person.
- Make the environment safe (secure the windows and lock the doors).
- Make sure each patient wears an identification bracelet or patch, and that it is fastened securely.
- Keep a recent photo of the patient in case the patient wanders off.
- Notify the physician, the administrator, the family, or the police department if the patient wanders away from his unit, facility, or home.
- Assign the patient brief tasks.
- Engage the patient in games, walks, swimming, and other activities if not contraindicated. These should be activities that enhance the patient's self-esteem.
- Use bean-bag seats and rocking chairs in the parlors of the nursing home or the patient's home.
- Care for the patient—watch for injuries.
- Engage the patient in conversations and in reality therapy or remotivation groups.
- Engage the patient in short-term activities. Realize that the patient's attention span is short. Thus, the patient needs rewards for short-term activities.
- Prevent the patient from becoming exhausted.
- Carefully monitor the patient's activities, because the agitated patient is at risk for falls and injuries.

Hypochondriasis

The patient suffering from **hypochondriasis** imagines or magnifies each physical ailment. Some authorities feel that hypochondriasis is an expression of depression and is one way these individuals reduce stress. These patients need reassurance and understanding but should not be encouraged to focus or believe in their supposed illnesses. However, the staff must be careful not to overlook real illness when it occurs, just because they have become used to hearing the patient complain. Nursing assistants should report all complaints and never make a judgment that a patient is a hypochondriac.

Paranoia

Paranoia is another extreme maladaptive response to stress. It is characterized by a heightened, false sense of self-importance and delusions of being persecuted. **Delusions** are false beliefs about oneself, other people, and events. People with paranoia believe that everyone is against them. When treating the paranoid patient, you should:

- Find ways to reduce the patient's feelings of insecurity and misunderstanding.
- Keep the person as involved as possible in reality activities.
- Report and document observed responses to medication and psychotherapy.
- Monitor nutrition and fluid balance—these patients often refuse to eat or drink for fear of poisoning.
- Observe sleep patterns—the person may be fearful of being harmed while sleeping.
- Be direct and honest in all interactions.
- Not support any misconceptions or delusions that the person exhibits.
- Never argue with anyone who has delusions. It can trigger a serious confrontation.

PROFESSIONAL BOUNDARIES

As a nursing assistant, you must stay within certain **professional boundaries** in the care of each patient. Boundaries are unspoken limits on the physical and emotional relationship with patients. They limit and define how a health care worker acts with patients. They involve using your best behavior, ethical practices, and good judgment when caring for patients. Respecting boundaries is one way that you will act appropriately when on the job.

It takes good judgment and experience to identify boundaries and keep from crossing them. When driving down the road, you do not see the boundary lines when you cross from one city to the next. Professional boundaries are the same way. They exist, but you cannot see them. You must be aware of boundaries and take active steps to avoid crossing them. You may cross them inadvertently or deliberately, thinking you are meeting a patient's need.

Being aware of boundaries is particularly important when caring for patients with emotional stress. Patients who are at risk of inappropriate relationships with health care workers usually have one or more of these risk factors:

- mental or emotional problems
- poor impulse control
- marital problems
- low self-esteem

- loneliness and/or need for caring

Health care workers who are at greatest risk for inappropriate relationships and boundary problems usually have one or more of these risk factors:

- family or marital problems
- näivete
- low self-esteem
- loneliness, feelings of isolation
- addiction (chemical or sexual)
- financial problems
- stress, burnout

To avoid crossing professional boundaries, strive to act professionally, as you were taught in class. Avoid putting yourself in a position in which you think and act as a family member or friend. You must use good judgment and determine the amount of contact and assistance that are right for the patient. Too much or too little contact can be unhealthy for both the assistant and the patient. Treat all patients professionally. Consult your charge nurse if you are uncertain.

Ethical Behavior with Patients and Families

As a nursing assistant, patients expect you to act in their best interests and treat them with dignity. You do this by not taking advantage of a patient's situation and by avoiding inappropriate involvement in the patient's personal and family relationships. Some relationships with patients and families are not healthy for the patient or the nursing assistant. It is not always easy to recognize unhealthy relationships until it is too late. Once you have crossed over a boundary line, it is difficult to turn back. Be aware of boundaries at all times, and strive to keep your relationships professional.

Actively work to find a balance in your relationships with patients and families. If any of the following occur, you are probably crossing professional boundaries and may be in a relationship danger zone:

- Discussing your personal problems with the patient or family members
- Being flirtatious with a patient, including making sexual innuendos, telling jokes that are sexual in nature, or using offensive language
- Discussing your feelings of sexual attraction with a patient
- Feeling that you may become involved in a sexual relationship with the patient
- Keeping secrets with a patient and becoming defensive when someone questions your relationship or involvement in the patient's personal life
- Thinking you are immune from having an unhealthy relationship with a patient
- Believing that you are the only nursing assistant who can meet the patient's needs
- Spending an inappropriate amount of time with the patient, including off-duty visits or trading assignments with others to be with the patient
- Reporting only partial information about the patient to your charge nurse, because you fear disclosing unfavorable information or secrets the patient has told you
- Feeling that you must protect the patient from other health care workers and always siding with the patient's position

Questions to ask yourself that will help you decide whether you are crossing a professional boundary line are listed in Table 30-2. If you have trouble staying objective, or think you may cross a boundary, seek help from your charge nurse, pastor, or another professional person whom you trust.

Consequences of Boundary Violations

Boundary violations lead to inappropriate relationships with patients or families. These cloud your clinical judgment, and may lead to serious consequences, such as inappropriate sexual relationships. They often carry over into your personal life. The improper relationship may cloud your judgment, causing you to do things that you would not ordinarily do (such as stealing from your employer). There are many serious personal, legal, and professional consequences to inappropriate relationships. For your own well-being, be aware that professional boundaries exist, and actively take steps to keep from crossing them.

TABLE 30-2 QUESTIONS TO ASK
• Is this in the patient's best interest?
• Whose needs are being served?
• Does this action benefit me rather than the patient?
• Will this affect the care I am delivering?
• Should I be concerned or consult with a colleague?
• How would the patient's family view this?
• How would I feel telling a colleague about this?
• Am I treating this patient differently from other patients?
• Does this patient mean something special to me?
• Am I taking advantage of the patient?
• Am I comfortable about documenting this in the medical record?
• Is this a violation of nursing assistant ethics?

Enabling

Enabling behavior is reacting to a patient in a manner that shields the person from experiencing the full impact or consequences of his or her actions or behavior. Enabling behavior differs from helping behavior in that it allows the person to be irresponsible. As a paraprofessional health care worker, the nursing assistant should be aware of enabling behavior and avoid it when caring for patients, particularly those with mental and emotional problems. By learning and respecting professional boundaries, you will avoid helping others inappropriately. Likewise, you must learn to set limits for yourself and prevent patients from crossing into your own personal territory. Enabling behavior with patients creates dependency rather than moving the patient toward independence and good mental health. Methods of enabling patients that you should avoid include:

- Protecting the patient from the natural consequences of his or her behavior
- Keeping secrets about a patient's behavior from others
- Making excuses for a patient's behavior
- Taking steps to get a patient out of personal trouble
- Blaming others for the patient's behavior
- Seeing the patient's problems as a result of something else
- Giving money to patients
- Attempting to control patients' lives and activities
- Doing things for the patient that she should do herself

Strive to keep your behavior in the zone of helpfulness (Figure 30-12) to avoid crossing professional boundaries and enabling patients.

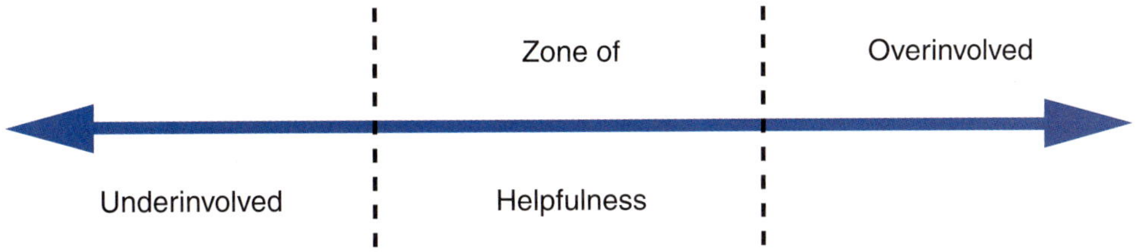

FIGURE 30-12 Keep your relationship with patients and families in the zone of helpfulness.

guidelines *for*

Assisting Patients with Behavior Problems

- Follow the care plan.
- Control your own responses and reactions.
- Be a good communicator.
- Avoid lying to the patient.
- Avoid making promises you cannot keep.
- Avoid discussing facility or staff problems with the patient. If the patient complains, inform the nurse or other appropriate person.
- Protect the safety of the patient and others.
- If the care plan tells you to respond to a specific behavior, apply the approaches when the behavior starts. Do not wait until the patient loses control.
- Use good communication and listening skills.
- Practice empathy.
- Attempt to learn the cause of the behavior. Communicate with other team members.
- Remove the cause (or trigger) of the behavior, if known.
- Let others know if you discover an approach that works.
- Modify your own behavior in response to the patient's behavior.
- Watch the patient's response to your approaches. Adjust your approach, equipment, routine, and other care, if necessary.
- Discuss family, friends, or other pleasant information with patients. This provides a source of strength, comfort, and support.
- Meet the patient's physical needs.
- Give patients as much control as possible. Offer choices in care and routines. Encourage them to direct their own care.
- Be patient. Control your reaction to the patient. Make sure your body language does not send the wrong message.
- Be happy. Smile. Make sure your body language sends a positive message. Positive behavior is contagious.

REVIEW

A. True/False.

Mark the following true or false by circling T or F.

1. T F Mental health refers to the adaptations a person makes to the multiple stressors of life.
2. T F Stressors are the physical and emotional problems that a person encounters throughout life.
3. T F Defense mechanisms are used only by mentally unhealthy persons.
4. T F If you know that the patient is wrong about something she is saying, it is proper to debate the issue with the patient.
5. T F The best way to handle the demanding patient is by trying to determine the underlying factors causing the patient's distress.
6. T F Very few senior adults use alcohol and even fewer become alcoholics.
7. T F The use of alcohol impairs mental alertness, judgment, reaction time, and physical coordination.
8. T F It is dangerous for a person to drink alcohol when taking other medications.
9. T F Alcohol is a drug.
10. T F When intoxicated, a person could choke on food.
11. T F Alcoholics have a poor chance for recovery.
12. T F Maladaptive behaviors reflect the failure of usual defense mechanisms.
13. T F Depression is the least common of the functional disorders in older people.
14. T F The depressed patient needs to be encouraged not to be overactive.
15. T F Dehydration can lead the patient into a state of disorientation.
16. T F The disoriented patient needs a stimulating environment.
17. T F It is best to give a disoriented patient one instruction at a time.
18. T F If a patient threatens suicide, you need not be concerned.
19. T F The white male who is over age 65 and living alone is at high risk for suicide.
20. T F It is the responsibility of only the licensed staff to guard against suicide attempts.
21. T F Suicides are attempted only by patients in psychiatric institutions.
22. T F The patient who is agitated may ask the same question repeatedly.
23. T F Agitation is a significant problem for the elderly, their families, and facility staff.
24. T F Paranoia is a maladaptive response that usually requires medication and psychotherapy.
25. T F Paranoid individuals believe that others are out to get them.

B. Matching.

Choose the correct word from Column II to match each phrase or statement in Column I.

Column I	Column II
26. ____ conscious refusal to recognize the reality of a situation	a. repression
27. ____ shielding a patient from the consequences of behavior	b. suppression
28. ____ blocking out painful or anxiety-producing events or feelings	c. projection
29. ____ involuntary exclusion of the awareness of reality	d. denial
30. ____ lack of awareness of reality	e. professional boundaries
31. ____ handling stressful situations	f. enabling
32. ____ attributing one's own failing to another	g. coping
33. ____ invisible lines that define relationships with patients	h. disorientation

C. Multiple Choice.

Select the one best answer for each of the following.

34. The patient tells you that her doctor says she has AIDS, but she knows that isn't possible. She most likely is using the defense mechanism of
    - a. repression.
    - b. displacement.
    - c. projection.
    - d. denial.
35. The best way to enhance the patient's capability to cope with an unpleasant situation that has developed with another patient is to
    - a. tell him to ignore it.
    - b. let him know he can talk to you safely.

c. tell him everyone has problems, his aren't so important.

d. suggest he discuss it with his clergyperson.

36. The patient who refuses to eat or drink because she is convinced that she is being poisoned is suffering from

a. paranoia.

b. depression.

c. agitation.

d. disorientation.

37. The patient is depressed. You can best help him by

a. pitying him.

b. keeping him from interacting with others.

c. agreeing that he probably deserves the way he feels.

d. stressing his continued value to society.

38. The best way to help the patient remain oriented to reality is to

a. keep glasses in the bedside stand so they will not be broken.

b. isolate the patient.

c. place a clock and calendar nearby.

d. explain things in detail.

39. The person holding a doll and acting as if it were a baby probably is experiencing

a. repression.

b. denial.

c. projection.

d. displacement.

40. Agitation may be demonstrated by

a. talking a lot.

b. boredom.

c. smiling for no reason.

d. repetitive questions.

41. Professional boundaries

a. apply only to licensed nursing personnel.

b. involve assisting patients with activities of daily living.

c. are set out in the job description.

d. are unspoken limits on relationships with patients.

42. Health care workers who are at risk of having inappropriate relationships with patients

a. are usually friendly and happy.

b. may have financial or marital problems.

c. exercise regularly to relieve stress.

d. occasionally drink alcoholic beverages.

43. Enabling behavior

a. is used when caring for patients who require total care.

b. involves orienting patients to person, place, and time.

c. is used to help patients relieve stress.

d. shields an individual from the consequences of his or her actions.

D. Nursing Assistant Challenge.

You are assigned to care for Mr. Simonson, who was recently diagnosed with diabetes. He is a top executive in a large corporation and has a wife and three adult children. He is learning how to administer his insulin, how to plan his diet, and how to test his blood sugar. He has been very quiet and keeps his eyes closed most of the time, although he is not sleeping. One day as you enter the room, he screams at you to get out and then picks up his water pitcher and throws it. Think about what you learned in this unit about human behavior as you consider these questions.

44. What examples of nonverbal communication is Mr. Simonson displaying?

45. Do you think he is using defense mechanisms to cope with his diagnosis? If so, which ones?

46. If Mr. Simonson displays this kind of behavior again, what would be an appropriate response from the nursing staff?

47. How would you document this episode?

48. How can the nursing staff show respect and concern for this patient?

EXPLORING THE WEB

Description	Location
About Alcoholism	*http://www.alcoholism.about.com*
American Council on Alcoholism	*http://www.aca-usa.org*
American Psychiatric Nurses' Association	*http://www.apna.org*
Enabling Behavior	*http://www.cita1.com*
—Early Warning Signs of Enabling	*http://shalomplace.com*
National Council on Alcoholism and Drug Dependence	*http://www.ncadd.org*
National Institute on Alcohol Abuse	*http://www.niaaa.nih.gov*
Nursing Specialties Psychiatric Nursing	*http://allnurses.com*
Online Dictionary of Mental Health	*http://human-nature.com/odmh*
Professional boundaries	*http://www.ncsbn.org*
—Maintaining Healthy Boundaries in Professional Relationships	*http://www.mnnurses.org*
—Professional Boundaries for Therapeutic Relationships	*http://www.crnm.mb.ca*
—Professional Boundaries—Guidelines	*http://www.nbv.org.au*
—Professional Boundaries in Health Care Relationships	*http://www.cpo.on.ca*
—Pushing the Limits of Professional Boundaries	*http://www.nurseweek.com*
Tools for Coping with Life's Stressors	*http://www.coping.org*

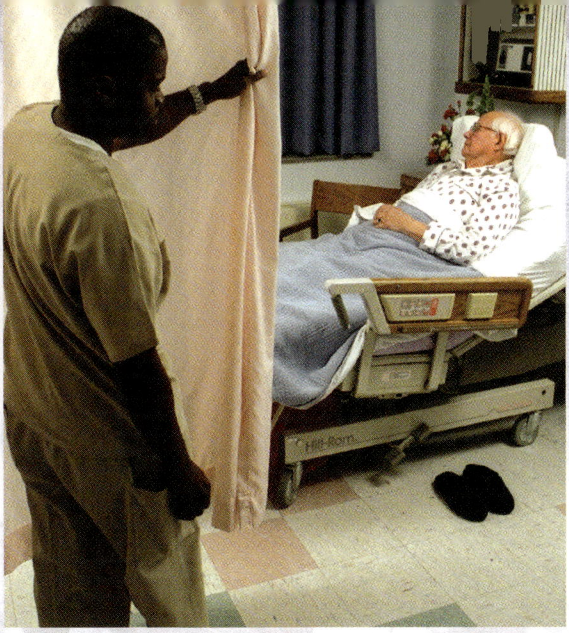

unit **31**

Death and Dying

objectives

After completing this unit, you will be able to:

- Spell and define terms.
- Describe how different people handle the process of death and dying.
- Describe the nursing assistant's responsibilities for providing supportive care.
- Describe the spiritual preparations for death practiced by various religious denominations.
- Describe the hospice philosophy and method of care.
- List the signs of approaching death.
- Demonstrate the following procedure:
  - Procedure 94 Giving Postmortem Care

vocabulary

Learn the meaning and the correct spelling of the following words and phrases:

acceptance
advance directive
anger
autopsy
bargaining
cardiac arrest
cardiopulmonary resuscitation (CPR)
critical list
denial
depression
DNR
durable power of attorney for health care
harvested
hospice care
life-sustaining treatment
living will
moribund
no-code order
postmortem
postmortem care
rigor mortis
Sacrament of the Sick
supportive care
terminal

INTRODUCTION

Death is the final stage of life. It may come suddenly, without warning, or it may follow a long period of illness. It sometimes strikes the young but it always awaits the old. As a nursing assistant, you will be providing care throughout the period of dying and into the after-death (**postmortem**) period. Accepting the idea that death is the natural result of the life process may help you respond to your patient's needs more generously.

The concept of death and dying is handled differently by different people (Figure 31-1). There are many reactions to the diagnosis of a **terminal** (life-ending) illness:

- Some patients may have had time to prepare psychologically for their deaths. They may accept or be resigned to the inevitable.
- Some may actually look forward to relief from the pain and emotional burden of a long illness and await death calmly.
- Some may be fearful or angry and demonstrate moods that swing from outright denial to depression.
- Others may reach out, trying to verbalize feelings and thoughts of an uncertain future.
- In others, despair and anxiety may give way to moments of active hostility or periods of searching, groping questions.

None of the reaction states are predictable and no patient falls into one rigid pattern or another. You must accept the patient's behavior with understanding, interpret the patient's very real need for family support, and support the family in meeting their own needs during this adjustment period.

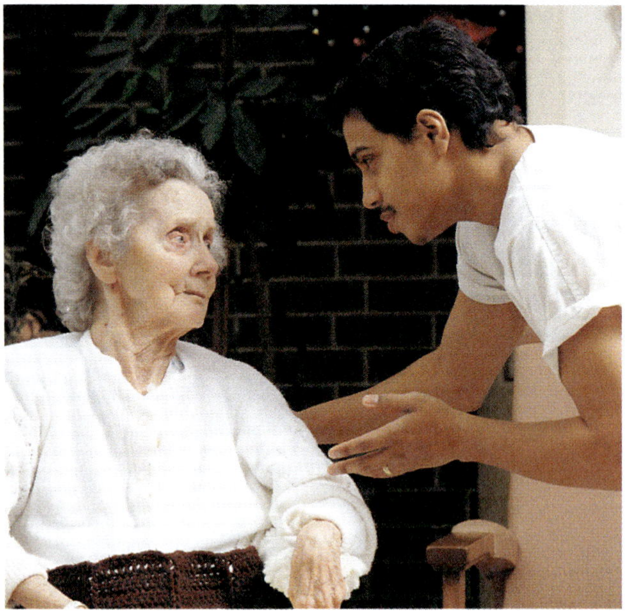

FIGURE 31-1 Each person handles death differently.

COMMUNICATION *Highlight*

Health care workers may feel helpless when caring for a dying patient. Remember that active listening is a means of therapeutic communication. Listening to a patient's concerns shows honest and caring concern for the patient. Using touch can also communicate caring and acceptance. When you are at a loss for words, consider these other means of showing the patient that you care.

FIVE STAGES OF GRIEF

Dr. Elisabeth Kübler-Ross identified five stages of grief that can occur in the dying patient. They are denial, anger, bargaining, depression, and acceptance (Table 31-1). If there is adequate time and support, some patients may be able to move psychologically through each stage to a point of acceptance of their illness and death.

- **Denial** begins when the person is made aware that he is going to die. He may not accept this information as truth, and may instead deny it. Making long-range plans that are not likely to be fulfilled may indicate that the patient is in the denial stage. Most people with a terminal illness must go through denial before they are able to eventually reach acceptance. This is a necessary and therapeutic stage. Other people should not try to convince the patient of his diagnosis or argue with the person. If denial begins to interfere with the person's adjustment, then professional counseling may be required.
- **Anger** comes when the patient is no longer able to deny the fact that she is going to die. The patient may blame those around her, including those who are giving care, for her illness. Added stresses, however small, are likely to upset the patient who is in the anger stage (Figure 31-2). Statements such as, "It's all your fault. I should never have come to this hospital," are typical of a patient in the anger stage. Remember, if the patient expresses anger, that she is angry about her diagnosis, not with you personally. Remain calm and avoid saying anything that may make her angrier. If you think the patient is angry about something other than the diagnosis, report this to the nurse so the situation can be remedied.
- **Bargaining** is the stage in the grief process in which the patient attempts to bargain for more time to live. He may ask to be allowed to go home to finish a task before he dies, or he may make private "deals" with

TABLE 31-1 EMOTIONAL RESPONSES TO DYING

Stages of Grief	Response of the Nursing Assistant
Denial	Reflect patient's statements, but try not to confirm or deny the fact that the patient is dying. **Example:** *"The lab tests can't be right—I don't have cancer."* *"It must have been difficult for you to learn the results of your tests."*
Anger	Understand the source of the patient's anger. Provide understanding and support. Listen. Try to meet reasonable needs and demands quickly. **Example:** *"This food is terrible—not fit to eat."* *"Let me see if I can find something that would appeal to you more."*
Bargaining	If it is possible to meet the patient's requests, do so. Listen attentively. **Example:** *"If only God will spare me this, I'll go to church every week."* *"Would you like a visit from your clergyperson?"*
Depression	Avoid clichés that dismiss the patient's depression ("It could be worse—you could be in more pain"). Be caring and supporting. Let the patient know that it is all right to be depressed. **Example:** *"There just isn't any sense in going on."* *"I understand you are feeling very depressed."*
Acceptance	Do not assume that, because the patient has accepted death, she or he is unafraid, or that she or he does not need emotional support. Listen attentively and be supportive and caring. **Example:** *"I feel so alone."* *"I am here with you. Would you like to talk?"*

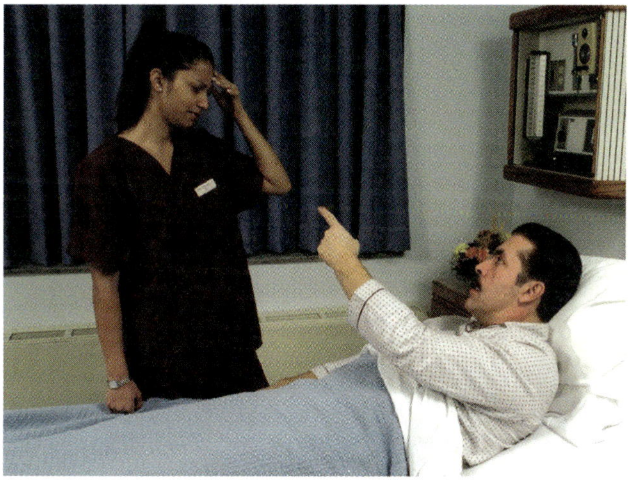

FIGURE 31-2 Patients may demonstrate feelings of frustration and anger.

God: "If you will let me live another two months, I promise I will try to be a better person." Bargaining frequently involves an important event that the patient has been looking forward to, such as a child's wedding or the birth of a grandchild. The patient in this stage is basically saying, "I know I'm going to die and I'm ready to die, but not just yet." This may be done in private and not stated verbally.

- **Depression** is the fourth stage identified in the grief process. During this stage, the patient comes to a full realization that he will die soon (Figure 31-3). He is saddened by the thought that he will no longer be with family and friends, and by the fact that he may not have accomplished some goals that he had set for himself. He may also express regrets about not having gone somewhere or done something: "I always promised my wife that we would go to Europe and now we'll never go."

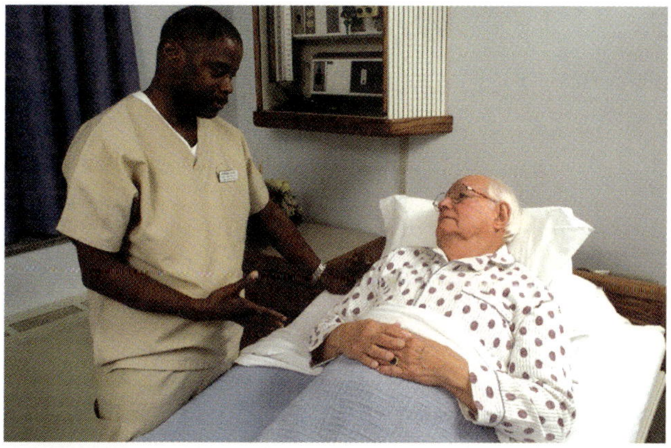

FIGURE 31-3 Depression is a normal part of the grieving process.

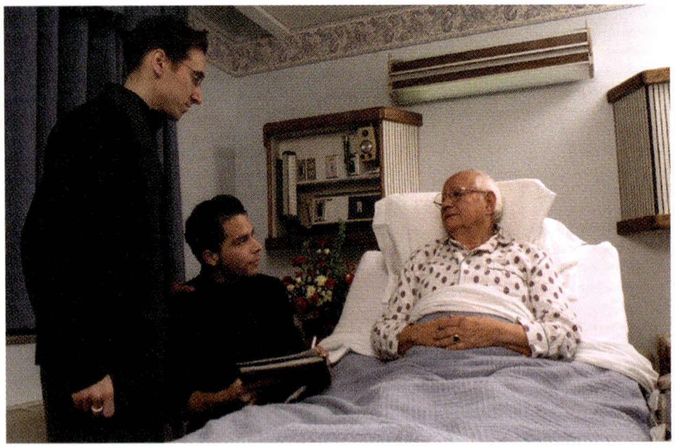

FIGURE 31-4 The patient may strive to complete unfinished business during the acceptance phase of the grieving process.

- **Acceptance** is the stage during which a patient understands and accepts the fact that he is going to die (Figure 31-4). During this stage, he may try to complete unfinished business. Having accepted his eventual death, he may also try to help those around him to deal with it, especially family members.

Not all patients progress through these stages in sequential order. Nor does movement from one level to the next mean that the previous level will be completely left behind. The staff must be aware of the possible psychological positions and be able to identify the patient's current reactions. For example, a patient who displays anger one day may be full of optimism and denial the next.

Denial frequently comes first, followed by anger and despair. Frustrated by feelings of helplessness, the person lashes out at those who are nearby. If each of these stages is expressed with some degree of success, the person is then able to move on to a level of grieving, for himself and for loved ones. When all five stages have been passed, it is believed that the patient is better able to accept the termination of life. If there is adequate time and support (Figure 31-5), many patients can be helped to reach a more accepting frame of mind.

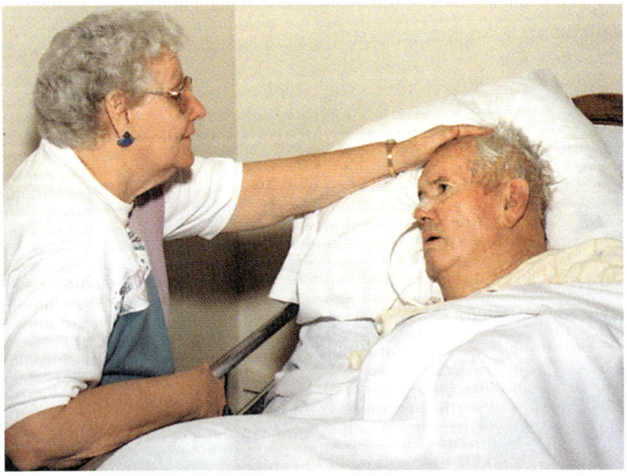

FIGURE 31-5 The support of family and friends is very important to the dying patient.

The family and staff move through these same stages, but not necessarily at the same time. It is particularly difficult when the patient is in one stage and the family is at another stage.

PREPARATION FOR DEATH

The knowledge of impending death comes to the patient directly from the physician or indirectly from the staff. A diagnosis of terminal illness is very difficult to conceal from the patient. The staff may, without realizing it, reveal the information by:

- Exhibiting false cheerfulness
- Being evasive
- Making fewer visits to the patient's room
- Spending less time with the patient

You must realize that most terminally ill patients do eventually come to accept that death is part of their near future. Keep the following in mind:

- Each patient reacts to this understanding in a unique way.
- How many feelings the patient wishes to share and with whom are very personal decisions.
- You should be available to listen, but do not force the issue.

Upon being told of the terminal diagnosis, the patient may proceed through several stages of emotional adjustment. Initially, the

- patient may react to the situation by denying the truth.
- patient may refuse all opportunities to discuss his illness with the staff or with family.
- patient's interpersonal relationships with family and staff may become greatly strained.
- patient may become defeated and full of despair, actively expressing a loss of hope.

THE PATIENT SELF-DETERMINATION ACT

The Patient Self-Determination Act of 1990 requires health care providers to supply written information about state laws regarding **advance directives**. An advance directive is a document that is put into effect if the patient later becomes unable to make decisions. All health care providers, including hospitals, long-term care facilities, and home health care agencies, must have policies and procedures covering these issues. The patient must be informed of the right to execute an advance directive before or at the time of admission. The patient may choose to execute an advance directive at the time of admission or at any time during his or her stay. Likewise, the patient may choose not to execute an advance directive.

Decisions often must be made when a patient is terminally or critically ill. These decisions involve provision of supportive care or life-sustaining treatment. The Patient Self-Determination Act was passed to assure patients and their families that their wishes will be followed. **Supportive care** means that the patient's life will not be artificially prolonged but that the patient will be kept comfortable physically, mentally, and emotionally. Supportive care includes:

- Oxygen to ease breathing if the patient needs it
- Food and fluids that the patient can consume by mouth
- Medications for pain, nausea, anxiety, or other physical or emotional discomforts
- The continuation of physical care such as grooming and hygiene, cleanliness, positioning, and range-of-motion exercises
- Caring and emotional support of staff

All patients deserve supportive care, but for terminally or critically ill patients, supportive care means the absence of life-sustaining treatment. **Life-sustaining treatment** means giving medications and treatments for the purpose of maintaining life. Life-sustaining treatments include all of the items listed under supportive care and may also include:

- Being placed on a ventilator to maintain breathing
- Receiving **cardiopulmonary resuscitation** (**CPR**) if **cardiac arrest** occurs (the heart and lungs stop functioning)
- Artificial nutrition through a feeding tube or hyperalimentation device
- Blood transfusions
- Surgery
- Radiation therapy
- Chemotherapy
- Other treatments that will maintain life

Note: Radiation therapy and chemotherapy may also be given to relieve pain, not to extend life.

There are basically two types of advance directives: the living will and the durable power of attorney for health care. The **living will** is a request that death not be artificially postponed if the patient has an incurable, irreversible injury, disease, or illness that the physician judges to be a terminal condition. A living will must be witnessed by two other individuals who do not stand to benefit because of the person's death.

The **durable power of attorney for health care** is a directive that assigns someone else the responsibility for making medical decisions for the patient if the patient becomes unable to do so himself. It must be signed by the *agent* (the person given the durable power of attorney) and by the *principal* (the person appointing the agent). It also must be signed by an adult witness. The durable power of attorney may indicate whether the person:

- Does not want his life to be prolonged and does not want life-sustaining treatment
- Wants his life prolonged and wants life-sustaining treatment to be provided unless the physician believes he is in an irreversible coma
- Wants his life to be prolonged to the greatest extent possible without regard to his condition

The durable power of attorney is one way to ensure that the wishes and rights of an individual will be followed and protected when the person is no longer able to make personal decisions. As a nursing assistant, you must be aware of the patient's status for supportive care or life-sustaining treatment. The person on supportive care will have a **no-code order** or **DNR** (do not resuscitate) order. This means that no extraordinary means, such as CPR to resuscitate the person, will be used to prevent death. This allows a person to die peacefully with maximum dignity. A no-code decision is reached after discussion by the patient with her family and physician. Once made, the no-code decision is entered in the patient's chart. All staff members are made aware of the decision, but it is kept confidential. If the patient changes her mind, the order in the chart is changed.

LEGAL *Alert*

Health care workers sometimes become confused about the meaning of a living will in which the patient specifies that no heroic procedures are to be undertaken if the patient is in terminal, irreversible condition. If the patient is not known to be in terminal condition, resuscitation will be done (unless otherwise ordered). For example, a 32-year-old patient in good health enters the hospital for a diagnostic procedure that involves the injection of contrast material into the veins. The patient has an allergic reaction to the contrast material and suffers a cardiac arrest. In this case, *CPR would be done*, because the patient is not known to be in terminal condition.

In another instance, an elderly patient enters the hospital for insertion of a central intravenous catheter to be used for pain management as part of terminal care for cancer. The patient is known to have inoperable cancer, as documented by two or more physicians. The patient experiences a complication during the procedure and has a cardiac arrest. In this case, the provisions of the living will would be observed, and *CPR would not be done*.

LEGAL Alert

The person designated as the agent in a durable power of attorney for health care should be familiar with the patient's wishes. The authority for making decisions takes effect only if the patient becomes physically or mentally unable to speak for herself. If the patient subsequently regains the ability to make decisions, the power of attorney and the agent's power are inactivated. Your facility will have a procedure for securing another person, usually a relative, to make decisions on the patient's behalf if she has not designated a durable power of attorney for health care. The durable power of attorney for health care covers only health care decisions, and only for the period of time during which the patient is unable to make decisions. It does not cover management of finances or other areas of the patient's life.

Witnessing Advance Directives

The nursing assistant must become familiar with facility policies and state laws for witnessing advance directives. In many states, persons who care for the patient are not permitted to witness advance directives. In most states, caregivers cannot legally be appointed to be the agent (medical decision maker) for a patient unless they are related by blood or marriage.

Withdrawing or Modifying Advance Directives

Patients may withdraw or modify their advance directives at any time. For example, a patient's advance directive states that he wants full life support if his heart and breathing stop. The patient later finds out that he has cancer, and wants only supportive care at the end of life. If a patient informs you of changes that affect the advance directive, notify the nurse promptly.

LEGAL Alert

Your facility may have designations for different levels of emergency care, ranging from comfort care to full advanced life support. Become familiar with the criteria for these levels. Many facilities have ethics committees made up of professionals from many disciplines. The committee meets to review some difficult care situations.

THE ROLE OF THE NURSING ASSISTANT

As a nursing assistant, you spend much time with the patient. You have a unique opportunity to be a source of strength and comfort. You must behave in a way that instills confidence in both the patient and the patient's family. Developing the proper attitude and approach for this type of situation is not easy. It will come with experience. There are some things to keep in mind:

- Your response should be consistent. It should be guided by the patient's attitude and the care plan.
- You must be open and receptive, because the terminal patient's attitude may change from day to day.
- Make sure you inform the nurse of incidents related to the patient that reflect moods and needs.
- Remember that each person's idea of death and the hereafter differs. You must be open to patients' ideas and not force your own upon them.
- Your own feelings about death and dying influence your ability to care for the dying patient. Honestly explore your feelings by talking about them with others until you can resolve any conflicts you may have. Your acceptance of death as a natural occurrence will enable you to meet patient needs in a realistic manner.
- Give your best and most careful nursing care, with special attention to comfort measures such as mouth care and fluid intake.
- You should be quietly empathetic and carry out your duties in a calm, efficient way.

When a patient's condition is critical, the physician will place his name officially on the **critical list**. Then the family and the chaplain will be notified.

Providing for Spiritual Needs

Many people find spiritual faith to be a source of great comfort during difficult times.

- Some religions have specific rituals that are carried out when a person is very ill or dying (Table 31-2). Your role is to cooperate with the patient, family, and clergyperson so that these rituals may be performed in a dignified, caring manner.
- Other religions do not have specific practices, but patients of those religions may spend time in prayer. Allow the patient and family privacy, but let them know you are close by if you are needed.
- Some patients may have no formal religious affiliation. This does not mean they do not have spiritual needs.

TABLE 31-2 BELIEFS AND PRACTICES RELATED TO DYING AND DEATH FOR MAJOR RELIGIONS

Religion	Autopsy	Organ Donation	Beliefs and Practices
Judaism (Orthodox)	Only in special circumstances	With consultation of rabbi	Visits to the dying are a religious duty. Witness must be present if death occurs, to protect family and commit soul to God. Torah and Psalms may be read and prayers recited. Conversation is kept to a minimum. Someone should be with the body after death until burial, usually within 24 hours. Body must not be touched 8 to 30 minutes after death. Medical personnel should not touch or wash body unless death occurs on Jewish Sabbath; then care may be given by nurse wearing gloves. Water is removed from the room. Mirrors may be covered at family's request.
Hinduism	Permitted	Permitted	Priest ties thread around neck or wrist of deceased and pours water in the mouth. Only family and friends touch body.
Buddhism	Personal preference	Permitted	Buddhist priest is present at death. Last rites are chanted at the bedside.
Islam (Muslim)	Only for medical or legal reasons	Not permitted	Before death, read Koran and pray. Patient confesses sins and asks forgiveness of family. Only family touches or washes body. After death, body is turned toward Mecca.
Roman Catholic	Permitted	Permitted	Sacrament of the Sick administered to ill patients, to patients in imminent danger, or shortly after death.
Christian Scientist	Unlikely	Not permitted	No ritual is performed before or after death.
Church of Christ	Permitted	Permitted	No ritual is performed before or after death.
Jehovah's Witness	Only if required by law	Not permitted	No ritual is performed before or after death.
Baptist	Permitted	Permitted	Clergy ministers through counseling and prayers.
Episcopalian	Permitted	Permitted	Last rites are optional.
Lutheran	Permitted	Permitted	Last rites are optional.
Eastern Orthodox Christian	Not encouraged	Not encouraged	Last rites are mandatory and are given by ordained priest.

They may request the services of a clergyperson and may not know who to call on. Relay this request to the nurse, because most health care facilities have chaplains to provide the services.

- Some patients do not believe in any higher spiritual being. This is their right and no one should try to change their feelings.

- Always respect the beliefs or nonbeliefs of any patient. Treat all religious items, such as holy books, medals, and rosaries, with respect.
- When a Catholic patient is ill, a priest may be called for the **Sacrament of the Sick** (Figure 31-6). It is preferable that the family be present and leave the room only while the confession is heard. The practicing Catholic and his family consider it a privilege to have the opportunity for confession. Many patients recover completely, but this hope should not prevent the reception of this sacrament if this is the patient's wish.
- A Bible or spiritual reading of the patient's faith, if requested, may be of some spiritual help through this crisis. Be courteous and provide privacy when the patient's clergyperson visits.

Be aware that dying is a lonely business, a journey each person must finish alone. Until the final moment comes, privacy, but not total solitude, should be the guiding rule (Figure 31-7).

It is important to remember the family and other loved ones when a patient is dying. Check the policies of your health care facility and assist in the following actions:

- Allow the family to be with the patient as they desire.
- Allow the family to assist with some of the care, if they wish to do so; for example, moistening the patient's lips or giving a backrub.
- Inform the family where they can get a cup of coffee or a meal.

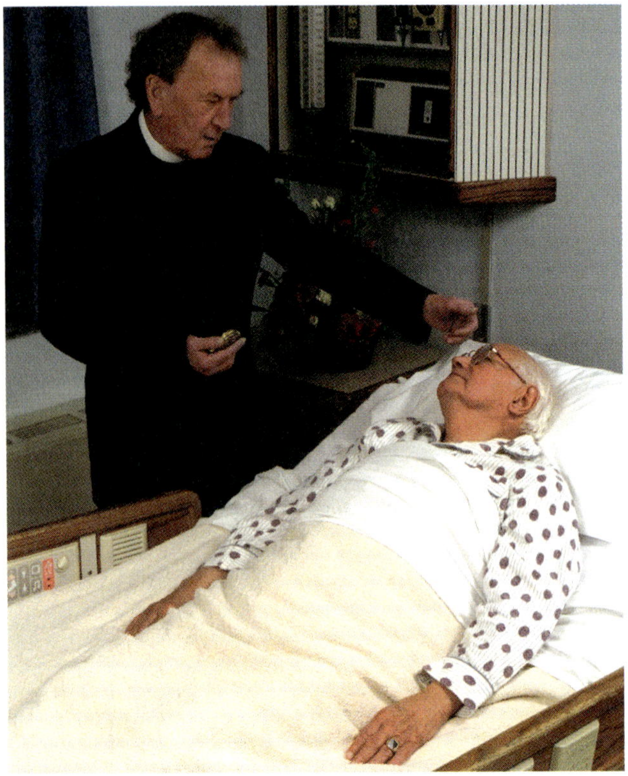

FIGURE 31-6 The Sacrament of the Sick may be administered to Roman Catholics who are gravely ill.

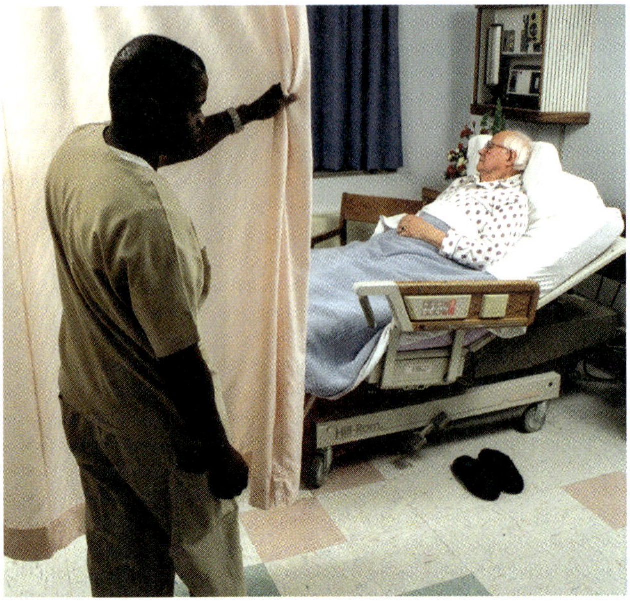

FIGURE 31-7 The dying patient needs privacy, but not total solitude.

- Show the family where they can use a telephone in private.
- If a family member stays during the night, offer a pillow and blanket. Some facilities provide recliners or cots for family members.
- Avoid being judgmental of family members. Remember that each person grieves in his or her own way. The emotions that others see are not necessarily an accurate indication of what the individual is feeling.

HOSPICE CARE

Hospice care has evolved around the philosophy that death is a natural process that should neither be hastened nor delayed and that the dying person should be kept comfortable. **Hospice care** is:

- Provided to terminally ill people with a life expectancy of six months or less
- Involved with direct physical care when needed
- Supportive to both the family and the patient
- Provided in special hospice facilities, in other care facilities, and at home
- Largely carried out by a home health assistant or a nursing assistant under the direction of professional health care providers
- Follow-up bereavement counseling to help survivors accept the death of a loved one
- A program in which volunteers play an important role, making regular personal visits to the patient and family

Hospice care is provided by teams who work in conjunction with the terminally ill person and his family. The team usually consists of a physician, professional nurse, nursing assistant, and other professionals (such as social workers and clergy) as needed and desired.

The goals of hospice care include:

- Control of pain so the individual can remain an active participant in life until death
- Coordinating psychological, spiritual, and social support services for the patient and the family
- Making legal and financial counseling available to the patient and family

Because hospice care is a philosophy, it becomes part of the guide for your actions when caring for the terminally ill. Hospice care is provided as you give your usual care. Some things to keep in mind, however, are:

- Report pain immediately and give close attention to comfort measures.
- Encourage the person to carry out as much self-care as possible.
- Be readily available to listen. Spend as much time with the patient as possible and desired by the patient.
- Get to know the family and be supportive to them.
- Give the same care you would if a terminal diagnosis had not been made.
- Carry out all activities with dignity and respect.

PHYSICAL CHANGES AS DEATH APPROACHES

As death approaches, there are notable physical changes. As these changes occur, report them immediately to the charge nurse.

- The patient becomes less responsive (Figure 31-8).
- Body functions slow down.
- The patient loses general voluntary and involuntary muscle control.
- The patient may involuntarily void and defecate.
- The jaw tends to drop.

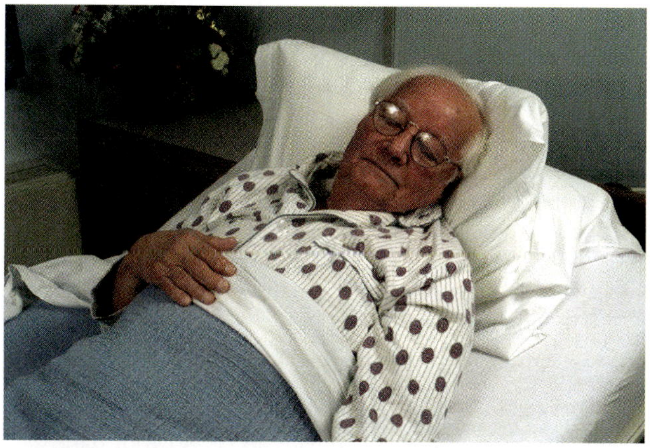

FIGURE 31-8 The patient becomes less responsive and body functions slow down as death approaches.

- Breathing becomes irregular and shallow.
- Circulation slows and the extremities become cold. The pulse becomes rapid and progressively weaker.
- Skin pales.
- The eyes stare and do not respond to light.
- Hearing seems to be the last sense to be lost. Do not assume that because death is approaching, the patient can no longer hear. You must be careful what you say.

In the period before death, the patient with a terminal diagnosis needs and receives the same care as the patient who is expected to recover. Attention is paid to physical as well as emotional needs.

As it becomes clear that death will occur very soon, you should call the nurse, who will supervise the care during the final moments of life.

Signs of Death

After death, changes continue to take place in the body. These changes are called **moribund** (dying) changes.

- Pupils become permanently dilated.
- There is no pulse or respiration.
- Heat is gradually lost from the body.
- The patient may urinate, defecate, or release flatus.
- Blood pools in the lowest areas of the body, giving a purplish discoloration to those areas.
- Within 2 to 4 hours, body rigidity, called **rigor mortis**, develops.
- Unless embalmed within 24 hours, there is indication of progressive protein breakdown.

POSTMORTEM CARE

The patient's body should be treated with respect at all times. Before death occurs, the limbs should be straightened and the head elevated on a pillow. The body should be cleaned by gently washing it with warm water. Discharges must be washed off and wiped away.

Care of the body after death is called **postmortem care** (Figure 31-9). This may be your responsibility. You may find it easier if you ask a coworker to assist.

- Use gloves when giving postmortem care. The body may continue to be infectious following death.
- Treat the body with the same dignity you would a living person.
- Some facilities prefer to have the patient left alone until the mortuary staff arrive. Your responsibility will be only to prepare the body for viewing by the family.
- Check the hospital procedure manual before proceeding with postmortem care.

The contents of morgue kits vary (Figure 31-10), but they usually include:

- A shroud of some kind (paper or cloth)

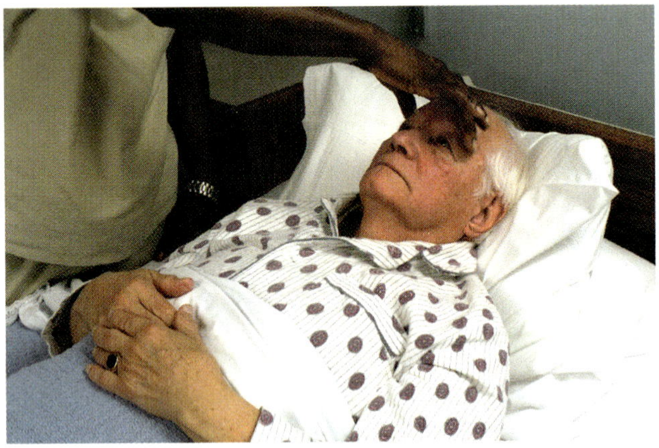

FIGURE 31-9 Postmortem care is given after death occurs.

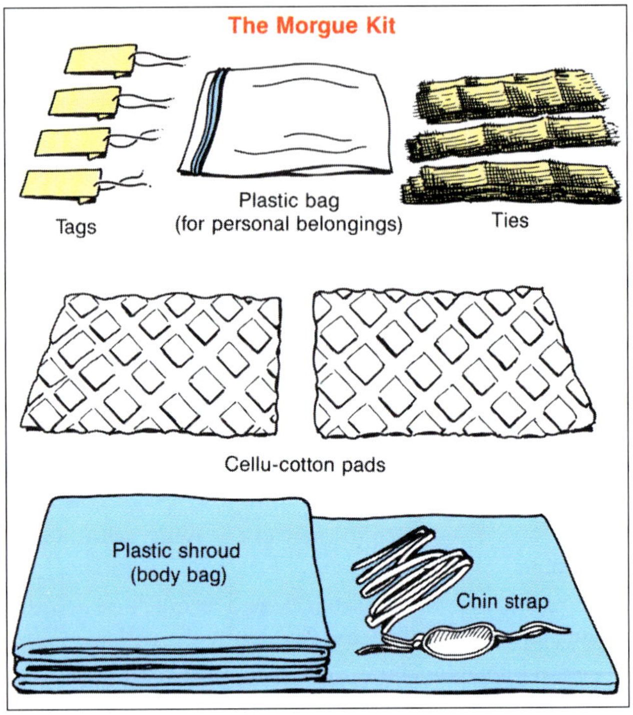

FIGURE 31-10 Supplies needed for postmortem care.

- A clean gown
- Tags used to identify the body
- Gauze squares for padding
- Safety pins

One procedure for postmortem care is described here (refer to Procedure 94). See also Figure 31-11 for instructions on using a shroud.

PROCEDURE 94

GIVING POSTMORTEM CARE

1. Carry out beginning procedure actions.
2. Assemble equipment:
   - shroud or clean sheet
   - basin with warm water
   - washcloth
   - towels
   - disposable gloves
   - identification tags
   - cotton
   - bandages
   - pads as needed
3. Put on disposable gloves.
4. Remove all appliances, tubing, and used articles, if instructed to do so.
5. Work quickly and quietly; maintain an attitude of respect.
6. With the bed flat, place the body on the back, with head and shoulders elevated on a pillow.
   a. Close the eyes by grasping the eyelashes, gently pulling the eyelids down, and holding shut for a few seconds.
   b. Replace dentures in the patient's mouth, if used. Replace an artificial eye, if used.
   c. The jaw may have to be secured with light bandaging.
   d. Pad beneath the bandage. Handle the body gently, as tight bandaging or undue pressure from your hands may leave marks.
   e. Straighten the arms and legs and place the arms at the sides.
7. Bathe as necessary. Remove any soiled dressings and replace with clean ones. Groom hair.
8. Place a disposable pad underneath the buttocks. If the family is to view the body:
   a. Put a clean hospital gown on the patient.
   b. Cover the body to the shoulders with a sheet.
   c. Remove disposable gloves and wash your hands.

continues

PROCEDURE 94

continued

d. Make sure the room is neat.
e. Adjust the lights to a subdued level.
f. Provide chairs for the family.
g. Allow the family to visit in private.

9. Return to the patient's room after the family leaves. Wash your hands and put on disposable gloves.
10. Collect all belongings and make a list. Wrap properly and label. Valuables remain in the hospital safe until they are signed for by a relative.
11. Fill out the identification cards or tags in the morgue kit and attach them as follows:
    a. Place one card on the right ankle or right great toe.
    b. Attach one card to the bag with the patient's valuables.
12. Put the shroud on the patient and attach an identification card or tag to the outside.
13. Transport the body to the morgue.
    a. Call an elevator to the floor and keep it empty.
    b. Close patient corridor doors.
    c. Empty the corridor.
    d. With an assistant, place the body on a gurney.
    e. Keep the patient supine, with a rubber head elevator under the neck.
    f. Cover the body with a sheet.
    g. Remove disposable gloves and discard according to facility policy. Wash your hands.
    h. Take the body to the morgue.
    i. Attach one identification card or tag to the morgue compartment.

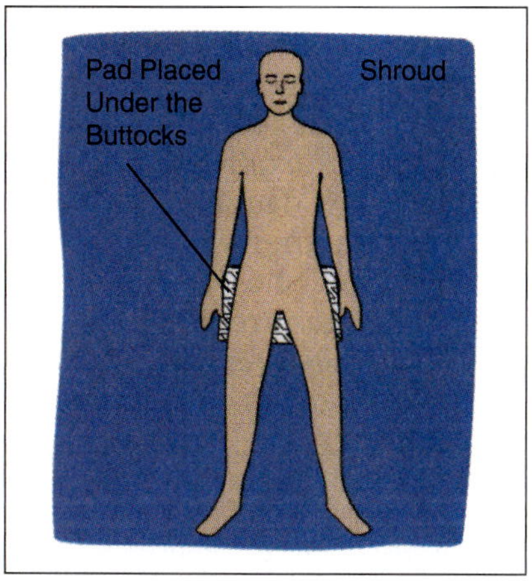

FIGURE 31-11A Position the shroud under the deceased with the pad under the buttocks.

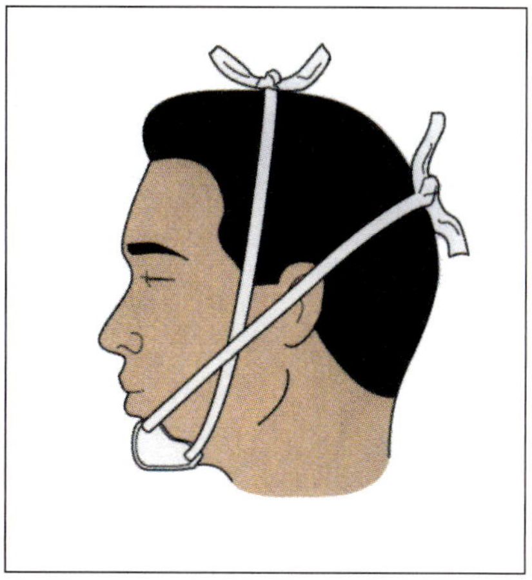

FIGURE 31-11B Apply the chin strap as shown to keep the mouth closed.

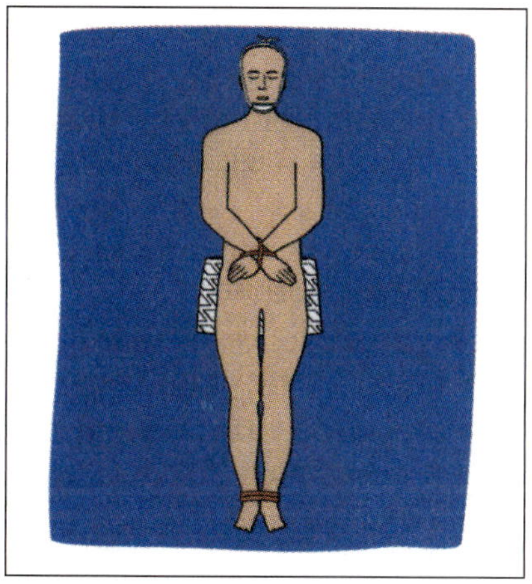

FIGURE 31-11C Fasten the wrists and ankles together with the ties. Use gauze sponges under the ties so they do not make marks on the skin.

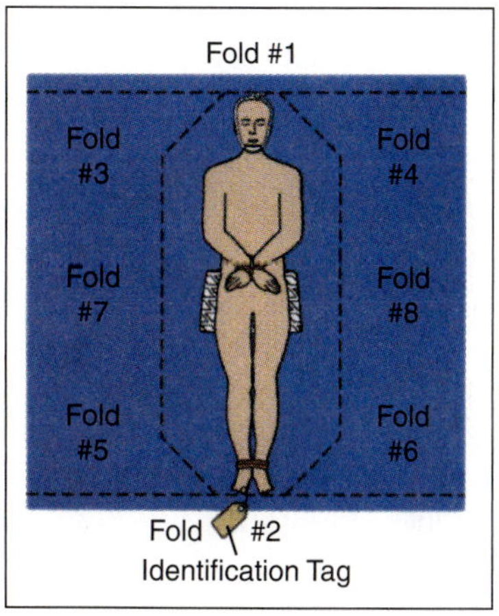

FIGURE 31-11D Fill out and attach four identification tags. Place one tag on the:
- right big toe or right ankle
- outside of the shroud
- patient's personal belongings (securely wrapped)
- compartment in the morgue

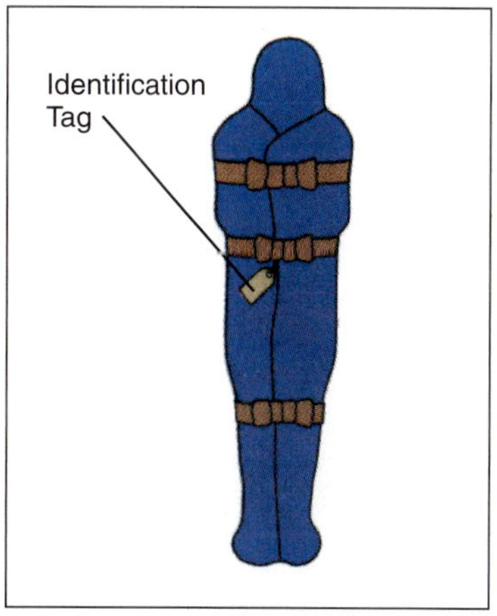

FIGURE 31-11E Fold the shroud around the body as shown. Use the long ties or tape to hold the shroud closed. Fasten a tag to the outside of the shroud.

ORGAN DONATIONS

Some people desire to share their organs with others after death. They use an organ donor card that is part of the driver's license. The card specifies if particular organs or the whole body is being donated. At times, because of a special need, the patient's family is asked for permission so that certain body organs may be removed and saved or removed and **harvested** (reused). Such a request is made by the physician or the nurse, never by the nursing assistant.

If the patient or family make their wishes known to you without your asking, it is important to report this to the nurse.

POSTMORTEM EXAMINATION (AUTOPSY)

In certain situations, the law requires a medical postmortem examination or **autopsy** of the body. At other times, the family and physician may desire such an examination to understand the reasons for the patient's death. It is possible that information learned from the examination can be used to protect other family members. As in the case of organ donations, however, requesting family permission for an autopsy is not part of the nursing assistant's responsibilities. The nursing assistant is responsible for being supportive of the family and the decision that has been made.

REVIEW

A. True/False.

Mark the following true or false by circling T or F.

1. T F All people respond to a terminal diagnosis in the same way.

2. T F Hearing is the first sense to be lost in the dying patient.

3. T F Death is the final stage of life.

4. T F The nursing assistant should call the physician when the patient dies.

5. T F Sometimes the staff, without realizing it, allow the patient to learn of a terminal diagnosis through their behavior.

6. T F The dying patient receives the same complete care that would be given to someone expected to recover.

7. T F The hospice philosophy has pain relief as one of its goals.

8. T F Permanent dilation of the pupils is a moribund sign.

9. T F Hospice-type care is only possible in the acute care facility.

10. T F The dying person needs a great deal of understanding and realistic support.

B. Matching.

Choose the correct word from Column II to match each phrase or statement in Column I.

Column I	Column II
11. C refusal to accept reality	**a.** moribund
12. E after death	**b.** rigor mortis
13. F covering for the body after death	**c.** denial
14. ____ stiffening of the body after death	**d.** hospice
15. ____ dying	**e.** postmortem
	f. shroud
	g. anger

C. Multiple Choice.

Select the one best answer for each of the following.

16. Organs from a dead person may be
- **a.** harvested without permission.
- **b.** obtained on an as-needed basis.
- **c.** donated with permission of the family at the time of death.
- **d.** donated only if listed in the patient's will.

17. Postmortem examinations
- **a.** are never performed.
- **b.** may provide valuable information.
- **c.** are arranged by the nursing assistant.
- **d.** are forbidden by law.

18. As death approaches, changes include
- **a.** constriction of the pupils.
- **b.** muscle spasm.
- **c.** slowing of circulation.
- **d.** skin develops a yellow hue.

19. Moribund changes include
  a. permanent pupil constriction.
  b. increased body heat.
  c. pulse and respiration increase.
  d. blood pools in the lower body.

20. A "no-code" order on a patient's chart means
  a. to start CPR immediately.
  b. do not resuscitate.
  c. begin postmortem care at once.
  d. to call the family if the patient seems in danger of dying.

D. Nursing Assistant Challenge.

Mrs. Goldstein is a patient in the hospital where you work. She was diagnosed with cancer of the ovaries two years ago. She has been at home but is admitted periodically for chemotherapy. You have taken care of her each time she has been in the hospital. The first time was right after Mrs. Goldstein was diagnosed. She seemed happy and made frequent comments like, "I'm glad I don't have cancer." The last time she was a patient, she refused to follow the suggestions of the nursing staff, but did allow her chemotherapy to be administered. When her family visited, she was irritated and hostile toward them. This time, she is agreeable with the staff on all matters and seems genuinely happy to see her family. She has told you that if she can live to see her granddaughter get married in two months, she will become a volunteer at the hospital so she can help other patients. She is not receiving chemotherapy anymore because the cancer is in an advanced stage. She is hospitalized for pain management now but plans to go home for hospice care. Consider these questions about Mrs. Goldstein:

21. Do you think she is preparing for her death?

22. How would you describe the stages of dying she has been experiencing?

23. What response is appropriate to her comments about the wedding?

24. Do you think hospice care will benefit Mrs. Goldstein? Give reasons for your answer.

25. Mrs. Goldstein is Jewish. What considerations must you give to her postmortem care?

EXPLORING THE WEB

Description	Location
Care of the dying patient	*http://ccm-l.med.edu*
Hospice and home care resources	*http://www.growthhouse.org*
Hospice Patient's Bill of Rights	*http://www.hospice-america.org*
Loss, grief, and death	*http://www.delmarhealthcare.com/olcs/white/pnotes.asp* (see Chapter 17) *http://www.delmarhealthcare.com/olcs/whiteduncan/pnotes.asp* (see Chapter 9)
Principles for end-of-life care	*http://www.milbank.org*
Resources for end-of-life care	*http://www.public-health.uiowa.edu*
Compassion in Dying	*http://www.compassionindying.org*
Hospice and Palliative Care Nurses Association	*http://www.hpna.org*
Last Acts	*http://www.lastacts.org*
National Hospice and Palliative Care Organization	*http://www.nhpco.org*
Nursing Specialties Hospice Nursing	*http://allnurses.com*
Oncology Nursing Society	*http://www.ons.org*
Partnership for Caring	*http://www.partnershipforcaring.org*
Project Grace	*http://www.p-grace.org*